Cardiac Ultrasound Workbook

CARDIAC ULTRASOUND WORKBOOK

M-Mode and Two-Dimensional Echocardiography

James V. Talano, M.D.

Associate Professor of Medicine
Northwestern University School of Medicine

Grune & Stratton

A Subsidiary of Harcourt Brace Jovanovich, Publishers

New York London
Paris San Diego San Francisco São Paulo
Sydney Tokyo Toronto

Library of Congress Cataloging in Publication Data

Main entry under title:
Cardiac ultrasound workbook.

Bibliography
Includes index.
1. Ultrasonic cardiography—Problems, exercises, etc.
I. Talano, James V. [DNLM: 1. Echocardiography.
WG 141.5.E2 C267]
RC683.5.U5C374 616.1′207543′076 81-20324
ISBN 0-8089-1437-5 AACR2

Grune & Stratton, Inc.
111 Fifth Avenue
New York, NY 10003

Distributed in the United Kingdom by
Academic Press Inc. (London) Ltd.
24/28 Oval Road, London NW 1

Library of Congress Catalog Number 81-20324
International Standard Book Number 0-8089-1437-5

Printed in the United States of America

Contents

Acknowledgments

I gratefully acknowledge the assistance of the following persons who so graciously helped in the preparation of this workbook: David Mehlman, M.D., for critical review of the entire manuscript; Carl Tommaso, M.D., for his assistance in the preparation, layouts, and design of exercises; Amy Light and Jean Salomon for assistance in obtaining the ultrasound studies; Joan Francis and Ray Luedtke for their help with the artwork and illustrations; Judith KinKaid and Janie Zimring for proofreading, and Melanie Merutka for designing and typing the text.

Preface

The *Cardiac Ultrasound Workbook* has been written for cardiac ultrasound specialists and physicians who require basic knowledge of M-mode and two-dimensional echocardiography. Its purpose is to teach common echocardiographic positions and two-dimensional cardiac anatomy, as well as performance and interpretation of diagnostic examinations.

The Workbook starts out with a discussion of the techniques and measurements used in echocardiography. Chapter 2, which discusses anatomy, contains precise tomograms of the heart to most closely represent two-dimensional echocardiographic positions. The remaining chapters are devoted to common cardiac disease states, and heavy emphasis is placed on echocardiographic illustrations of the conditions that are discussed. Each chapter is supplemented by M-mode and two-dimensional illustrations to emphasize normal or marked anatomy. The two-dimensional studies are illustrated in diastole or systole to define not only anatomy but also function. The illustrations have been chosen for clarity; however, some anatomical detail is always lost in changing from a dynamic real-time image to a static image. At the end of each chapter, figures with exercises are presented to reinforce principles and highlight an occasional clinical point. Answers to these exercises are provided in Appendix H. The exercises can be used either as a pretest to determine knowledge of a specific area or as a post-test to be taken after reading the material.

Each contributor to the Workbook was asked to introduce a specific topic, describe normal anatomy, and highlight common cardiac abnormalities. I then expanded upon this framework, wrote the exercises, selected the illustrations, and worked closely with the artist in executing the labelled diagrams.

Additional information is to be found in the eight appendices at the back of the Workbook. Appendix F lists common abbreviations used in the test; additional and uncommon abbreviations are explained in the figure legends. Terms defined in the Glossary (Appendix G) are in boldface when first mentioned in the test. Additional information and detailed study of specific disease entities can be obtained by consulting the Selected Additional References (Appendix E).

All criteria and standards for the *Cardiac Ultrasound Workbook* have been adopted from the Committee on Nomenclature and Two-Dimensional Echocardiography of the American Society of Echocardiography.

Contributors

IVAN D'CRUZ, M.D., F.A.C.C., Chief, Echocardiographic Section, Cardiovascular Institute, Michael Reese Hospital; Associate Professor of Medicine, Pritzker School of Medicine, University of Chicago, Chicago, Illinois.

CHARLES GANOTE, M.D., Attending Physician, Northwestern Memorial Hospital; Professor of Pathology, Northwestern University Medical School, Chicago, Illinois.

JULIUS GARDIN, M.D., Director, Cardiac Non-Invasive Laboratory, Assistant Professor of Medicine, University of California; Irvine Medical Center, Orange, California.

WILLIAM R. JACOBS, M.D., F.A.C.C., Chief, Cardiac Graphics Section, Veterans Administration Hospital, Hines, Illinois; Assistant Professor of Medicine, Loyola University Stritch School of Medicine, Maywood, Illinois.

DAVID KOENIGSBERG, M.D., Instructor in Medicine, Northwestern University Medical School; Veterans Administration Lakeside Hospital, Chicago, Illinois.

DAVID J. MEHLMAN, M.D., F.A.C.C., Associate Director, Cardiology Graphics Laboratory, Northwestern Memorial Hospital; Assistant Professor of Medicine, Northwestern University School of Medicine, Chicago, Illinois.

JAMES V. TALANO, M.D., Associate Professor of Medicine, Northwestern University School of Medicine; Director of Cardiology Graphics Laboratory, Northwestern Memorial Hospital, Chicago, Illinois.

CARL L. TOMMASO, M.D., Assistant Professor of Medicine, Department of Cardiology, University of Maryland Hospital, Baltimore, Maryland.

Carl L. Tommaso

1

Echocardiographic Techniques and Measurements

Echocardiography has become a useful diagnostic tool for the diagnosis, quantitation, and follow-up of cardiac diseases. Its usefulness is compounded by its capability of supplying data easily and reproducibly, without risk to the patient. The purpose of this chapter is to introduce the types of echocardiography commonly used, to describe the instrumentation and techniques of each type, and to acquaint readers with the interpretation of echocardiograms through a description of the methods used to identify and quantitate cardiac structures.

TYPES OF ECHOCARDIOGRAPHY

All diagnostic ultrasound uses sound waves with a frequency above the audible range to visualize structures of interest. Three forms of echocardiography are currently in use, the most familiar of which is the **M-mode** or **time-motion echocardiogram** (Figure 1-1). In this technique, cardiac structures are viewed as if through an ultrasonic "ice-pick" inserted through the heart. The M-mode echocardiogram records the motion over time of the cardiac structures in its path, hence the designation time-motion. Recordings are usually on a **strip chart,** with the vertical axis representing the distance of structures from the transducer, and with the horizontal axis representing time. The latter is recorded at a rate of 10 to 100 mm/sec, the usual recording speed being 50 or 75 mm/sec. By redirecting the M-mode transducer, the operator is able to identify and record the various cardiac structures (Figure 1-1).

In M-mode echocardiography, the transducer is usually placed first on the anterior chest wall in the fourth **intercostal space,** 1 to 2 cm to the left of the **sternum** and directed straight posteriorly; this usually records the characteristic motion of the mitral valve (Figure 1-2). If the mitral valve cannot be found, it may be necessary to reposition the transducer several centimeters medially or laterally, or to move it to one interspace above or below, in order to find the proper **window** for recording the echocardiogram. From this position, angulation of the transducer (superiorly, inferiorly, medially, or laterally) is usually all that is necessary to record the other cardiac structures (Figure 1-2). The aortic valve can be recorded by pointing the transducer medially and superiorly (towards the right shoulder). The left ventricle can be examined by directing the transducer inferiorly and

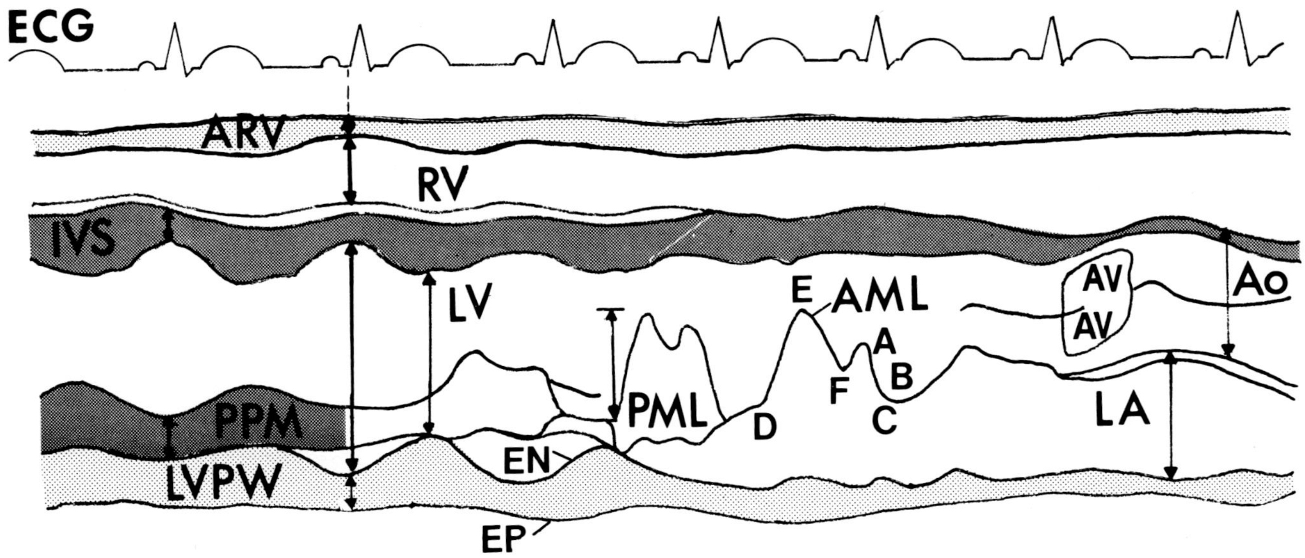

Figure 1-1

Diagrammatic M-mode echocardiogram depicting a low-speed scan from the left ventricle in the standard position to the aorta. A – F signify identification points of mitral valve motion on M-mode echocardiography. (Adapted from Sahn et al.[3])

laterally (towards the left hip). The tricuspid and pulmonic valves are sometimes difficult to record in the absence of abnormalities; the tricuspid valve can be recorded by directing the transducer medially from the mitral valve position, and the pulmonic valve can be recorded by directing the transducer superiorly from the mitral valve. **Scans** of the heart can be recorded by visualizing one area of the heart (e.g., the body of the left ventricle) and then directing the transducer through other areas (e.g., the mitral valve) to a final location (e.g., the aortic valve); this generally is done with a slow paper speed — 25 mm/sec (Figure 1-1). Scans are extremely valuable in identifying the interrelationships of various cardiac structures.

Two-dimensional echocardiography, also referred to as sector scanning, cross-sectional echocardiography, real-time echocardiography, or two-D, is another commonly used form of ultrasonic cardiac imaging. The type may vary with the instrumentation used; the purpose is the same, however: to record a planar

Figure 1-2

Echocardiographic windows. Direction of transducer movement for recording various cardiac structures.

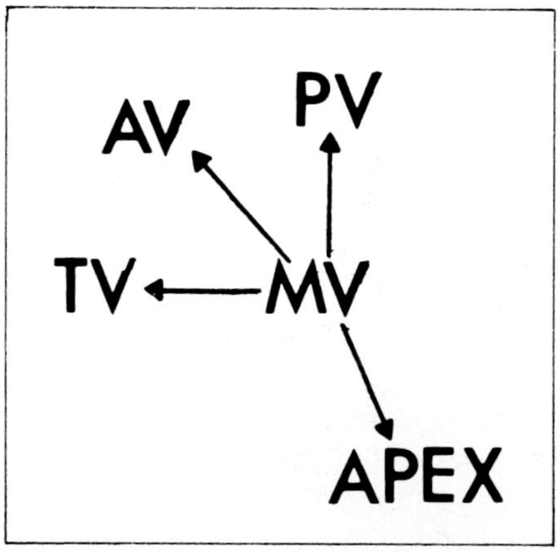

rather than an "ice-pick" view of the heart. This is accomplished by moving the ultrasound beam either mechanically (sector scan) or electronically (phased-array) through cardiac structures and displaying the resultant ultrasonic plane on a video screen. It differs from an M-mode echocardiography in that it produces a two-dimensional image (or tomogram) and gives a **real-time display** of the heart that can be recorded on videotape for future playback.

Because two-dimensional echocardiography records a plane, or tomogram, of the heart, the transducer usually is repositioned several times to visualize the heart from different locations, with several distinct orientations. It may be positioned in the **parasternal** area (similar to the location for M-mode echocardiography) on either the left or right side of the sternum; it may be positioned under the **xiphoid (subxiphoid)** or in the xiphoidal notch **(subcostal);** it may be positioned at the apex of the left ventricle **(apical)** in the area where the cardiac impulse is felt; or it may be positioned in the notch above the sternum **(suprasternal)** (Figure 1-3).

Three different orientations can be attained, depending on the rotation of the

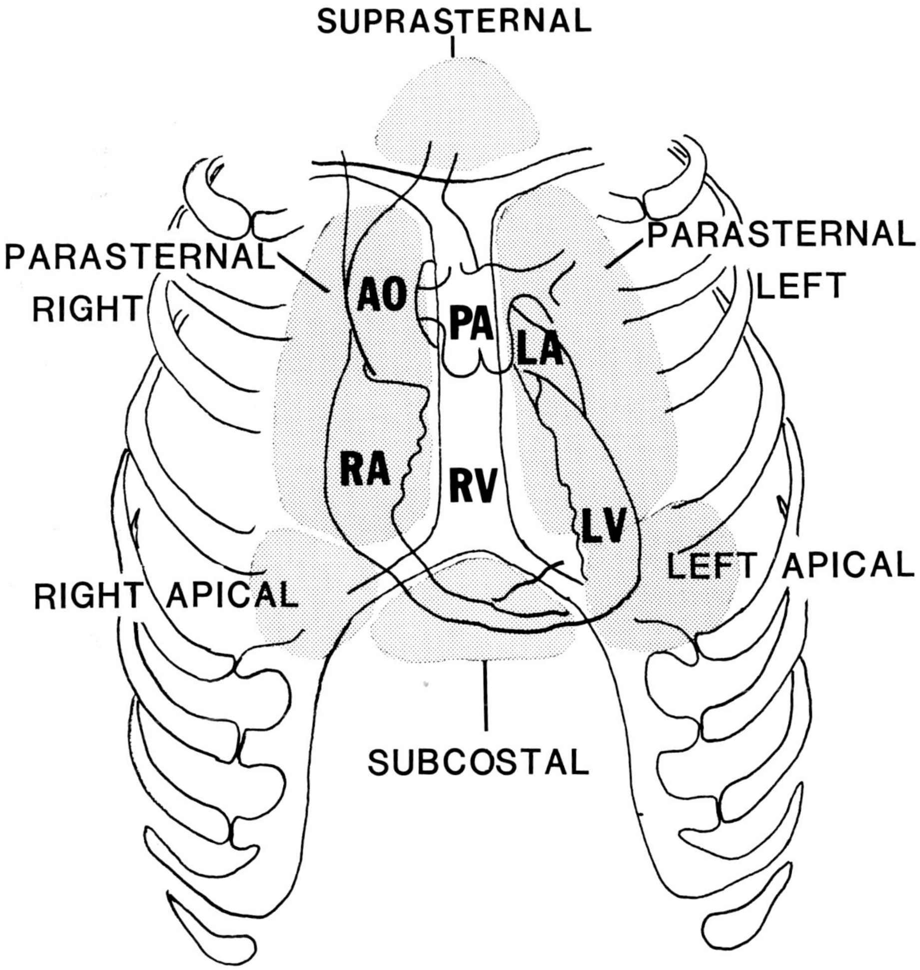

Figure 1-3
Transducer positions (shaded area) for various echocardiographic windows.

transducer. An orientation parallel to the long axis of the heart (base to apex) is called the **long-axis view.** Rotation of the transducer 90° from the long-axis position gives a **short-axis view.** Placing the transducer at the apex of the left ventricle or in the subcostal location in a plane parallel to the chest wall gives an **apical four-chamber** or **subcostal four-chamber view** (Figure 1-4).[1] The anatomy of these locations and orientations will be discussed in Chapter 2.

The third format of echocardiography currently in use analyzes alterations in the frequency of reflected sound from moving objects (e.g., blood flowing), known as the **Doppler principle.** This is similar to the technology used by police to detect speeders. It has been demonstrated useful in detecting and quantitating regurgitant valvular lesions, such as mitral regurgitation, and is currently under study for the quantitative assessment of cardiac output.

INSTRUMENTATION

Proper instrumentation is essential for a complete echocardiographic examination. Progress in the development of instrumentation has been rapid during the

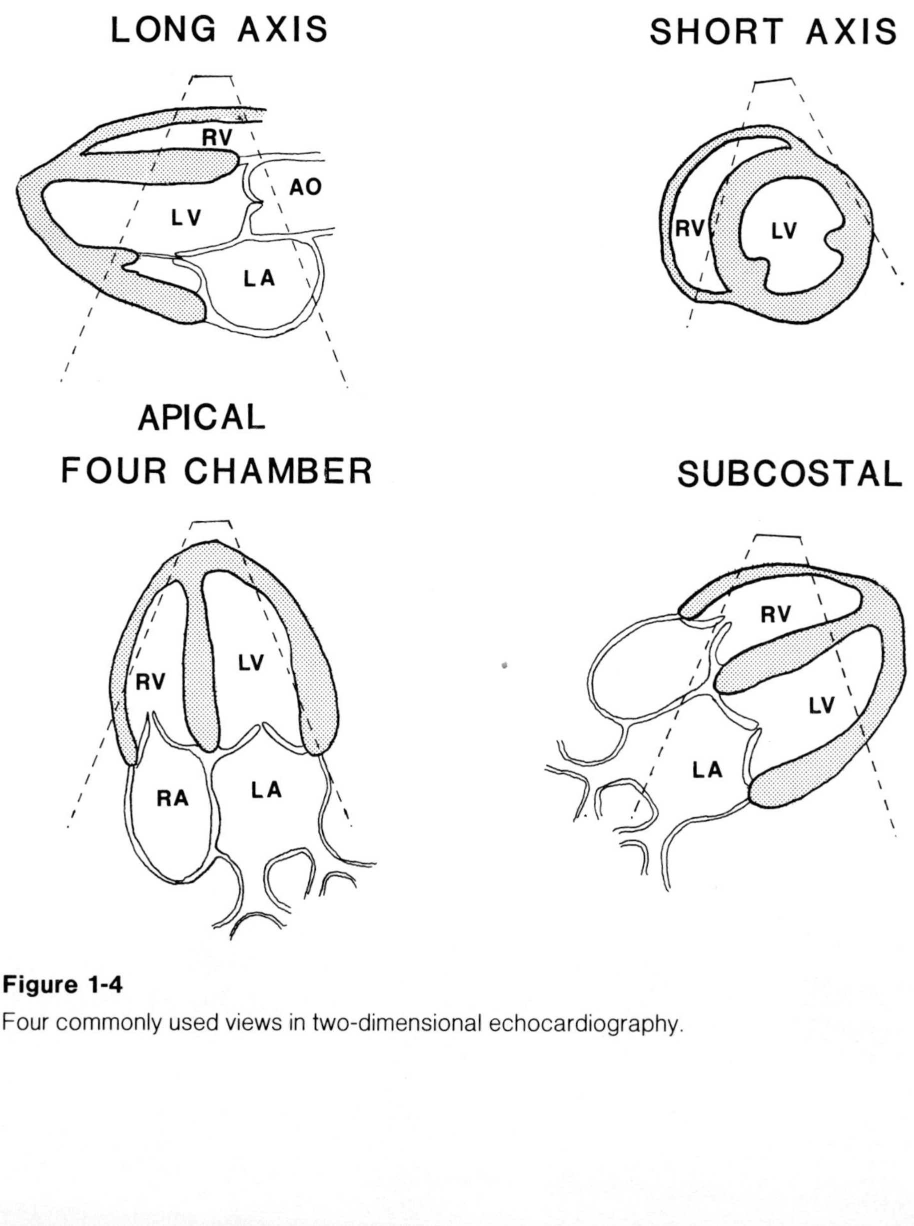

Figure 1-4
Four commonly used views in two-dimensional echocardiography.

past few years, so that, with present equipment, a properly trained person can perform a complete echocardiographic study within a reasonably short period of time and obtain satisfactory results in the majority of patients. The echocardiographic record can be easily stored. The following sections outline the instrumentation needed to perform M-mode and two-dimensional echocardiography.

M-Mode Echocardiography

The minimal instrumentation required for M-mode echocardiography is as follows:

- An echocardiographic scope providing oscilloscopic display of **A-mode** as well as M-mode, with schematic representation of **depth compensation.** The oscilloscope for M-mode display should be of the long-persistence type.
- Focused, partially focused, or nonfocused transducers approximately 1 cm in diameter with focal lengths from 5 to 15 cm (0.6 cm in diameter in pediatric usage).
- A strip-chart recorder capable of continuous recording speeds of 10, 25, 50, 75, and 100 mm/sec. If simultaneous echocardiographic and phonocardiographic recordings are to be obtained, a 100 mm/sec recorder will be necessary.
- An electrocardiographic recording channel.
- Calibrated time and distance markers.
- A foot switch to activate the recorder drive (optional, but desirable).
- Auxillary recording channels, such as a phonocardiogram, external pulse channel, and respiration channels (optional, as desired).

Echoscope Controls

Delay. Delay postpones the oscilloscope scan for a certain distance after the ultrasound pulse is transmitted, and thus controls the depth at which the scan begins; it is used to eliminate display echoes from the most anterior structures. The control is normally set so that chest-wall echoes are the most proximal ones recorded.

Depth. This control is used to adjust the distance displayed from the crystal artifact of the transducer. It determines the maximum extent of the display as measured from the chest wall, with the heart interposed between it and the lung. The control is usually adjusted by the operator to point 2 cm beyond the strong echoes of the posterior left ventricular wall. For a normal subject, 15 cm is the extent of the **depth display.**

Depth compensation (time-compensated gain). Normally, echoes returned from structures in close proximity to the chest wall (e.g., the right ventricle) will appear very strong, whereas those received from more distal structures (e.g., the posterior left ventricular wall) will be relatively weak. This occurs because the signal must pass through a greater amount of tissue before reaching the posterior structures; much of the ultrasound beam is absorbed and deflected by the intervening and a proportionately weaker signal results. Depth compensation counteracts this phenomenon by suppressing the signals from near the transducer and amplifying signals from more distant structures. By setting the depth compensation to the appropriate level, the operator is able to highlight an echo of particular interest. It is important that the echoscope provide a visual representation of depth compensation on the A-mode display, as this greatly facilitates proper setting of the control. Variable time-depth compensators are available for suppression or enhancement of echoes at various depth levels from the transducer.

Near gain (initial gain) and coarse gain (overall gain). Near gain controls the amplification of ultrasound waves reflected from a region extending from the chest wall to the point where depth compensation takes effect. Coarse gain controls the amplitude of all received ultrasound signals equally. If the control is set too high, desired proximal structures (e.g., the right and left sides of the interventricular septum) will be poorly imaged because ultrasound waves that are not essential are overamplified and recorded. If, on the other hand, the control is set too low, desired distal structures (e.g., the left ventricular posterior wall) will appear fragmented and poorly defined. Thus, the combination of overall gain (or coarse gain), depth compensation, and near gain allows selection of two amplification levels: one for anterior (near gain) and the other for posterior structures (coarse gain).

Damping (pulse power). Damping controls the power of the transmitted ultrasound impulse. A strong pulse will generate strong echoes; a weak pulse will generate weak ones. Reducing pulse power (damping) is sometimes desirable to reduce reverberation, or ringing, in a transmitter and thus to improve the resolution of distant structures. When weak echoes are obtained, however, it is usually best to decrease the damping, that is, to use a more powerful ultrasound pulse.

Reject. This control entirely eliminates low-amplitude ultrasound impulses from the system. If it is set too low, many echoes of very low amplitude will occupy the ventricular chamber between the left interventricular septum and the left ventricular endocardium. The control serves to eliminate the weakest echoes from the display and eliminates many ultrasound artifacts.

Transducer. Transducers are generally of various frequency ranges—quantitated in megahertz (MHz) — and are focused or nonfocused. Most transducers can be focused at 5.2 cm for a 2.25 MHz transducer and at 11.6 cm for a 5.0 MHz transducer. The current transducers have a frequency of 2.25 or 3.5 MHz, and are 13 mm in diameter. For small children and patients with small intercostal spaces, a 3.5 MHz transducer 7 mm in diameter is commonly used. For newborn infants, a 5.0 or 7.5 MHz transducer can be utilized, and, for premature infants, a 7.5 MHz transducer is used. **Resolution** is defined as the ability to distinguish echoes from structures in close proximity, such as the pericardium and epicardium. In selecting a transducer, it must be remembered that the *lower* the frequency, the *longer* the wavelength and, therefore, the *greater* the penetration into tissue. However, the *lower* the frequency, the *poorer* the resolution will be. At higher frequencies, the wavelength will be shorter and the ability to penetrate tissue diminished, but the resolution will be improved. New quarter-wave transducers have much improved resolution.

Echoscope Recorder Controls

Paper speed. Paper speed should usually be linked to the M-mode display so that the speeds of the oscilloscopic display and of the recording paper will correspond. For most purposes, 50 mm/sec is ideal; recorders should have the capacity for a range of speeds, however — from 10 mm/sec for slow-speed scans to 100 mm/sec for simultaneous echocardiographic and phonocardiographic studies.

Echo display position. This control allows the M-mode picture to be positioned on the recording paper at the desired level.

Echocardiographic size. This control adjusts the vertical height of the echocardiographic recording. The recording may cover the entire width of the paper or, if other parameters are also being recorded, may be adjusted to cover a smaller area. The control should be reset for each patient to include the heart and some posterior lung, while allowing space, as needed, for other parameters.

Trace contrast. This control, included on some recorders, allows the operator to adjust the density of the tracing independent of the **overall contrast level,** which controls the contrast of the entire echoscope display.

ECG lead, amplitude, position. An ECG lead showing both atrial and ventricular depolarization (lead II of the electrocardiogram) should be utilized. The ECG recording should be positioned so that it does not interfere with the echocardiographic picture; it is generally placed either at the top or at the bottom of the record.

A phonocardiographic, or pulse, recording may be desirable at times. The echocardiographic display size should be reduced accordingly, to allow space at the top or bottom of the paper for the phonographic recording.

Time marker. Time-marker lines should be displayed at the top or bottom of the paper, or, for more precise measurements, they can be displayed over the entire record.

Coupling gel. Coupling gel, or jelly, ensures air-free contact between the patient's skin and the transducer. One should use commercially available gels that do not stain clothing, are hypoallergenic, and will not melt at slightly elevated body temperatures or in an isotonic solution such as skin perspiration.

Clip (intensity control). Clip controls the intensity of individual echoes. A high setting causes blooming or clouding around each echo. As a consequence, echoes lying in close proximity will bleed into each other, resulting in loss of lateral resolution.

Two-Dimensional Echocardiography

Two-dimensional echocardiography can be divided into three basic types: mechanical echocardiography, phased-array echocardiography, and linear-array echocardiography. The following sections briefly discuss the instrumentation each requires.

Mechanical Echocardiography

Mechanical two-dimensional echocardiography includes use of a transducer, generally an oscillating one with one element or a rotary one with three or four elements, that is sealed in a fluid-filled housing (Figure 1-5). Weight of the

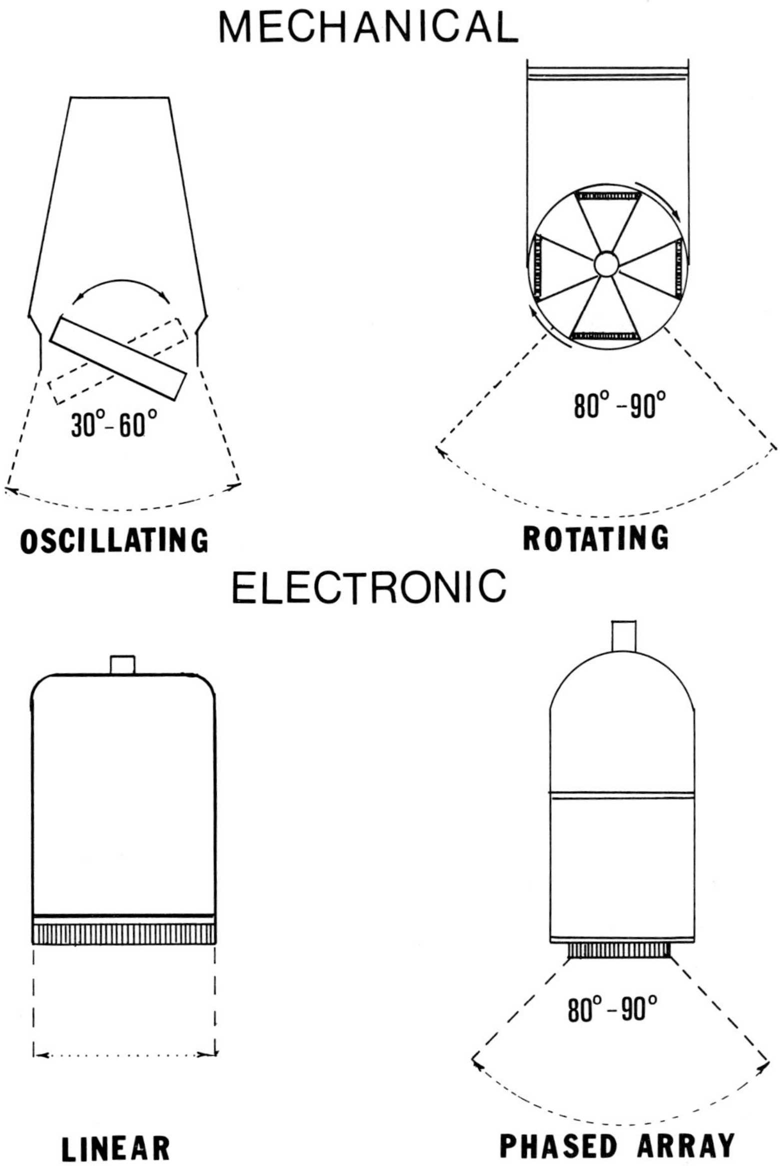

Figure 1-5
Different types of mechanical and phased-array two-dimensional transducers.

probe head is relatively light. The ultrasound specifications include a transducer with a frequency of 2.25 or 3.5 MHz, a transducer diameter of 12 mm or less, and display arc from 30° to 90°. For children, 3.5 and 5.0 MHz transducers are used. Other instrumentation includes an interface module, a videocassette recorder, a display monitor, a foot switch for the recorder, a camera, a strip-chart recorder, and an electrocardiographic display.

The mechanical two-dimensional system usually can provide either M-mode or two-dimensional real-time images, or in some cases, both. The images can be displayed on a large X - Y monitor, a **cathode-ray tube** (CRT) display for photographs, or a strip-chart recorder. A videocassette recorder is an integral part of the system; it records the ultrasonic images on videotape and plays them back on the X - Y display monitor, thereby permitting later analysis of echocardiographic data. A hand-held-probe creates a two-dimensional, 30° to 90° image for display; a time-motion (M-mode) display is obtained by either stopping the probe scan (switching to M-mode format) or by selecting any desired line of the two-dimensional scan. With some systems, a line-selected M-mode display can be obtained on one scope, while simultaneous two-dimensional display is obtained on another. The M-mode display can be recorded on a strip-chart recorder. Controls are provided to vary the tissue depth presented on display for either mode.

The videocassette recorder may be activated by a foot switch. With the videocassette recorder switched to "play," the system should automatically switch into the mode that is consistent with the tape-recorded data. The foot switch can be used to start the videocassette recorder or the strip-chart recorder, or both simultaneously.

Phased-Array Echocardiography

Phased-array echocardiography employs multiple-element transducers in which a series of delays is programmed into the firing of individual elements so that an ultrasonic wave front is created at an angle to the transducer. The activation sequence of the individual elements is alternated by a small microprocessor, producing a beam that is swept electronically through a sector of from 60° to 90°. The result is a two-dimensional electronic scanner than can cover a wider angle than is possible with two-dimensional mechanical scanners. There are generally thirty-two transmitters with 16 to 24 receiver boards for wide-angle ultrasonic imaging, enhanced image qualities, and target resolution.

The phased-array system also has the capability of electronically focusing the ultrasound beam to a greater degree than is possible with the current lenses of traditional transducers. This application also requires newer, more advanced electronic mini-computers or microprocessors. To date, the phased-array ultrasonograph has provided a wider field of imaging with less distortion. However, definition of finely detailed cardiac structures is not substantially improved over that obtained with mechanical systems. These systems are inherently more costly due to added research and development costs and to the need for frequent adjustments.

Linear-Array Echocardiography

In **linear-array echocardiography,** a multielement transducer arranged in a linear system is utilized to obtain a cross-sectional, linear scan of the heart. This multihead transducer has 20 small transducer elements, approximately 3 mm in diameter, which are activated in rapid sequence. Virtually simultaneous firing of the transducer will create a linear scan of the heart.

With **interlacing,** or reduplicating of lines of information, forty lines of information are presented, giving a composite image of the heart and great vessels. Although the two-dimensional image produced is potentially larger, interference of the transducer heads with the adult rib cage limits the size of the image actually obtained. This two-dimensional system was one of the earliest, and prompted a greater degree of interest and investigation in real-time, cross-sectional imaging of the heart. It has been developed and utilized largely in European medical centers.

ECHOCARDIOGRAPHIC MEASUREMENTS

Several factors influence the accuracy of echocardiographic measurement, perhaps the most important of which is the resolution of the echocardiographic instrumentation. At the frequency of sound waves commonly used, distinction can be made between objects that are approximately 1 mm apart. Resolution is further limited by the fact that the echo beam has a finite width and will diverge at a distance from the transducer: since the signal in the lateral edges of the ultrasonic beam will be weaker, objects in the periphery may not be visualized as well and resolution will be poorer than in the center of the beam.

Because of these problems of resolution and because of a certain amount of arbitrariness in the choice of where echocardiographic measurements are made, the American Society of Echocardiography has devised a set of standards for M-mode measurements, presented below.[2] All measurements are taken using the **"leading-edge" method.** Since the border of any structure is likely to have a finite width, it was decided that measurements would be from the most anterior margin of a line representing the anterior surface of the structure to the most anterior margin of a line representing the posterior surface of that structure (Figure 1-1).

To date, quantitative measurements of chamber dimensions or wall thicknesses are best made from M-mode echocardiograms; however, quantitative assessment of chamber volumes and orifice size (particularly the mitral valve area in mitral stenosis) are best made from two-dimensional echocardiograms.

Proper measurement in echocardiography provides the opportunity to reevaluate the completeness and comprehensiveness of the procedure. The following measurements are adopted from the American Society of Echocardiography's recommendations for M-mode echocardiograms.[2]

Aortic Root

The **aortic root** should be measured by the leading-edge method — from the most anterior (outer) portion of the anterior aortic wall to the most anterior (inner) boundary of the posterior aortic wall. To reduce the potential for angulation error, measurements should be made only after a mitral - aortic sweep in the area of the recording has visualized at least two aortic cusps. The aortic tracing should be marked on the record by the technician at the time he or she completes the sweep and finds his or her hand perpendicular to the chest wall. Because, due to angulation, aortic interfaces are often less clear in **systole,** and because the expansion of the aortic root in systole is variable, the aortic root should be measured at **end diastole,** at the onset of the first rapid deflection of the QRS complex of the ECG.

Left Atrium

A sweep from the left ventricle to the aorta is first performed to demonstrate which line in the left atrium is in continuity with the left ventricular posterior wall (Figure 1-1). Once this line has been located, the left atrial dimension can be measured, at the **end of ventricular systole** (at the end of T-wave of ECG), to include the thickness of the posterior aortic wall.

Timing of End Diastole

There is considerable variability in the pinpointing of end diastole and in the morphology of the QRS complex. The peak of the R wave occupies a variable portion of the ECG, depending on the lead selected, and any arbitrary delay after the onset of the QRS must take into account the age of the patient and the heart rate. Therefore, although it does not represent the real end of diastole, the onset of the first defection of the QRS complex of the ECG is recommended as the most reasonable point at which measurements should be made.

Cavities and Walls — Definition of the Standard Plane

With regards to the measurement of **cavities** and **walls,** it has been shown that the mitral leaflets occupy a larger portion of the left ventricular cavity in a small heart than in the adult heart. In young children and infants, therefore, the **standard plane** for measuring right and left ventricular cavity dimensions and wall-thickness measurements is at the level of the mitral leaflets. In older children, adolescents, and adults the structures can be measured at the level of the chordae tendineae. The transducer should be perpendicular to the chest wall or pointed slightly inferiorly and laterally. Measurements should be made only after a long-axis sweep has been obtained.

Right Ventricular Anterior Wall

The **right ventricular anterior wall** can be measured, but only on echocardiograms in which the epicardial and endocardial surfaces have been brought out by use of damping and a high-frequency transducer. It should be measured at the onset of the QRS complex, in a plane passing through standard plane of the left ventricle.

Right Ventricular Cavity Dimension

The **right ventricular cavity dimension** should be measured only when the right side of the septum and the endocardium of the right ventricular anterior wall have been clearly visualized. Measurements should be made in the usual plane passing through the left ventricle — at the level of either the chordae tendineae or the mitral valve, depending on the patient's age. **Switch gain** and / or damping may be utilized to avoid confusion of chordal echoes on the right septal surface. The right ventricle should be measured specifically in the portion of the echo marked by the technician at the end of expiration of the respiratory cycle.

In some patients, even when the right ventricular wall is not imaged clearly, it may be useful to try to estimate the size of the right ventricular cavity. It is recommended that such a measurement be called a right ventricular dimensional *estimate* and that it be performed at end expiration, at the onset of the QRS, from the right septal surface to the point most closely approximating the right ventricular anterior wall echo. Care should be taken to avoid left lateral decubitus positioning during this portion of the echo, since this position alters the right ventricular dimensional estimate, and the right ventricular dimension itself.

Left Ventricular Septum, Posterior Wall Thickness, and Left Ventricular End-Diastolic Cavity Dimension

With good septal visualization of both the right and left septal surfaces at the onset of the QRS, one may measure the **left ventricular septum,** the **posterior wall thickness,** (if endocardial and epicardial surfaces are imaged clearly), and the **left ventricular end-diastolic cavity dimension.** In all these measurements, switch gain or damping should be used to decrease the thickness of the endocardial and epicardial lines and to separate chordal structures. Wall and cavity measurements should be made according to the leading-edge method and using the thinnest continuous echo lines (from the front edge of endocardial lines of the septum to the front edge of endocardial lines of the posterior wall). Although this will require that cavity measurements extend slightly into the septum for the left ventricle, or into the right ventricular anterior wall for the right ventricle, it avoids the **gain dependence** inherent in the position of the trailing edge of echo lines.

Left Ventricular Systolic Dimension

There appears to be little difference between measurements of the **left ventricular systolic dimension** taken at the peak of the posterior wall motion and those taken at the **nadir** of septal motion. Because of its closeness in time to end systole, it is recommended that the nadir of septal motion be the point of measurement in patients in whom septal motion is normal. In patients in whom septal motion is abnormal or paradoxical at the level of the chordae tendineae (standard plane), however, left ventricular systolic dimension, should be measured at the peak of the posterior wall motion.

Fractional Shortening

Fractional shortening is the percentage of minor-axis shortening of the left ventricle during systole. It can be calculated using the following formula:

$$\% FS = \frac{EDD - ESD}{EDD} \times 100$$

where FS = fractional shortening
EDD = left ventricular end-diastolic dimension
ESD = left ventricular end-systolic dimension

Mitral Valve

The mitral valve should be measured as a D - E excursion in an area derived from a standard sweep in which both the anterior and posterior leaflets are imaged.

In addition to the basic measurements made from the echocardiogram, several indices of left ventricular function and extrapolations to left ventricular volume can be made. These include:

Left Ventricular End-Diastolic Volume (*EDV*):

$$EDV = \left(\frac{\pi}{3}\right) (EDD)^3$$

or

$$= (EDD)^3$$

or

$$= \left(\frac{7.0}{2.4 + EDD}\right) (EDD)^3$$

Left Ventricular End-Systolic Volume (*ESV*):

$$ESV = \left(\frac{\pi}{3}\right) (ESD)^3$$

or

$$= (ESD)^3$$

or

$$= \left(\frac{7.0}{2.4 + ESD}\right) (ESD)^3$$

Mean Velocity of Circumferential Shortening ($\bar{V}_{cf}$):

$$\bar{V}_{cf} = \left(\frac{EDD - ESD}{EDD}\right) ET$$

where ET = left ventricular ejection time (measured from the onset of opening to closure of the aortic valve or from systolic time intervals)

Left Ventricular Ejection Fraction (*EF*):

$$EF = \frac{SV}{EDV} = \frac{EDV - ESV}{EDV}$$

where SV = stroke volume

ECHOCARDIOGRAPHIC REPORTS

Echocardiographic reports are likely to be as varied as the personalities and backgrounds of the physicians interpreting echocardiograms. Experience, however, has made it possible to offer guidelines that facilitate communication with the referring physician.

Information from the Requesting Physician

In some instances, a specific question will be asked: for example, whether there is any evidence of mitral valve disease. Knowledge of history or physical findings usually will not affect interpretation but will provide direction for the performance of the test and wording of the interpretation. An echocardiogram performed in the absence of any signs or symptoms of heart disease is much less likely to detect any abnormality. Dating the request will help to monitor the delay between request, testing, and interpretation.

Patient Data

The most important patient data after the name, identification number, and date of examination is the patient's height and weight. Height, weight, age, and gender should be reported for both children and adults. In children, the importance of age and / or height and weight is self-evident; in adults, it is equally necessary to know these parameters. A 5.5-cm left ventricle belonging to a large, 2.5-m^2 man may be normal; belonging to a small 1.6-m^2 woman, however, it would be markedly abnormal. Normal adult echocardiographic values have been found to change with advancing age. Blood pressure at the time of echocardiography is used by some echocardiographers for the estimation of aortic valve gradients. Transducer position (e.g., parasternal, subxiphoid, suprasternal, or right sternal border) and patient position (e.g., left lateral) should be noted on the request forms or on the echocardiogram. The latter is preferred if more than one patient position or transducer location is used for an examination. Some echocardiographers may wish to know whether the examination was performed in the department or at the bedside.

Measurements

Measurements reported may be simple or brief (including the right and left ventricular internal dimensions, left ventricular posterior wall, septal thickness, and aortic, aortic root, and left atrial dimensions) or all-inclusive. Inclusion of every possible echocardiographic value or index makes the report cumbersome and may confer little additional benefit to the requesting physician. Highly detailed report forms require frequent updating as well.

Cardiac chamber size and wall thickness are often measured from the M-mode echocardiogram, even when two-dimensional echocardiographic studies are also performed. The timing of intracardiac events is more easily accomplished with M-mode echocardiography than with two-dimensional studies. Direct measurement of the left ventricular volumes or mitral valve area, on the other hand, is better with two-dimensional echocardiography. Qualitative study of segmental abnormalities in the motion of the left ventricular wall is possible with two-dimensional echocardiography. Routine calculation of left ventricular volume and ejection fraction by two-dimensional echocardiography requires good demonstration of the endocardium, careful transducer positioning, and a light pen or digitizer (see Chapter 12).

Interpretation

The most important recommendation regarding interpretation is that it be conservative. If a structure is not clearly imaged, it is preferable to repeat the examination or to omit a measurement rather than to guess.

If the patient's physician has posed a specific question, a clear answer should be included in the interpretation. Echocardiographic jargon like "B-bump" or "diastolic mitral fluttering" will mean little to a nonechocardiographer unless the physiologic significance is explained. Synthesis of echocardiographic findings must also be approached with caution: for example, although a combination of rheumatic mitral disease, left ventricular enlargement, and increased septal and posterior wall motion would suggest predominant mitral regurgitation, undetected aortic regurgitation must be considered as an alternate diagnosis.

SAFETY OF ECHOCARDIOGRAPHY

Widespread clinical experience with pulsed ultrasound, as utilized in echocardiography over the past 25 years, has demonstrated it to be a safe procedure without significant risk to either the patient or the operator. Although no untoward reactions directly resulting from this technique have been reported, its benefit-risk ratio requires continual reevaluation. The biologic effects of ultrasound are complex and poorly understood. Among the most obvious is the production of heat. Most commercially available M-mode equipment delivers a maximal intensity of approximately 50 w/cm^2. However, the short signal transmission period (1/1000 of the time) reduces actual delivered intensity to about 5 mw/cm^2, which appears quite safe for clinical purposes. Additionally, it has been estimated that only 10 percent of transmitted sound energy actually penetrates the skin to enter cardiac structures. Although initial reports suggested that ultrasound may cause chromosomal aberrations, other studies have not substantiated these findings.

Numerous types of instrumentation, with many modifications, are currently available. All newly acquired equipment must undergo performance as well as safety testing by the manufacturer prior to usage. Subsequently, periodic quality control testing must be continued by the medical facility electronics technician. Specifically, current leakage from the chassis through the power line ground and transducer should be checked. As most available systems are transportable to areas where access of direct electrical stimulation to the heart is possible (intensive care areas, catheterization laboratories), the need for strict safety standards is obvious. With the newer two-dimensional systems that have been developed, additional safety modifications have been undertaken.

REFERENCES

1. Henry WL, DeMaria A, Gramiak R, King DL, Kisslo JA, Popp RL, Sahn DJ, Schiller NB, Tajik A, Teichholz LE, Weyman AE: Report of the American Society of Echocardiogra-

phy Committee on Nomenclature and Standards in Two-dimensional Echocardiography. Circulation 62:212–215, 1980

2. Committee on Nomenclature and Standards in Two-dimensional Echocardiography: Recommendations Regarding Quantitation in M-mode Echocardiography. Indianapolis: American Society of Echocardiography, 1978
3. Sahn DJ, DeMaria A, Kisslo J, Weyman A: Recommendations regarding quantitation in M-mode echocardiography: Results of a survey of echocardiographic measurements. Circulation 58:1073–1978

ADDITIONAL ILLUSTRATIONS AND EXERCISES

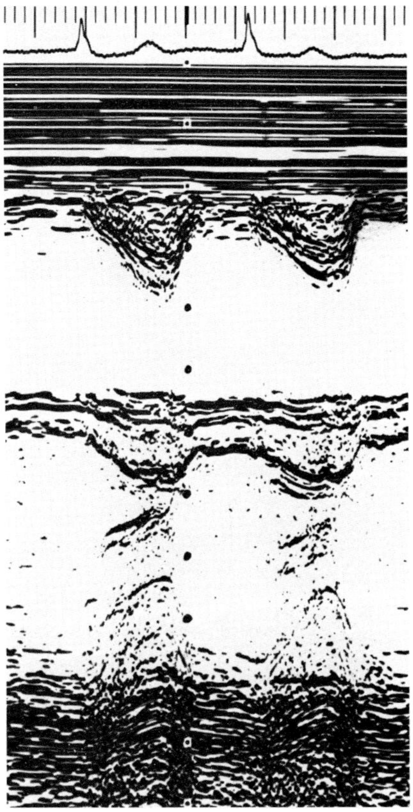

Figure 1-6

M-mode echocardiogram taken at the minor or short axis of the left ventricle. Anterior chamber is the right ventricle.*

1-6.1. Identify and measure the following dimensions in centimeters:

Right ventricle	______
Left ventricular diastolic dimension	______
Left ventricular systolic dimension	______
Interventricular septal thickness	______
Posterior wall thickness	______

1-6.2. Calculate the:

Percent fractional shortening	______
Ejection fraction	______

*The distance between one calibration dot and the next represents 1 cm.

Figure 1-7

M-mode echocardiogram taken at the aortic root, just at the level of the aortic leaflets. Note the large chamber behind the aorta.*

1-7.1. Identify and measure the:

Left atrium ________

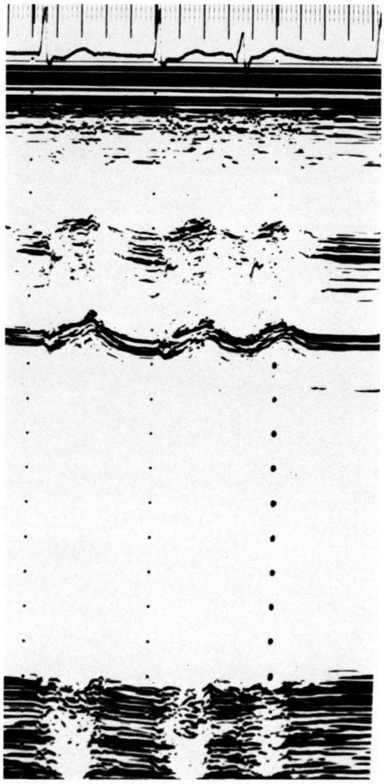

Figure 1-8

M-mode echocardiogram of the left ventricle of a patient with long-standing severe hypertension.*

1-8.1. Measure the following:

Interventricular septal thickness ________

Left ventricular posterior wall thickness ________

Left ventricular diastolic dimension ________

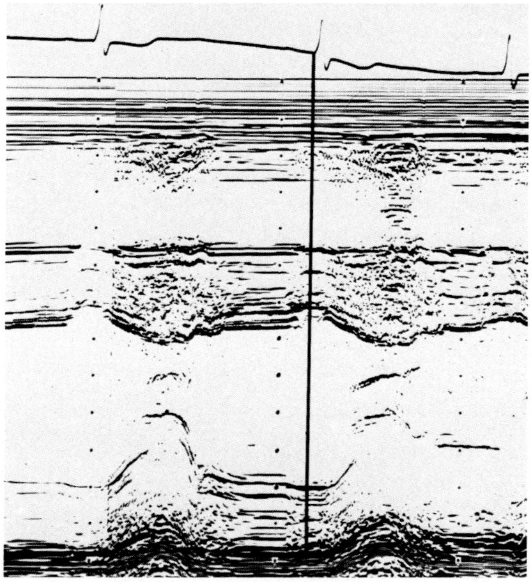

*The distance between one calibration dot and the next represents 1 cm.

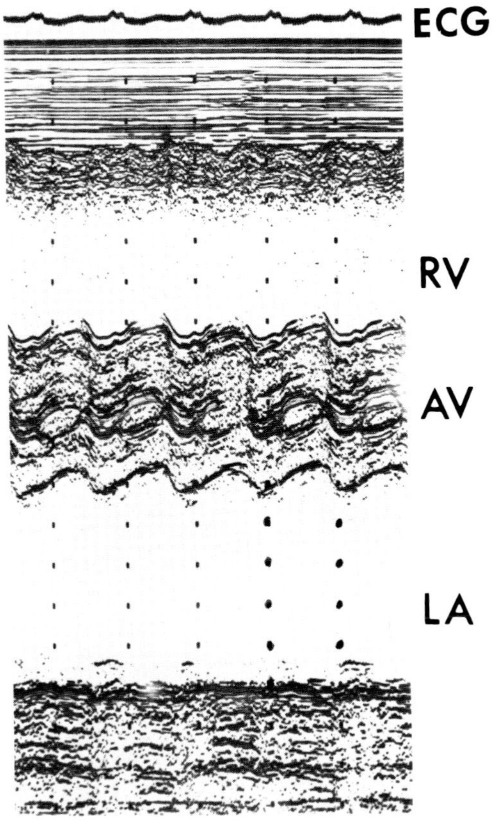

Figure 1-9

M-mode echocardiogram taken at the aorta in a patient with syncope and a harsh aortic systolic murmur. Note the thickened aortic leaflets.*

1-9.1. Measure the:

Left atrium ________

Aortic root ________

1-9.2. What is the probable diagnosis? ________

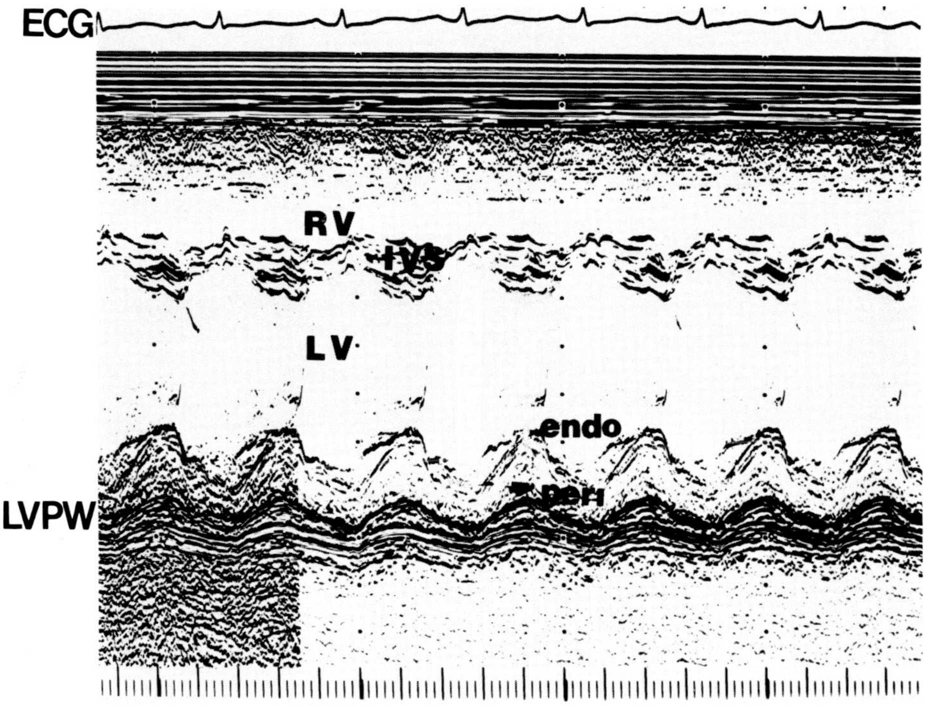

Figure 1-10

M-mode echocardiogram taken at the minor axis of the left ventricle.*

1-10.1. What is the left ventricular end-diastolic dimension?

A. 4.6 cm
B. 4.1 cm
C. 3.1 cm
D. 2.8 cm

1-10.2. What is the left ventricular end-systolic dimension?

A. 4.6 cm
B. 4.1 cm
C. 3.1 cm
D. 2.8 cm

1-10.3. What is the calculated fractional shortening?

A. 38%
B. 35%
C. 33%
D. 29%

*The distance between one calibration dot and the next represents 1 cm.

Figure 1-13

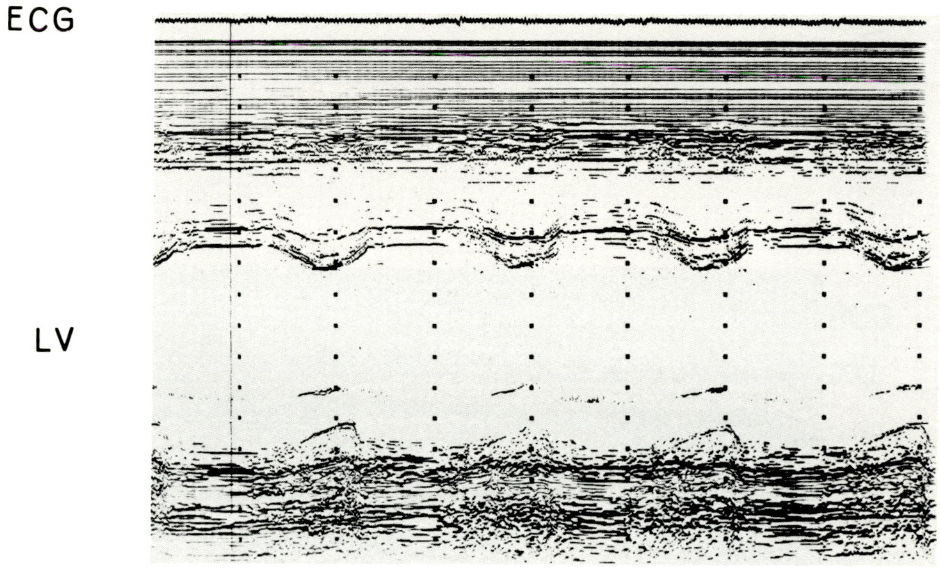

1-13.1. What is the left ventricular end-diastolic dimension?*
A. 5.0 cm
B. 6.5 cm
C. 6.8 cm
D. 7.0 cm

1-13.2. What is the left ventricular end-systolic dimension?
A. 4.9 cm
B. 6.4 cm
C. 6.8 cm
D. 7.0 cm

1-13.3. What is the percent fractional shortening?
A. 16%
B. 25%
C. 28%
D. 33%

1-13.4. Are these values normal or abnormal?
A. Normal
B. Abnormal

Figure 1-14

Slow-speed M-mode scan from the aorta to the left ventricle.*

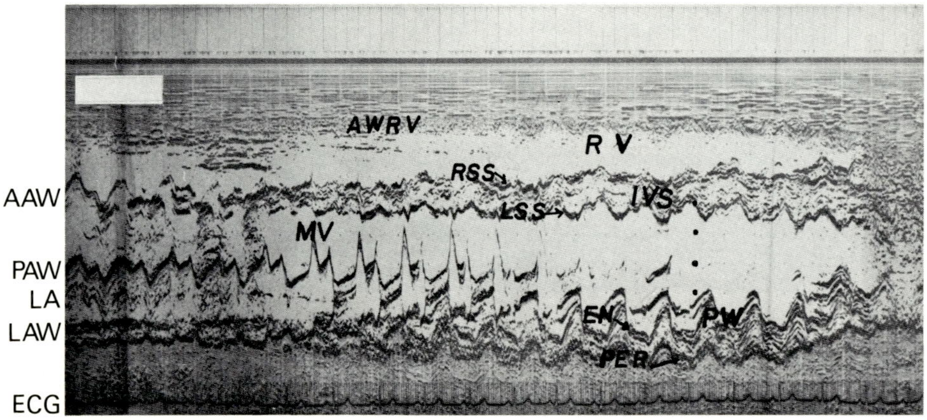

1-14.1. The motion of the interventricular septum is:
A. Normal
B. Abnormal

1-14.2. The motion of the posterior wall is:
A. Normal
B. Abnormal

1-14.3. Is pericardial effusion present?
A. Yes
B. No

*The distance between one calibration dot and the next represents 1 cm.

David I. Koenigsberg
Charles Ganote

2

Anatomy of the Heart as Related to Two-Dimensional Echocardiography

Hearts obtained at postmortem examination never exactly duplicate the size or configuration of hearts during life. This is because normal intravascular and intracavitary pressures are no longer present. With cessation of blood flow, hearts become globally ischemic, undergo ischemic contracture, and, finally, enter a state of rigor or stiffening analogous to rigor mortus in skeletal muscle.

Because of ischemic contracture and rigor, hearts after death assume a ventricular cavity size and wall thickness approximating that of cardiac systole during life. Hearts in failure or with elevated end-systolic intracavitary volumes during life retain dilated atria and ventricles after death, superficially resembling normal hearts in the diastolic phase of the cardiac cycle. Only fortuitious circumstances, however, would generate a heart that at postmortem examination exactly duplicated a heart at any particular instant during a normal cardiac cycle. Despite these limitations in the extent to which living and fixed hearts correspond, there are also limitations in the extent to which they can differ.

It is often difficult, even impossible, to section a heart specimen so as to correspond exactly to an analogous echocardiographic tomogram made during life. Nevertheless, attempts to correlate sectional views of fixed hearts with two-dimensional echocardiograms can lead to a greater understanding of normal and pathologic anatomical relationships among structures in normal and diseased hearts.

The two-dimensional echocardiograms illustrated in this chapter were obtained using a SmithKline mechanical two-dimensional scanner (SmithKline Instruments, Sunnyvale, Calif.) with a 90° transducer and a Varian 3400 phased-array ultrasonograph (Varian Medical Ultrasound Division, Salt Lake City, Utah). Where instructive, the two-dimensional echocardiograms in both systole and diastole are demonstrated. A still-frame picture of a two-dimensional echogram does not do justice to the real-time videotape of the entire cardiac cycle. In addition, still photographs of mechanical two-dimensional echocardiograms require double exposure of film, since still frames do not interlace with the mechanical sector system. Some resolution is thereby lost. Nevertheless, sufficient information is present on still photographs of two-dimensional echocardiograms for comparison with pathologic specimens.

LEFT VENTRICLE—PARASTERNAL LONG-AXIS VIEW

Anatomical Specimen

The section in Figures 2-1 A and B, oriented to correspond to a parasternal long-axis view, shows the right portion of the cut heart facing the interventricular septum (IVS) and the left side of the atrial septum (LA). The anterior wall of the right ventricle (RV) appears at the top of the photograph. The plane crosses the interventricular septum, and the aortic valve is sectioned across the right coronary cusp (RCC) and the left coronary cusp (LCC). The membranous septum (MS) is located just below the junction of the right coronary cusp and the noncoronary cusp (NCC) of the aortic valve.

The section passes near the middle of the anterior (AML) and posterior

Figure 2-1 A

Parasternal long-axis view of the heart—anatomical specimen.

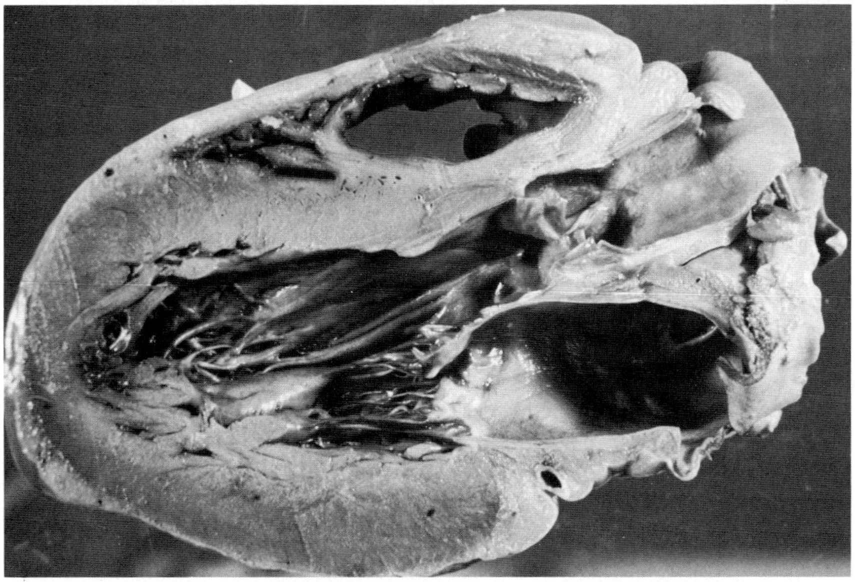

Figure 2-1 B

Labelled diagram of Figure 2-1 A

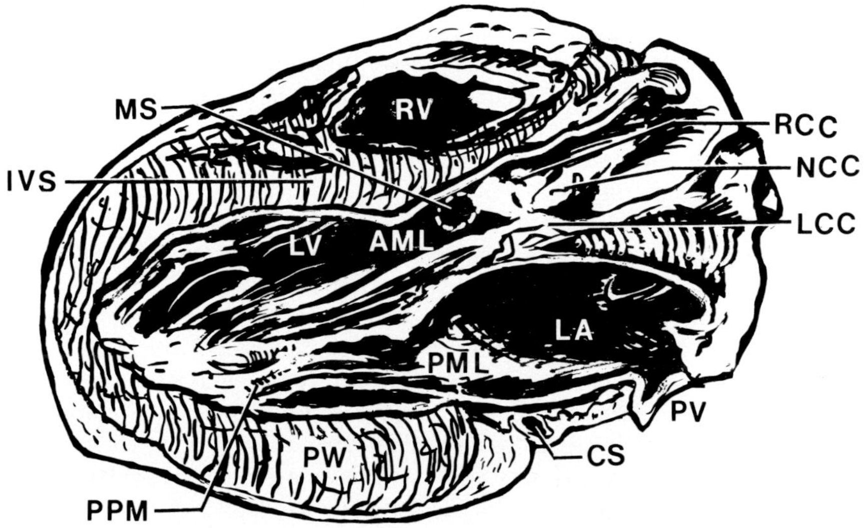

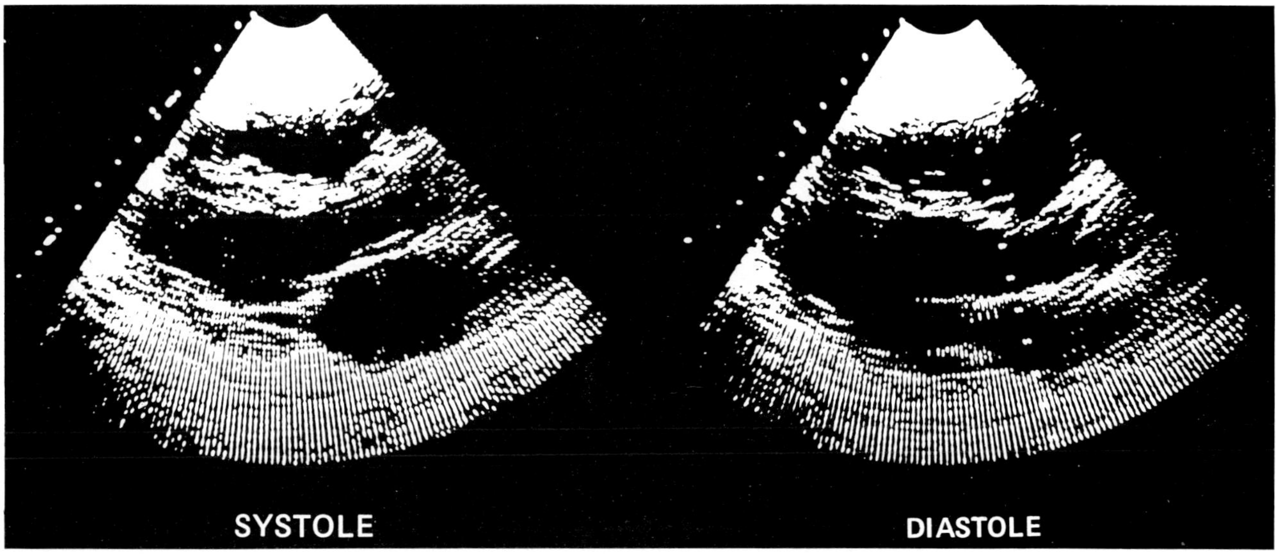

Figure 2-1 C

Parasternal long-axis views of the heart in systole and diastole—two-dimensional echocardiogram.

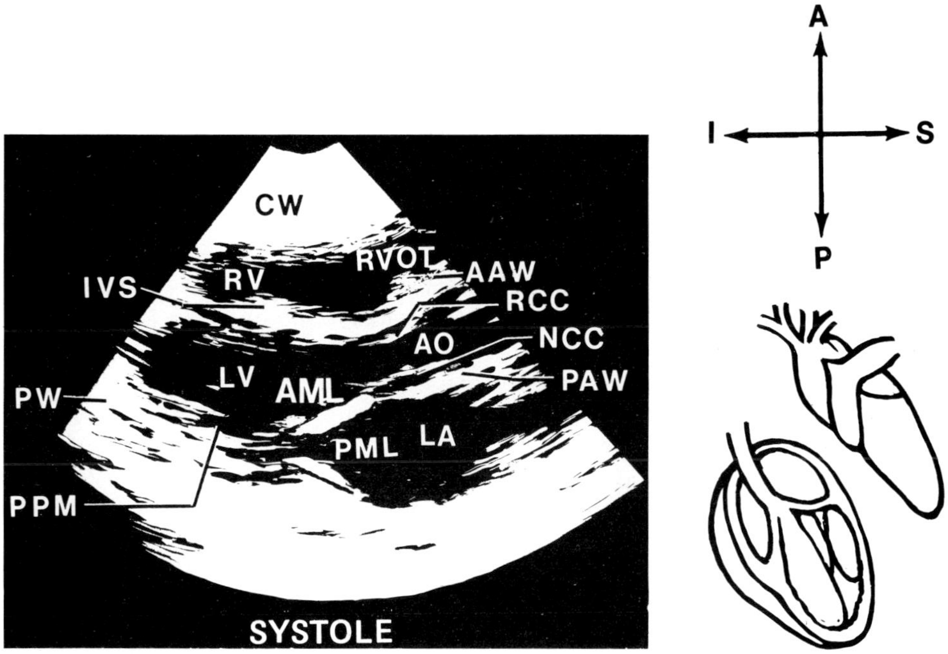

Figure 2-1 D

Labelled drawing of heart in systole from echocardiogram in Figure 2-1 C.

(PML) leaflets of the **mitral valve.** The posteromedial **papillary muscle** (PPM) of the mitral valve lies at the junction of the septum (IVS) and posterior wall of the left ventricle (PW) and sends **chordae tendineae** to the medial halves of both the anterior (AML) and posterior (PML) mitral leaflets. The posterior wall of the left atrium is continuous with the posterior wall of the left ventricle, and there is a smooth line between the cavities of the left atrium and ventricle. The posterior wall of the left ventricle forms a rounded shelf that bulges somewhat in the area posterior to the wall of the left atrium; the **atrioventricular sulcus** (groove) thus formed is filled with fat and contains the **coronary sinus** (CS). A pulmonary vein (PV) opens into the left atrium.

Two-Dimensional Echocardiogram—Systole and Diastole

In the echocardiogram of the heart during systole (Figures 2-1 C, D) the coapted leaflets of the mitral valve appear in the form of a "Y" on its side. The anterior mitral leaflet (AML) and posterior mitral leaflet (PML) form the two arms of the "Y"; the chordae tendineae form the leg. The anterior leaflet of the mitral valve is seen to be continuous with the posterior aortic wall (PAW). The left atrium (LA) is posterior to the aorta. Both the right coronary cusp (RCC) of the aortic valve (anterior cusp) and the noncoronary cusp (NCC) of the aortic valve (posterior cusp) are seen in an open position. The right ventricular outflow tract (RVOT) is anterior to the aorta (AO). The left ventricle is seen in its long axis, with the interventricular septum (IVS) and right ventricle (RV) anteriorly, and the posterior wall (PW) and posteromedial papillary muscle (PPM) posteriorly. The apex of the left ventricle is located inferior to the papillary muscle.

In echocardiogram taken during diastole (Figure 2-1 C), the anterior mitral leaflet and posterior mitral leaflet have opened. The left atrium has consequently decreased and the left and right ventricles have consequently increased in size.

RIGHT VENTRICLE—PARASTERNAL LONG-AXIS VIEW

Anatomical Specimen

To view the right atrium and right ventricle in the long-axis view, a section has been made tangential to the heart, almost parallel to the chest wall. Figure 2-2 A (the right side of the heart viewed from the right) shows the plane of section. Medial to the plane of section (viewed clockwise) are the superior vena cava, the aorta, the right atrial appendage, the septal leaflet of the tricuspid valve, and the coronary sinus opening. The section cuts across the anterior and posterior tricuspid valve leaflets, the inferior vena cava, and the right coronary artery. The cutaway section at the bottom becomes the long axis view of the right ventricular inflow tract.

The specimen shown in Figures 2-2 B and C is the long-axis view of the right ventricular inflow tract, facing toward the right side of the atrium (RA) and ventricle (RV). The section passes across the anterior (ATL) and posterior leaflets (PTL) of the tricuspid valve and the opening of the inferior vena cava (IVC). The anterior (APM) and posterior (PPM) papillary muscles of the tricuspid valve are present. The right coronary artery (RCA) lies in fat near the atrioventricular sulcus. This section is oriented to correspond to echocardiographic views in which the portion of the heart nearest the transducer is at the top of the image.

Two-Dimensional Echocardiogram—Systole

The right atrium appears at the bottom of this echocardiogram (Figure 2-2 D). The anterior leaflet of the tricuspid valve (ATL) and posterior leaflet of the tricuspid valve (PTL) have coapted. The anterior wall of the right ventricle (RVW) is seen near the top of the echocardiogram.

ASCENDING AORTA AND PULMONARY ARTERY—PARASTERNAL SHORT-AXIS VIEW

Anatomical Specimen

The heart shown in Figure 2-3 A has been sectioned in the short-axis view from above and then reassembled. The most superior section (base of the heart) has been laid back, as though opening a book. This section is viewed as if looking from the apex toward the base of the heart. Seen in the remaining heart are the main pulmonary artery (MPA) and its branching into the right (RPA) and left (LPA) pulmonary arteries. The section crosses the pulmonic valve (PV), the superior portion of the right atrium, and the ascending aorta. (These structures are labeled in Figure 2-3 C.)

The section shown in Figures 2-3 B and C, taken from the specimen above, has been reoriented in the anteroposterior position as the heart lies in the chest cavity. It shows the ascending (top) and descending (bottom) portions of the aorta (AO), which straddle the right (RPA) and the left (LPA) pulmonary arteries, the pulmonic valve (PV), and the right atrium (RA).

Two-Dimensional Echocardiogram—Systole

The two-dimensional echogram in Figure 2-3 D is oriented 30° counterclockwise from Figure 2-3 B and C, with the right ventricular outflow tract (RVOT) at the top of the screen. The aorta (AO) is in the center of the field, with the main pulmonary artery (MPA) located anteriorly and the right (RPA) and left (LPA) pulmonary arteries located to the left of the aorta. The right atrium (RA) is to the right.

AORTIC VALVE—PARASTERNAL SHORT-AXIS VIEW

Anatomical Specimen

The heart shown in Figure 2-4 A has been sectioned in short axis in a plane at the level of the aortic valve. The top section is laid back and is viewed from the apex toward the base of the heart. The plane crosses portions of the tricuspid, aortic, and pulmonic valves.

Figures 2-4 B and C show the top section from Figure 2-4 A. The section passes through the right ventricular outflow tract (RVOT) and includes portions of the pulmonic valve (PV), the right (RCC), left (LCC), and noncoronary (NCC) cusps of the aortic valve, as well as the anterior leaflet of the tricuspid valve (ATL). Other structures seen are the coronary sinus (CS), the left atrium (LA), the right atrium (RA), and the left atrial appendage (LAA). The left anterior descending coronary artery (LAD) is seen passing between the left atrial appendage and the pulmonic valve.

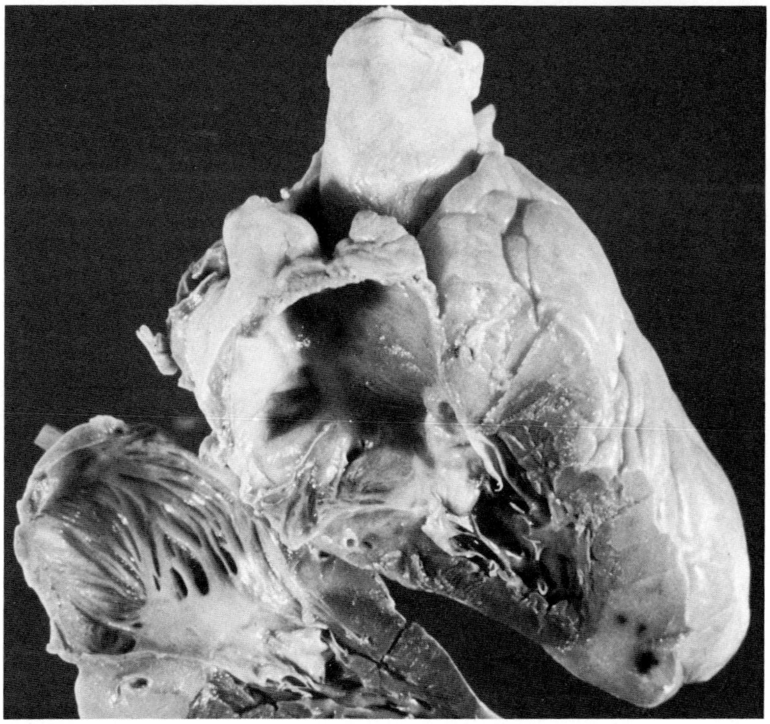

Figure 2-2 A

Whole heart opened to show the plane of section along the axis of the right ventricle. The heart is viewed looking from the right towards the left, as in a right anterior oblique view.

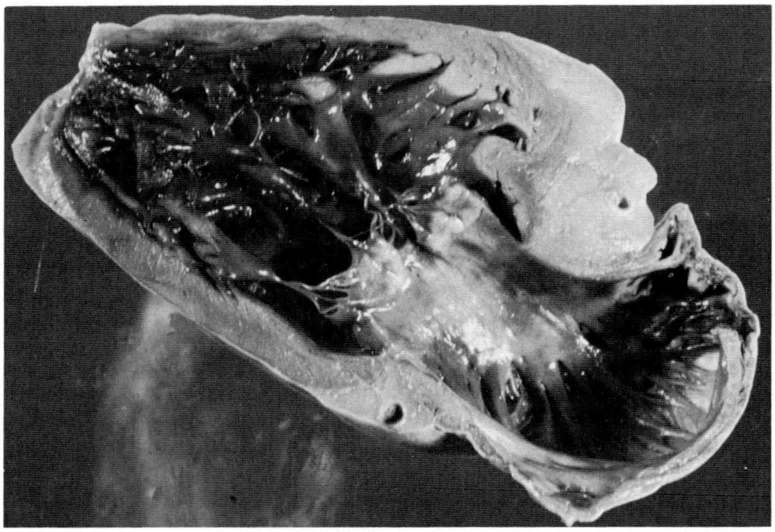

Figure 2-2 B

Long-axis section of right ventricle oriented with the anterior wall at the top of the picture and the posterior wall of the right ventricle at the bottom. The view is of the free wall of the right ventricle showing the large anterior papillary muscle and one of the smaller posterior papillary muscles.

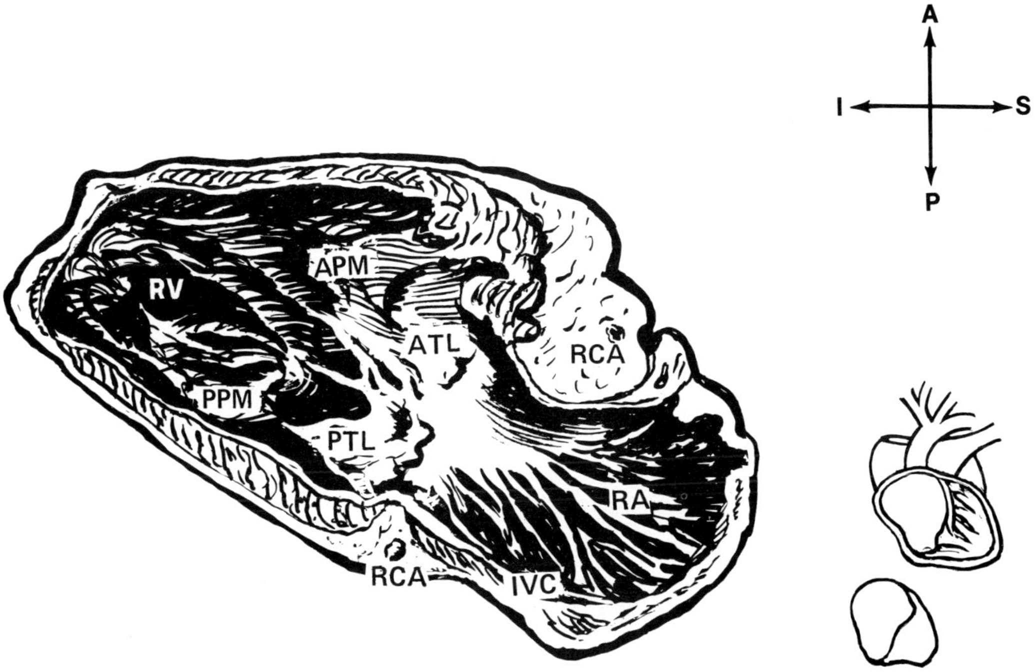

Figure 2-2 C

Labelled drawing of Figure 2-2 B.

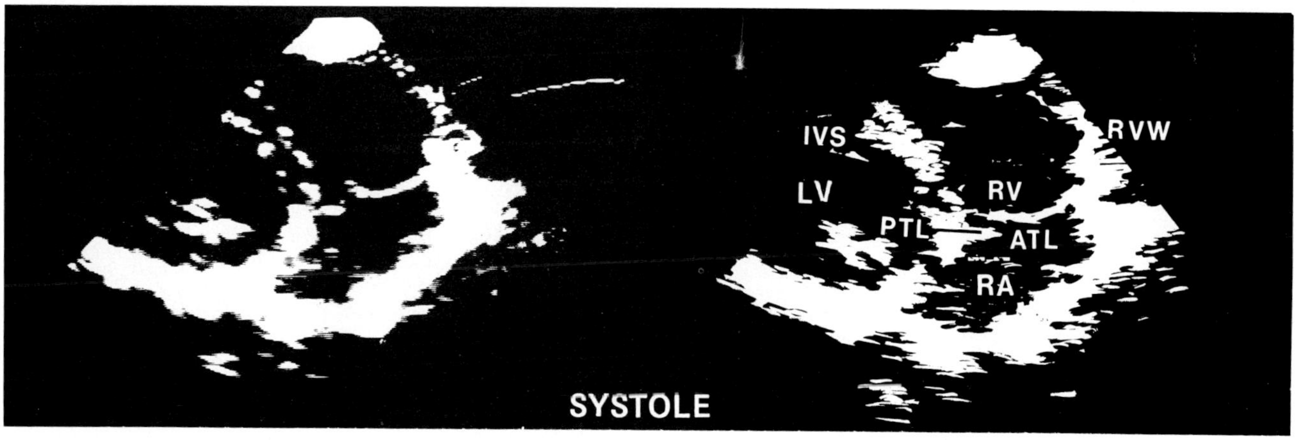

Figure 2-2 D

Parasternal long-axis view of the right ventricle in systole—two-dimensional echocardiogram to the left, diagrammatic drawing to the right.

Figure 2-3 A

Parasternal short axis plane—anatomical specimen.

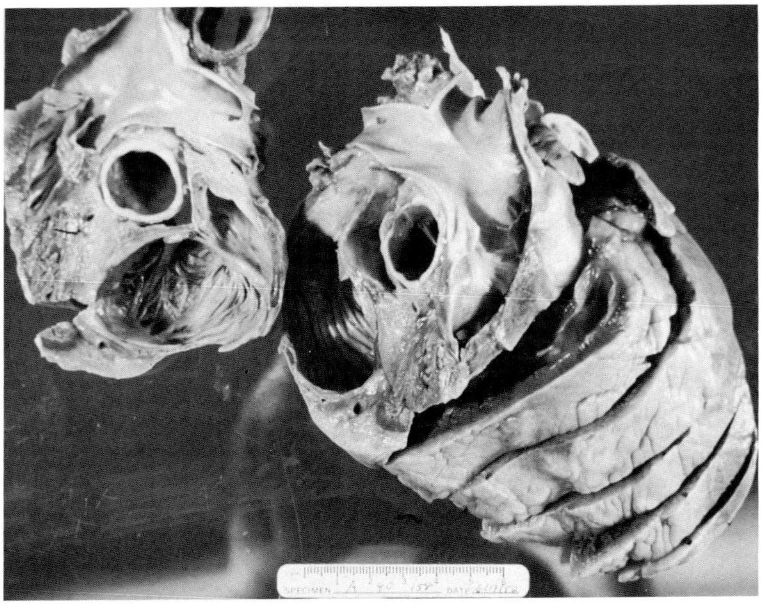

Figure 2-3 B

Parasternal short-axis view of the heart, pulmonary artery level—anatomical specimen.

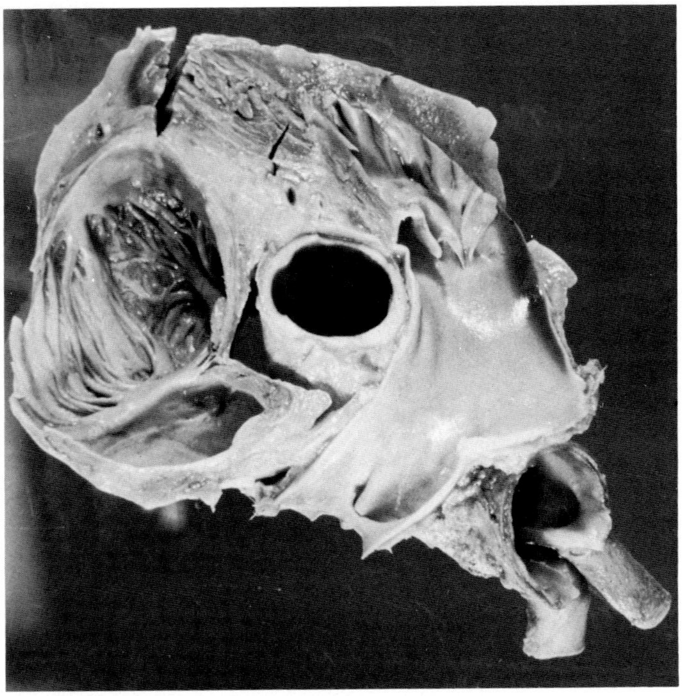

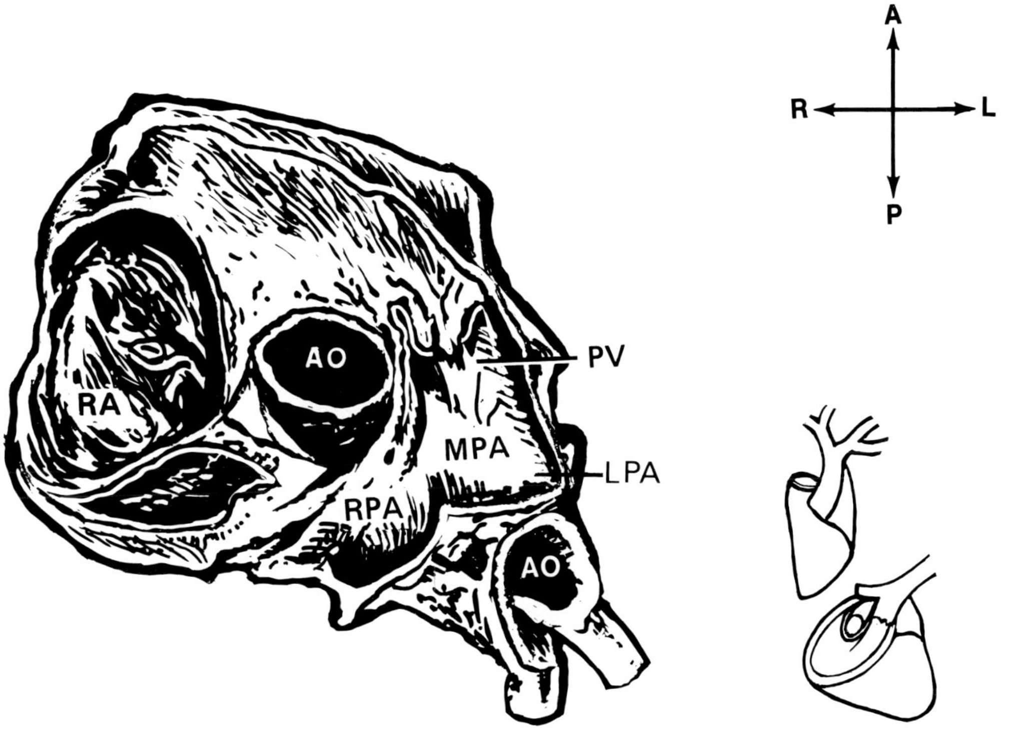

Figure 2-3 C
Labelled drawing of Figure 2-3 B.

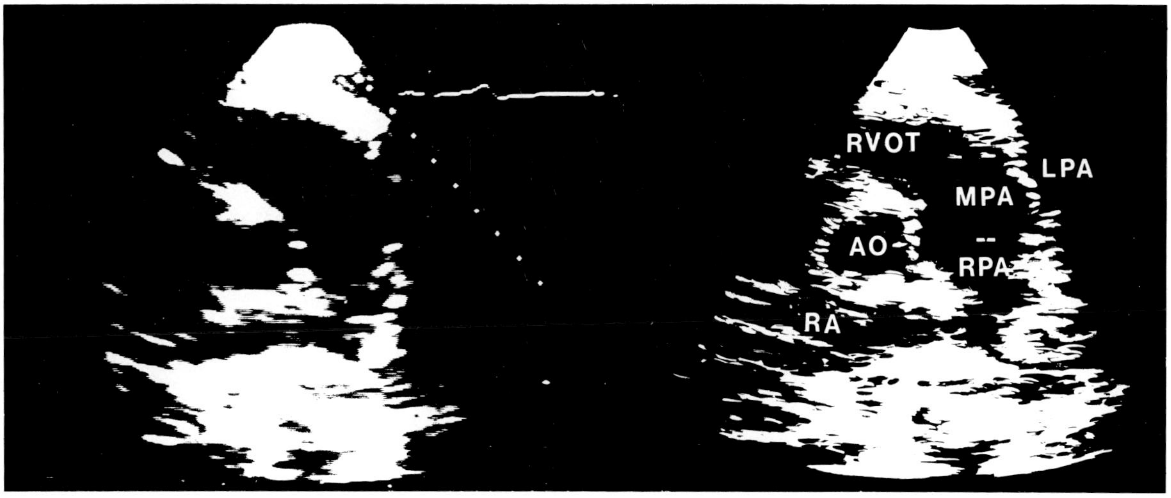

Figure 2-3 D
Parasternal short-axis view of the heart in systole, pulmonary artery level—echocardiogram to the left, diagrammatic drawing to the right.

Figure 2-4 A

Whole heart in short-axis plane—anatomical specimen.

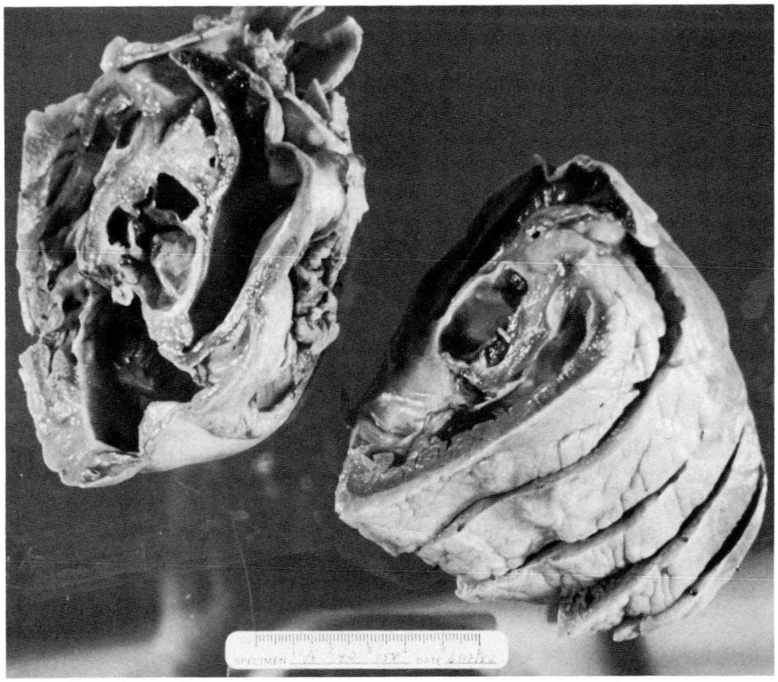

Figure 2-4 B

Parasternal short-axis view of the heart, aortic valve level—anatomical specimen.

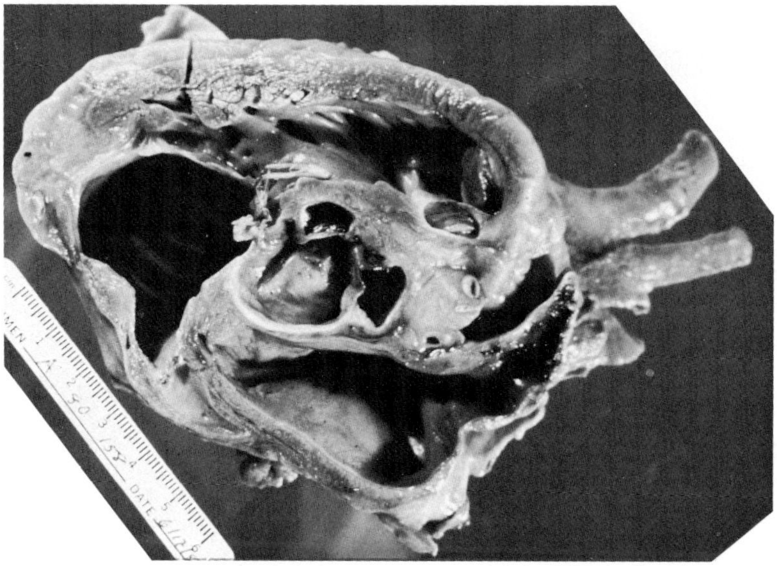

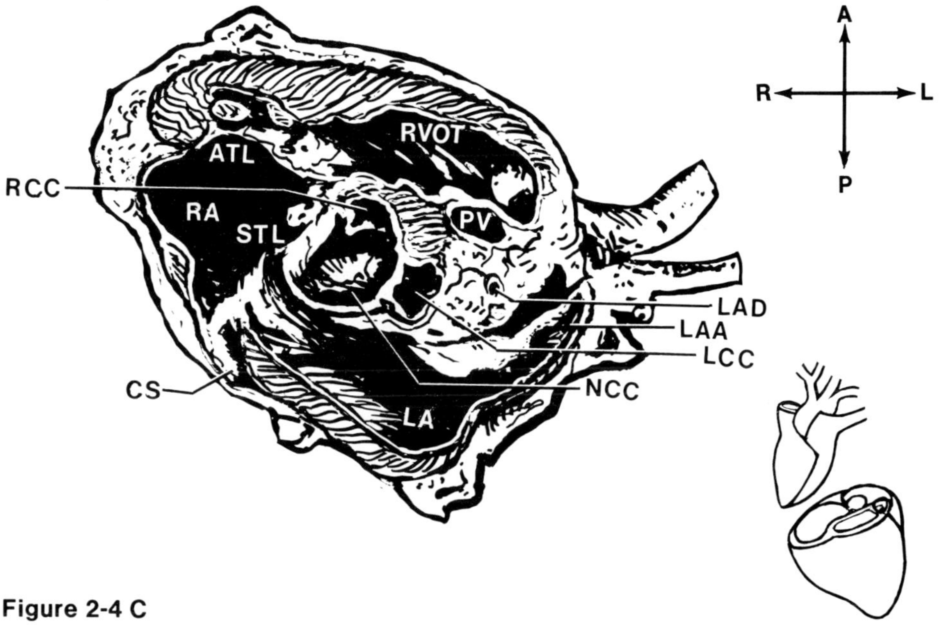

Figure 2-4 C

Labelled drawing of Figure 2-4 B.

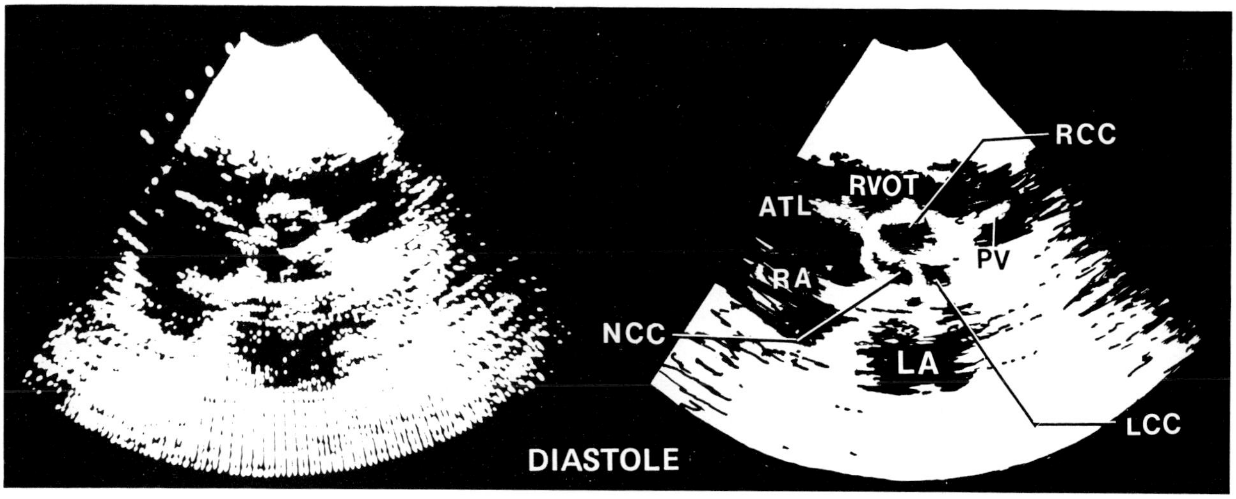

Figure 2-4 D

Parasternal short-axis view of the heart in diastole, aortic valve level—echocardiogram to the left, diagrammatic drawing to the right.

Two-Dimensional Echocardiogram—Diastole

In the echocardiogram in Figure 2-4 D, the three leaflets of the aortic valve can be seen in an inverted "Mercedes Benz" sign, with the three cusps of the aortic valve forming the components. The posterior cusp of the pulmonic valve (PV) is seen to the left of the aorta. The anterior tricuspid leaflet (ATL) is to the right of the aorta. The left atrium (LA), right atrium (RA), and interatrial septum appear at the bottom of the echocardiogram.

MITRAL VALVE—PARASTERNAL SHORT-AXIS VIEW

Anatomical Specimen

A section passing near the base of the heart (Figures 2-5 A and B) shows the tricuspid valve (TV) and anterior (AML) and posterior (PML) leaflets of the mitral valve. The interventricular septum (IVS) separates the right ventricular (RV) and left ventricular cavities. The left anterior descending artery (LAD) lies in the groove at the junction of the right and left ventricles.

Two-Dimensional Echocardiogram—Systole and Diastole

In the echocardiogram taken during systole (Figure 2-5 C), the mitral valve leaflets have coapted. The left ventricular outflow tract (LVOT), interventricular septum (IVS), and right ventricle (RV) are seen anterior to the mitral valve (AML). The anterolateral wall of the left ventricle is to the left of the mitral valve and the posterior wall (PW) of the left ventricle is below it. (Structures are labelled in Fig. 2-5 D.)

During diastole, both leaflets of the mitral valve open and the appearance of the valve orifice is akin to a fish mouth (Figures 2-5 C, D).

PAPILLARY MUSCLE—PARASTERNAL SHORT-AXIS VIEW

Anatomical Specimen

Figures 2-6 A and B show a section taken at the standard plane in the mid-portion of the ventricular cavities. The section shows the anterior (APM) and posterior (PPM) papillary muscles of the tricuspid valve (top of specimen) and the anterolateral (APM) and the posterior medial papillary muscles (PPM) of the mitral valve in the left ventricle (LV). Note also the moderator band (MB). The specimen is oriented to correspond to an echocardiographic short-axis view taken with the subject slightly left lateral.

Two-Dimensional Echocardiogram—Systole and Diastole

In the echocardiograms shown in Figure 2-6 C and 2-6 D, the posteromedial papillary muscle of the mitral valve (PPM) is seen in the lower right portion, and the anterolateral papillary muscle (APM) is seen in the lower left portion of the left ventricle (LV). The interventricular septum (IVS), right ventricle (RV), and anterolateral free wall of the left ventricle (ALW) are seen near the top of the echocardiogram. The difference in size of the left ventricle during systole and diastole is easily appreciated.

APICAL FOUR-CHAMBER VIEW (OPTION 2)

Anatomical Specimen

This four-chamber view (Figures 2-7 A and B) is oriented according to option 2 of the American Society of Echocardiography's Committee on Nomenclature and Standards in Two-Dimensional Echocardiography.[1] The specimen is viewed with the posterior portion of the heart removed, looking toward the anterior surfaces of the cardiac chambers. The right atrium (RA) is to the right and the left atrium (LA) is to the left. The section cuts across the septal leaflet of the tricuspid valve (STL). Fat is present in the interatrial septum (IAS), and scarring is present in the ventricular septum (IVS). The anterior leaflets of the tricuspid valve (ATL), the mitral valve (AML), and the anterolateral papillary muscle of the mitral valve (APM) are anterior to the plane of section. The left circumflex coronary artery (LCA) and ostia of the pulmonary veins (LPV and RPV) are seen.

Two-Dimensional Echocardiogram—Systole

The echocardiogram in Figures 2-7 C and D, also oriented according to option 2, shows the interventricular septum separating the right (RV) from the left ventricle (LV) and the interatrial septum separating the left (LA) from the right atrium (RA). Note that there is normally some dropout of echoes in the interatrial septum, so that this does not necessarily imply that there is a defect in the atrial septum. The anterior and septal leaflets of the tricuspid valve (TV) and the anterior mitral leaflet (AML) can be seen separating the right ventricle from the right atrium and the left ventricle from the left atrium, respectively. Note that the tricuspid valve attachment to the septum is closer (inferior) to the apex than is the mitral valve.

APICAL FOUR-CHAMBER VIEW WITH AORTA (OPTION 2)

Anatomical Specimen

The section shown in Figures 2-8 A and B, slightly anterior to that in Figure 2-7 A, shows, in addition to the structures pointed out earlier, the left ventricular outflow tract—located between the septum (IVS) and the anterior mitral valve (AML)—the ascending aorta (AO), the openings of the superior vena cava (SVC), and the left atrial appendage (LAA). The section cuts across the anterolateral papillary muscle of the mitral valve (APM), the anterior leaflet of the mitral valve (AML), and part of the membranous septum (IVS). This view is sometimes called the five-chamber view.

Two-Dimensional Echocardiogram—Pre-Systole

The view in Figures 2-8 C and D is of similar orientation as the four-chamber view but includes the aorta and could be labelled as a five-chamber view. The aorta is seen at the junction formed by the interventricular septum, interatrial septum, mitral valve, and the tricuspid valve. The left atrial appendage and superior vena cava are not seen here.

Figure 2-5 A

Parasternal short-axis view of the heart, mitral valve level—anatomical specimen.

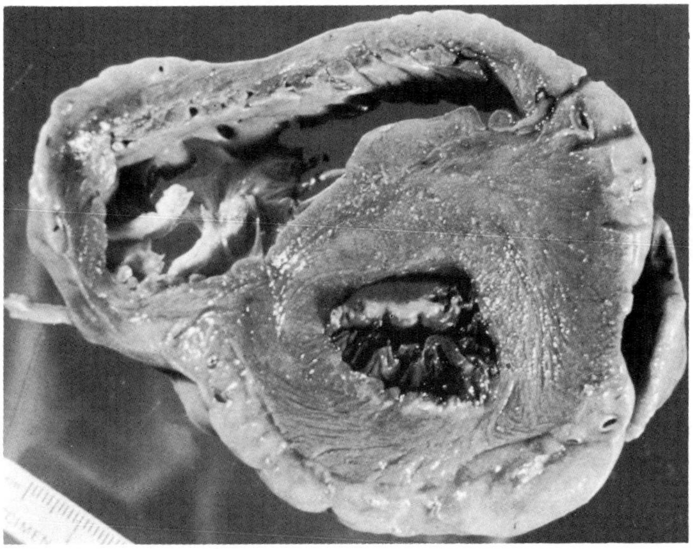

Figure 2-5 B

Labelled drawing of Figure 2-5 A rotated 30° clockwise.

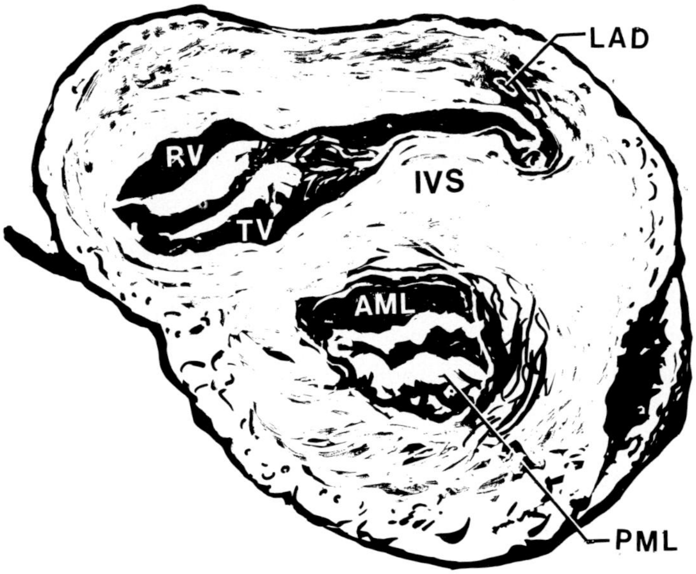

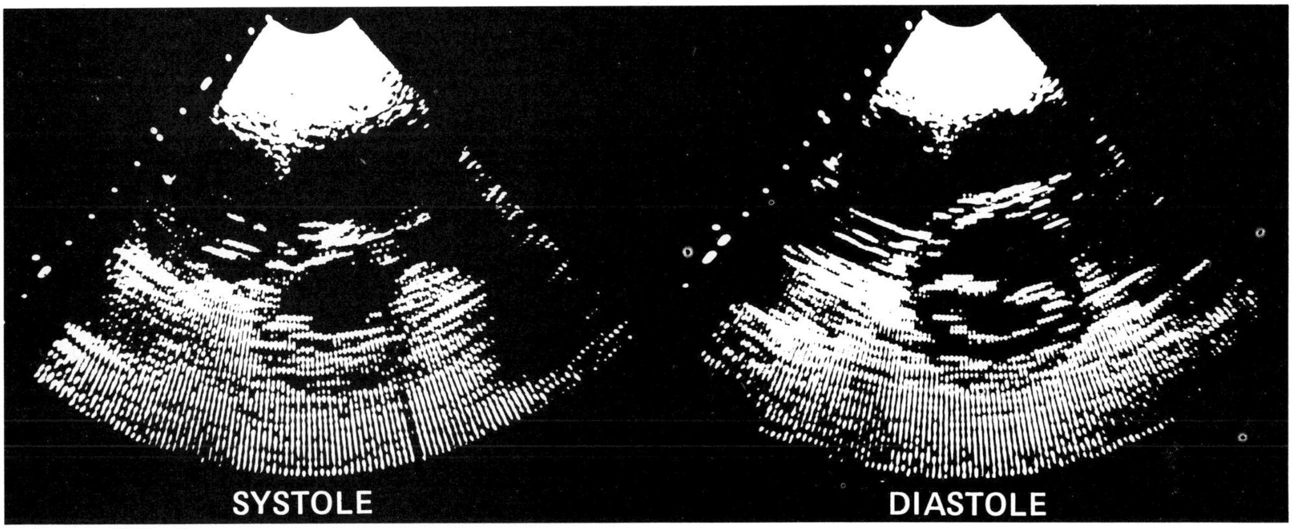

Figure 2-5 C
Parasternal short-axis view of the heart in systole and diastole, mitral valve level—two-dimensional echocardiogram.

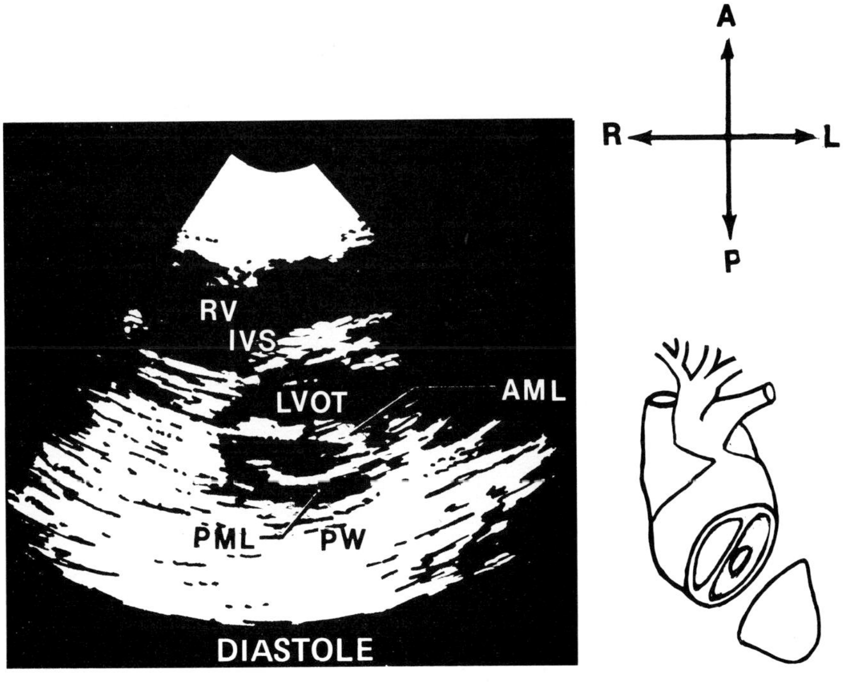

Figure 2-5 D
Labelled drawing of heart in diastole from Figure 2-5 C.

Figure 2-6 A

Parasternal short-axis view of the heart, papillary muscle level—anatomical specimen.

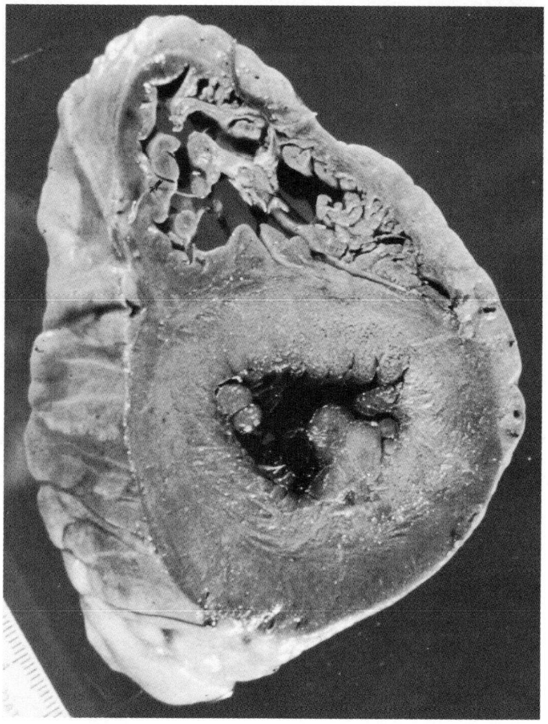

Figure 2-6 B

Labelled drawing of Figure 2-6 A.

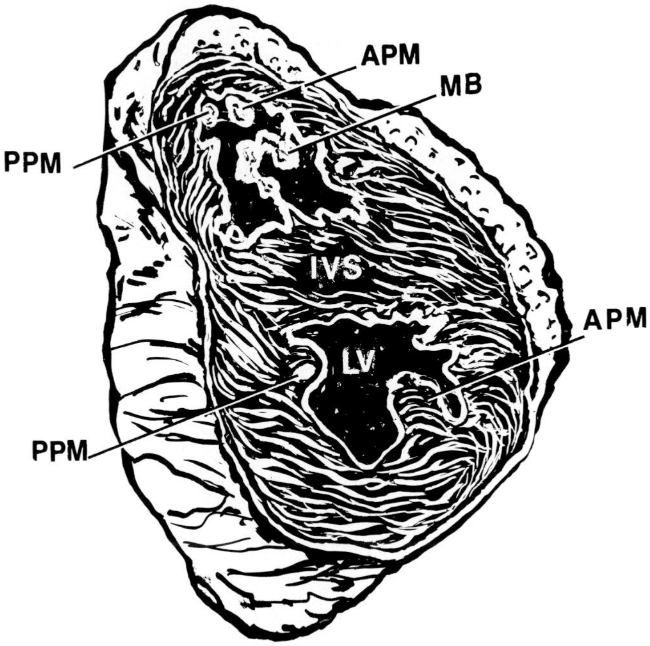

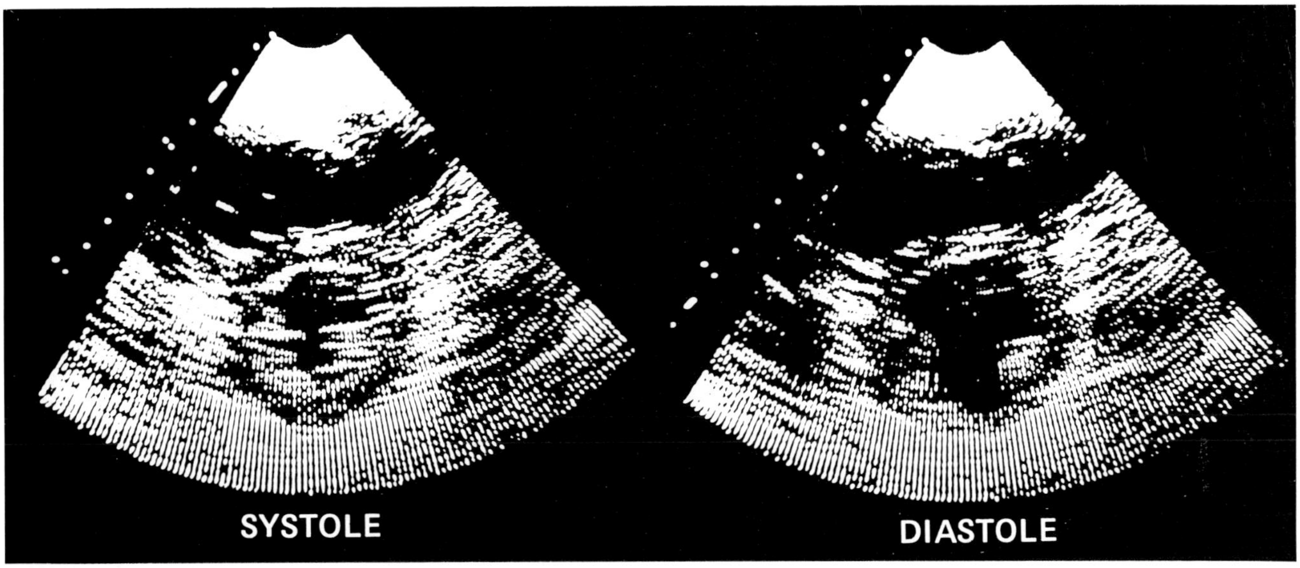

Figure 2-6 C

Parasternal short axis view of the heart in systole and diastole, papillary muscle level—two-dimensional echocardiograms.

Figure 2-6 D

Labelled drawing of heart in diastole shown in Figure 2-6 C.

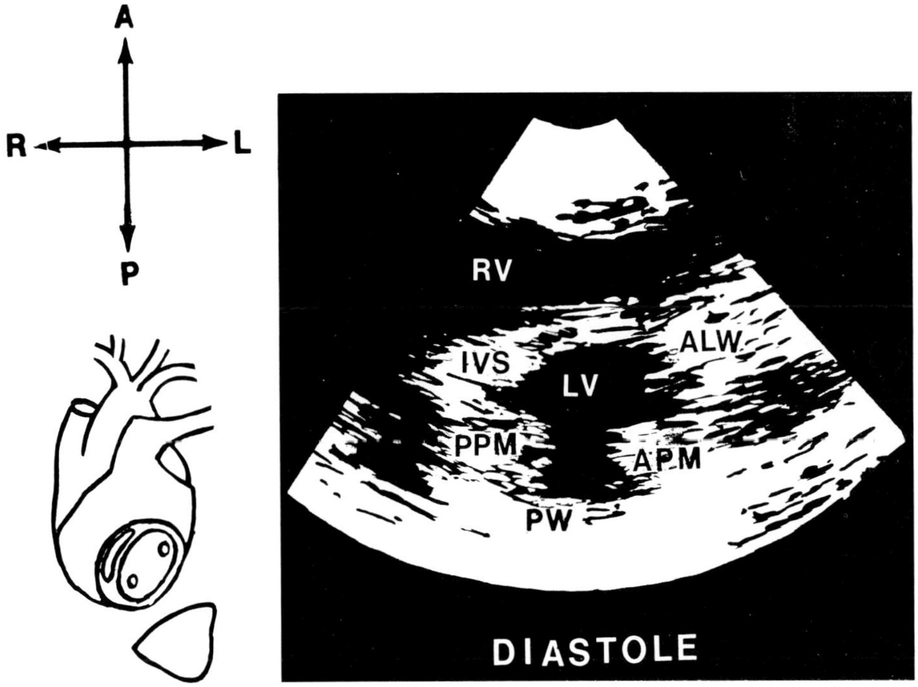

Figure 2-7 A

Four-chamber view of the heart—anatomical specimen.

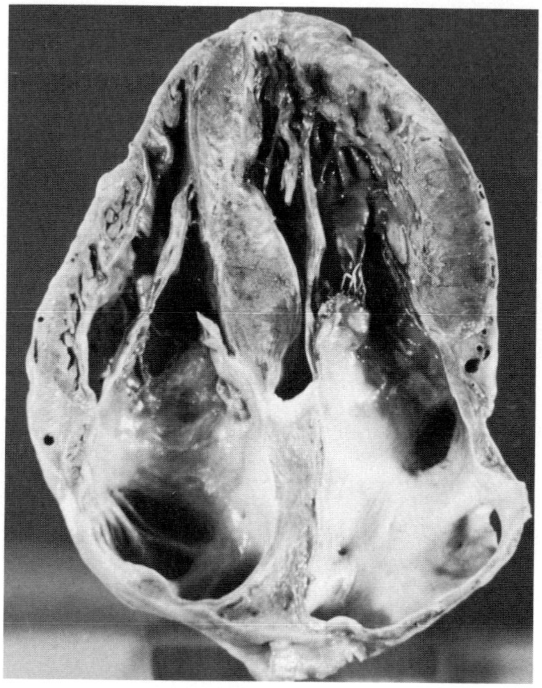

Figure 2-7 B

Labelled drawing of Figure 2-7 A

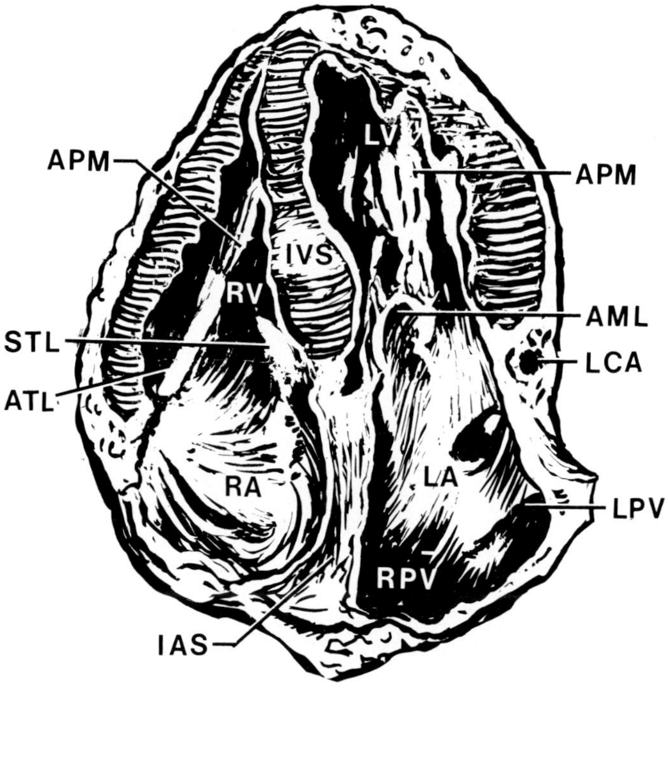

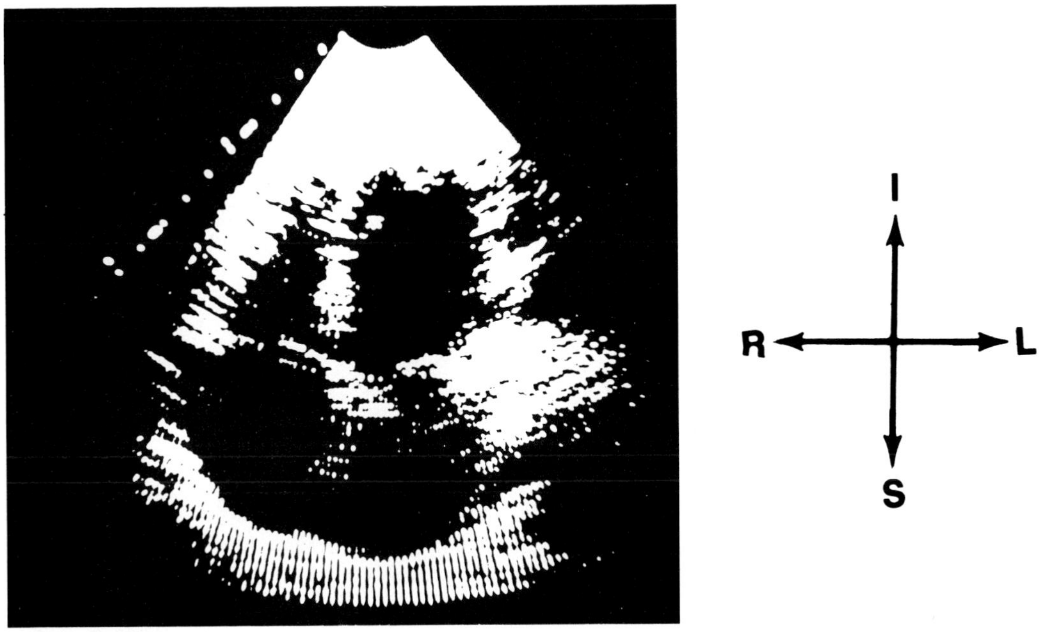

Figure 2-7 C
Apical four chamber-view (option 2)—echocardiogram.

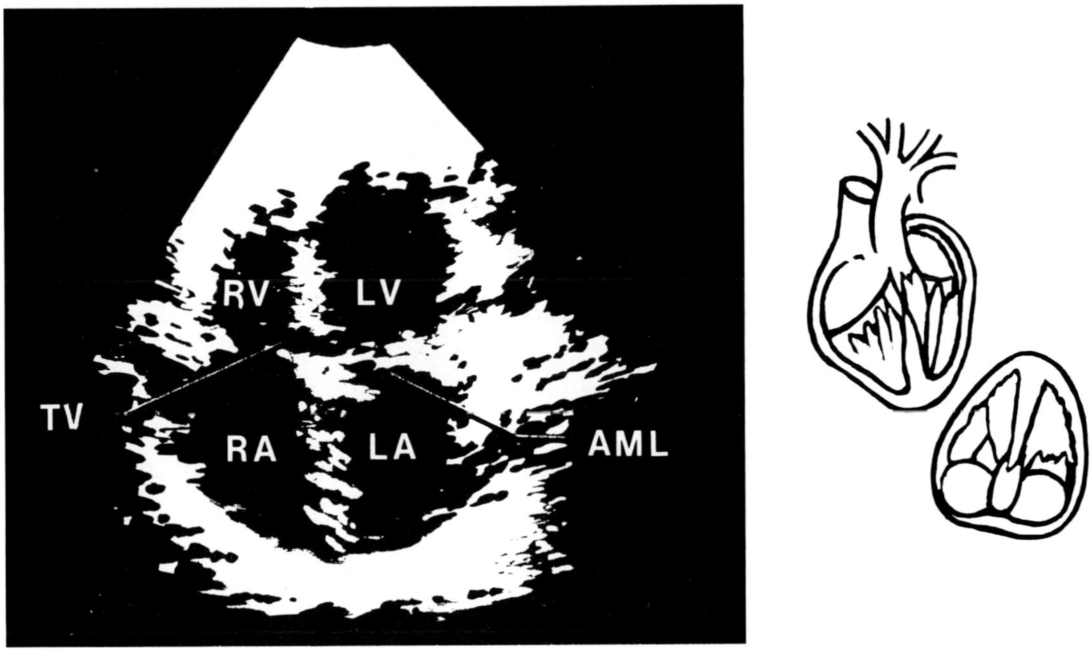

Figure 2-7 D
Labelled drawing of Figure 2-7 C.

Figure 2-8 A

Four-chamber view of the heart and aorta (five-chamber view)—anatomical specimen.

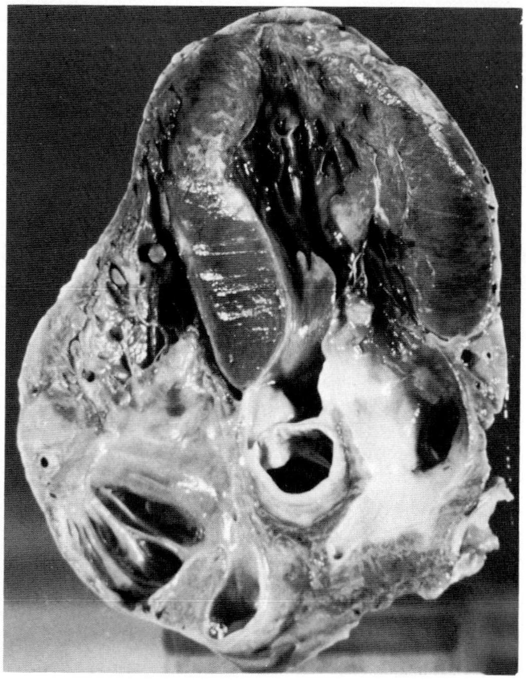

Figure 2-8 B

Labelled drawing of Figure 2-8 A.

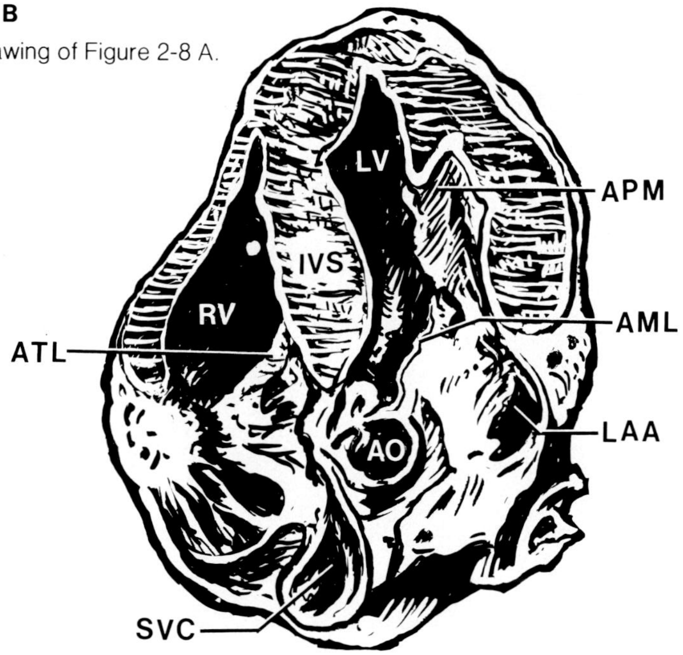

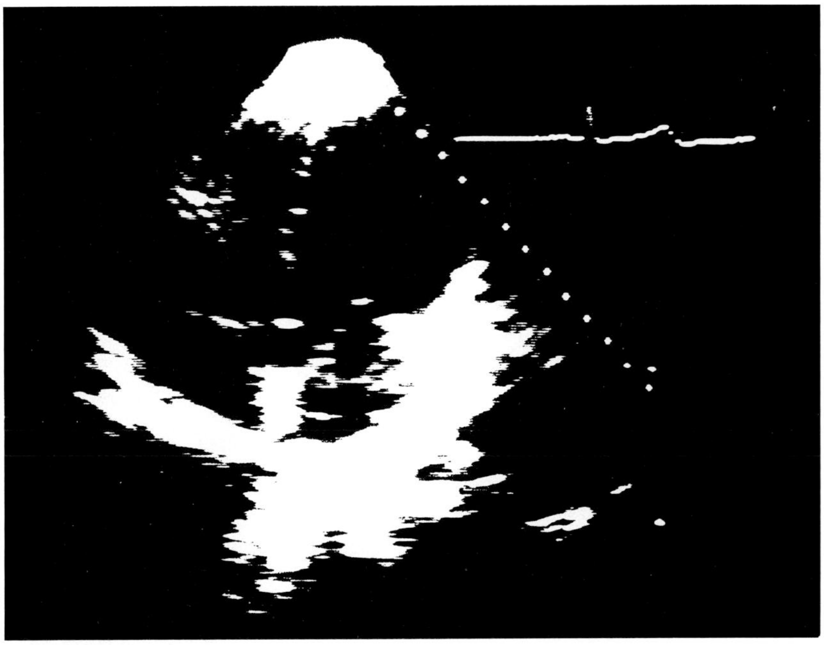

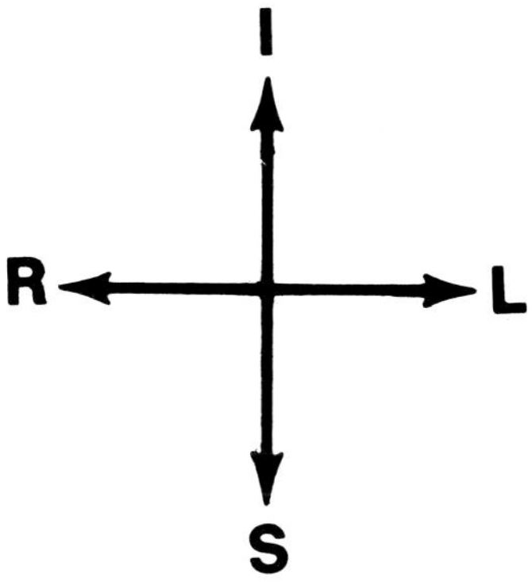

Figure 2-8 C

Apical four-chamber view of heart with aorta (option 2)—echocardiogram.

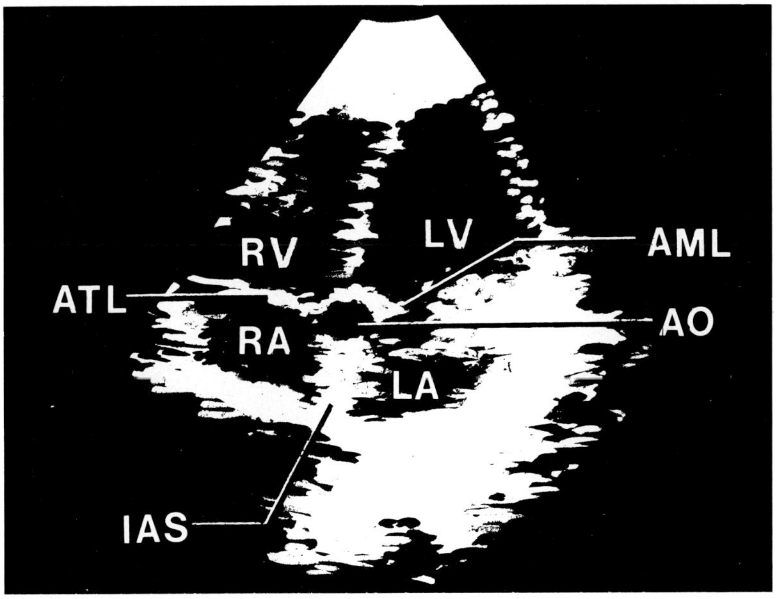

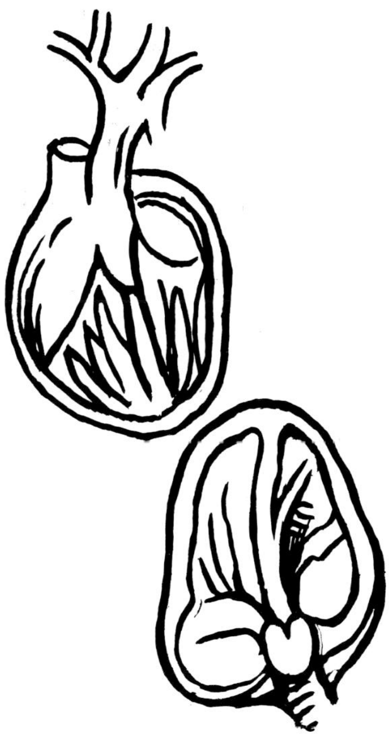

Figure 2-8 D

Labelled drawing of Figure 2-8 C.

Figure 2-9 A

Subcostal four-chamber view of the heart—anatomical specimen.

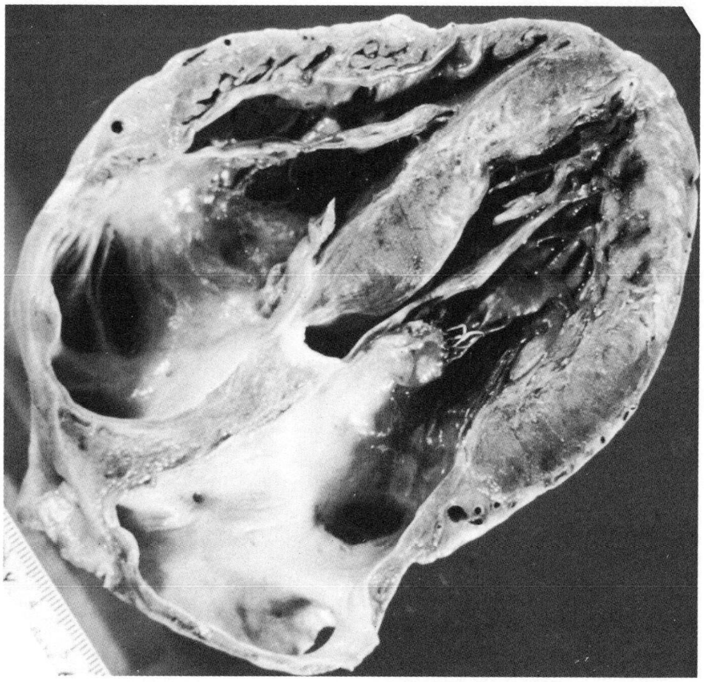

Figure 2-9 B

Labelled drawing of Figure 2-9 A.

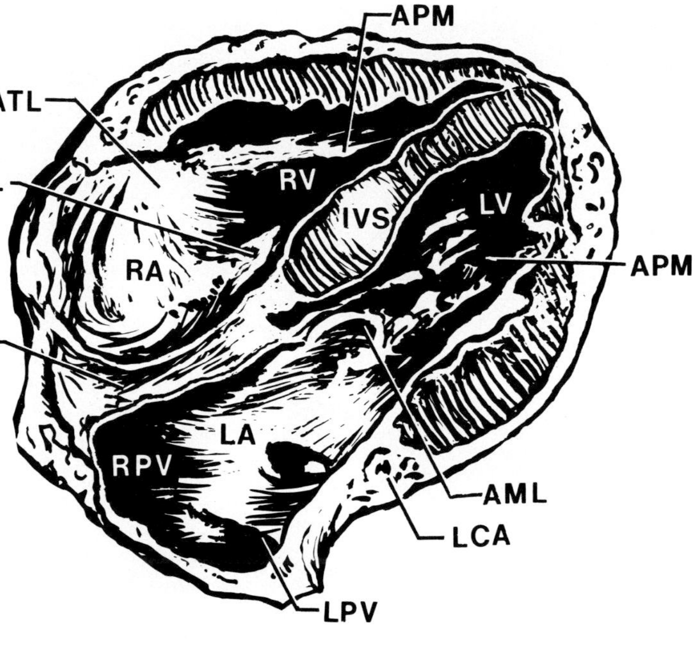

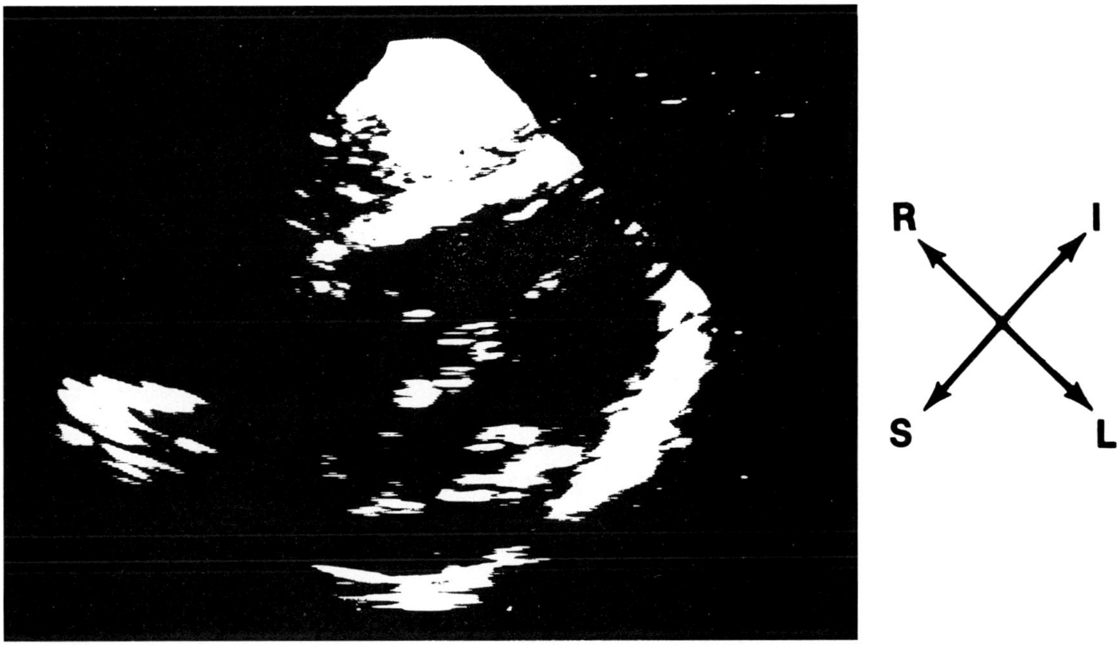

Figure 2-9 C
Subcostal four-chamber view of heart with aorta (option 2)—echocardiogram.

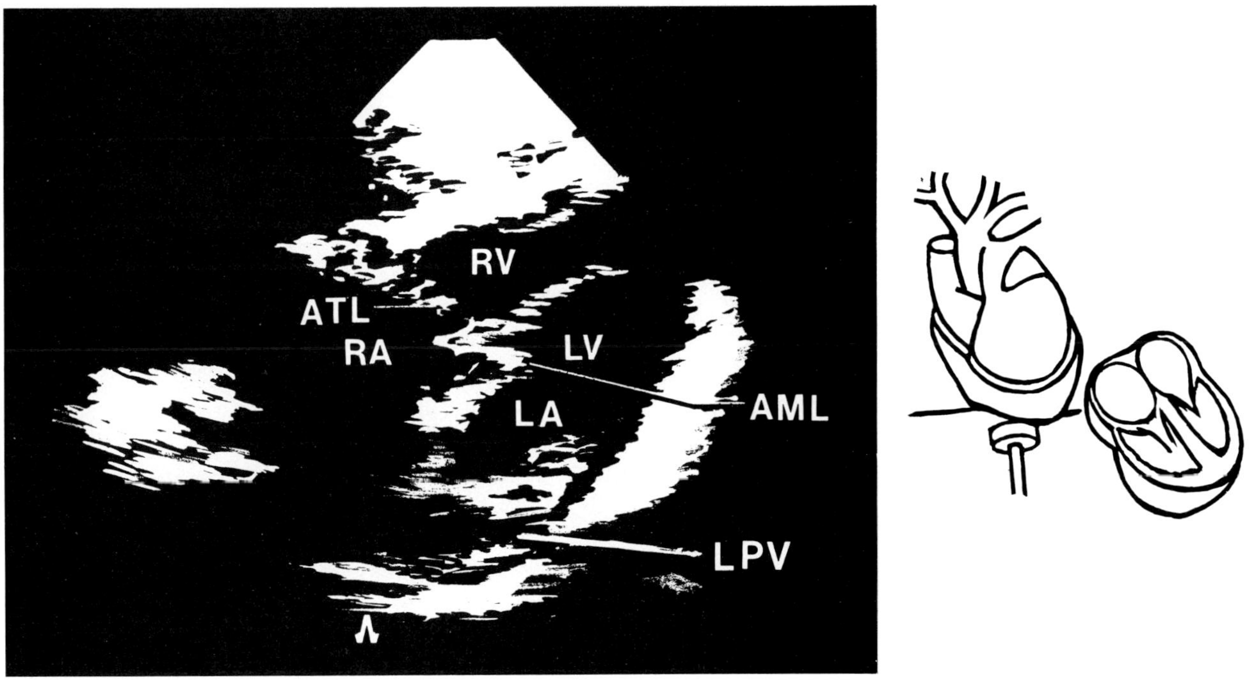

Figure 2-9 D
Labelled drawing of Figure 2-9 C.

SUBCOSTAL FOUR-CHAMBER VIEW

Anatomical Specimen

The anatomical specimen shown in Figures 2-9 A and B is the same as in Figure 2-7, but from a subcostal approach. This view is oriented 45° clockwise from the apical four-chamber view. The right atrium and right ventricle are at the top of the figure. Note that in this view the right (RPV) and left (LPV) pulmonary veins are seen.

Two-Dimensional Echocardiogram—Systole

Figures 2-9 C and D show an echocardiogram taken from the subcostal approach in systole. At the top of the figures, the liver–diaphragm interface with the right ventricular wall is seen. Note that the right (RPV) and left (LPV) pulmonary veins are seen superior and posterior to the left atrium (LA).

REFERENCE

1. Committee on Nomenclature and Standards in Two-dimensional Echocardiography: Recommendations Regarding Quantitation in M-mode Echocardiography. Indianapolis: American Society of Echocardiography, 1978.

Julius Gardin

3

Mitral Valve Disease

The image produced by the mitral valve is one of the most distinctive features of the echocardiogram and often is the reference point used for locating other structures. The anterior leaflet moves in an "M"-shaped configuration during diastole, while the posterior leaflet, moving in an antiparallel path, inscribes a "W"-shaped pattern (Figure 1-11). The leaflets come together at the conclusion of diastole (C point) and, during systole, exhibit a single, gradually upsloping line (C-D line). This is interrupted with the onset of the next diastole (D point), at which time the leaflets again move away from each other. The characteristic shape of the mitral valve echo is due to the valve's rapid opening — corresponding to the early rapid filling of the left ventricle — at this time. The filling of the left ventricle then slows, causing the mitral valve leaflets to come together gradually (the characteristic E-F slope). The valve subsequently reopens with atrial systole (A wave).

The mitral valve generally is located by positioning the transducer along the left sternal border, in the third or fourth intercostal space. The goal is to image the "M"-shaped motion of the anterior mitral leaflet, and then to tilt the transducer slightly, inferiorly and laterally, to image the "W"-shaped motion of the posterior leaflet. The valve is best imaged when the ultrasound beam is perpendicular to its leaflets. If the valve cannot be imaged from this original position in the third or fourth intercostal space, the transducer should be moved systematically over the precordium and, if necessary, to the subxiphoid position. Improper imaging can result in erroneous diagnoses, such as mitral leaflet thickening (and even stenosis) and mitral valve prolapse.

Mitral stenosis was one of the first disorders of the mitral valve to be diagnosed using echocardiography.[1] The characteristic echocardiographic findings include leaflet that are denser and thicker than normal, a reduced E-F slope, a reduced initial opening of the valve (D-E excursion), and loss of the antiparallel motion of the posterior leaflet (i.e., the posterior leaflet may follow directly the motion of the anterior leaflet during diastole) (Figure 3-1). In addition, loss of the A wave may occur if the patient remains in sinus rhythm.[2-4]

Although the E-F slope (velocity of the mitral valve's closing in early diastole) was initially felt to be an accurate indicator of the severity of mitral stenosis, it is now appreciated that this is not the case. The motion of the posterior leaflet in diastole either parallel or opposite to that of the anterior leaflet (antiparallel) is likewise known to be a poor predictor. In fact, "parallel" or "antiparallel" motion of the leaflets may merely depend on whether the ultrasound beam traverses the leaflets at their fused tips — in which case the motion would be parallel — or through their bodies — where the motion would be antiparallel. The degree of leaflet separation is more useful in estimating severity, but this, too, has limitations. In general, the M-mode echocardiogram is a good tool for establishing the diagnosis, although not the severity, of mitral stenosis. It also is useful in preoperative assessment for determining whether a **mitral commissurotomy** is feasible; dense echoes in the mitral region, signifying marked calcification of the valve, argue against the feasibility of a commissurotomy and tend to predict the necessity of mitral valve replacement.

Two-dimensional echocardiography, on the other hand, has proved quite accurate in estimating the severity of mitral stenosis by permitting measurement of the mitral valve orifice area.[3-6] Proper technique must be observed, however, so that the orifice is imaged in short axis just above the level of the papillary muscles and artifacts arising from improper ultrasound-beam angulation, signal intensity (e.g., "blooming"), or mitral orifice edge planimetry are avoided (Figures 3-11, 3-13).

The diagnosis of **mitral regurgitation** may be impossible to make on the basis of M-mode echocardiography. Certain findings may be present, such as left ventricular dilatation (with or without increased excursion of the septum and left ventricular posterior wall), left atrial enlargement, and increased early diastolic (D-E) excursion of the mitral valve. In acute mitral regurgitation, exaggerated motion of the posterior left atrial wall also may be seen. However, none of these findings is sensitive, let alone specific, for mitral regurgitation.[7] Even the use of two-dimensional echocardiography has not enhanced the diagnosis or estimation of the severity of mitral regurgitation. A number of causes of mitral regurgitation can be detected by M-mode echocardiography, however, including infective endocarditis, ruptured chordae tendineae, mitral valve prolapse, rheumatic mitral valve disease, and mitral annular calcification.

The diagnosis of **mitral valve prolapse,** to be discussed in detail in Chapter 4, is one of the more common applications of echocardiography. Attention to transducer angulation is of paramount importance in this diagnosis, since angulation of the beam caudad to the mitral leaflets may produce a hammock-like pattern mimicking prolapse. Other possible causes of **pseudo-mitral valve prolapse** include a large pericardial effusion (with a **swinging heart**) and mitral stenosis. Occasionally, multiple echoes may be seen behind the posterior mitral leaflet during diastole, simulating a myxoma, or flail leaflet. These multiple echoes most likely originate from an unusually large posterior leaflet that is folded onto itself, assuming a relatively vertical orientation. Other findings that may be noted in mitral valve prolapse syndrome include excessive mitral valve echoes from the leaflets, thought to be due to myxomatous changes, and a wide opening (D-E) excursion.

Although the two conditions may occur independently, infective endocarditis is a common cause for ruptured chordae tendineae (with a flail mitral leaflet). The mitral valve in such cases may exhibit a nonuniform mass of echoes on its anterior or posterior leaflet; this mass may represent a vegetation or merely a flail leaflet (secondary to ruptured chordae) — without a definite vegetation (Figure 3-2). The characteristic finding is erratic systolic and diastolic motion of the leaflet (Figure 3-3). The leaflet may also be seen as a mass of echoes in the left atrium behind the aorta during systole (Figure 3-4). A scan from the left atrium to the mitral valve may be helpful in further differentiating vegetation from ruptured chordae; the two conditions frequently coexist, however, so that this distinction is often impossible.[8-10]

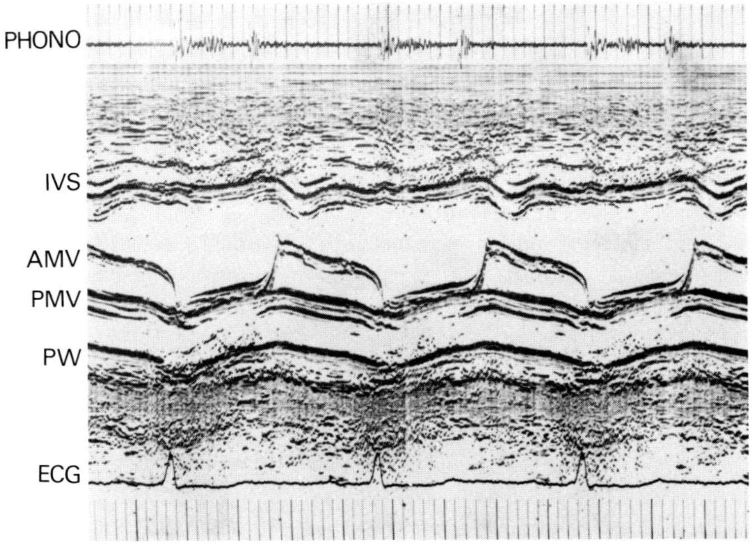

Figure 3-1

Phonocardiogram, taken at the apex of the heart, of the mitral leaflet in a patient with normal sinus rhythm.

3-1.1. The A wave of the anterior mitral leaflet is:

A. Absent
B. Present

3-1.2. The posterior or mitral leaflet motion is:

A. Normal
B. Abnormal

3-1.3. The diagnosis in this patient is:

A. Mitral valve prolapse
B. Mitral stenosis
C. Mitral chordal rupture
D. Mitral regurgitation

Another abnormality of the mitral valve that may be diagnosed by echocardiography is **systolic anterior motion** of the mitral valve and/or chordae tendineae. In this abnormality, commonly seen in the obstructive form of hypertrophic cardiomyopathy, portions of the anterior mitral leaflet move anteriorly during systole, often contacting the interventricular septum (Figure 3-5). The mitral valve is a dynamic structure, and the extent and duration of apposition of the mitral

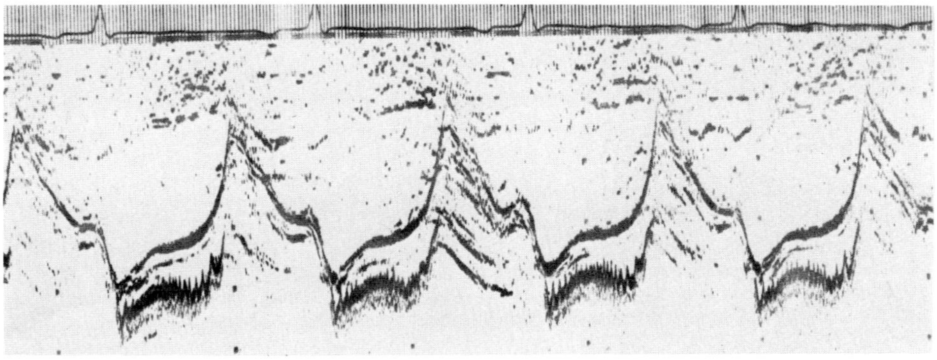

Figure 3-2

Echocardiogram of the mitral valve.

3-2.1. The abnormality noted is:

A. Vibration of anterior mitral leaflet
B. Vibration of posterior mitral leaflet
C. Abnormal motion of the anterior mitral leaflet
D. Abnormal motion of the posterior mitral leaflet

3-2.2. The most likely abnormality of this valve is:

A. Flail posterior mitral leaflet
B. Flail anterior mitral leaflet
C. Mitral stenosis
D. Mitral annulus calcification

leaflets and/or chordae to the septum have been shown to correlate to some degree with the left ventricular outflow gradient; in other words, to the degree of outflow tract obstruction. Various maneuvers, such as the Valsalva maneuver, induction of a premature ventricular beat, and administration of amyl nitrite, have been utilized to provoke or increase the systolic anterior motion in hypertrophic cardiomyopathy. The abnormality must be differentiated from the **pseudo-systolic anterior motion** sometimes seen in instances of vigorous left ventricular contraction. In pseudo-systolic anterior motion, the motion of the systolic portion of the mitral valve is parallel to the vigorous left ventricular posterior wall contraction (Figure 3-6), whereas, in true systolic anterior motion, the leaflet and/or chordae

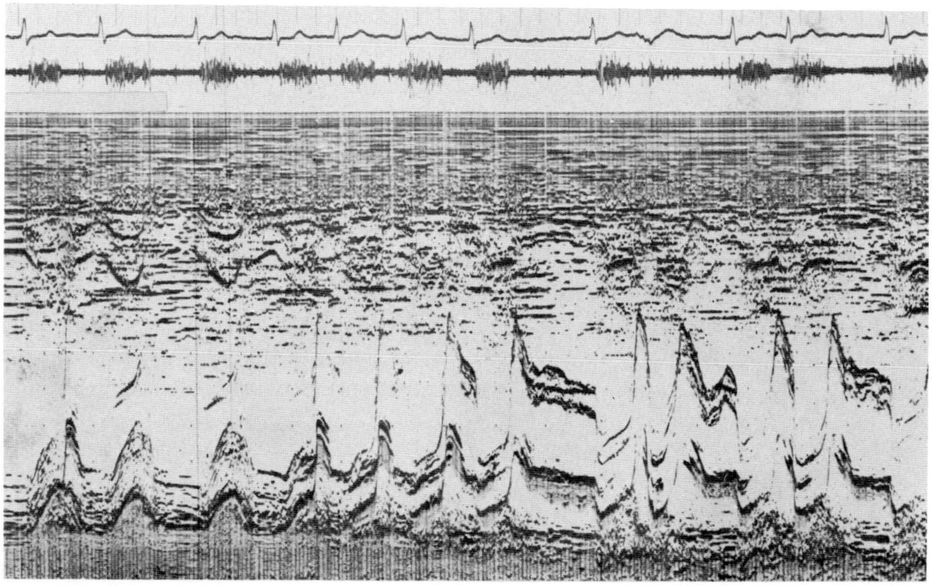

Figure 3-3

Echocardiogram taken at the level of the left ventricle scanning upwards towards the anterior and posterior mitral leaflet. An ECG appears at the top of the figure and, below that, a phonocardiogram taken at the apex of the heart. The patient is in atrial fibrillation with a variable ventricular response.

3-3.1. The leaflet of the mitral valve that has abnormal anterior diastolic motion is:

A. Anterior
B. Posterior

3-3.2. The soft, light-grey "smudgy" echoes on the posterior mitral leaflet most likely originate from:

A. Mitral annular calcium
B. Posterior leaflet calcium
C. Vegetation of the posterior leaflet
D. Vegetation of the anterior leaflet

3-3.3. The most likely cause of this patient's pansystolic murmur is:

A. Ventricular septal defect
B. Mitral regurgitation
C. Idiopathic hypertrophic subaortic stenosis
D. Aortic stenosis

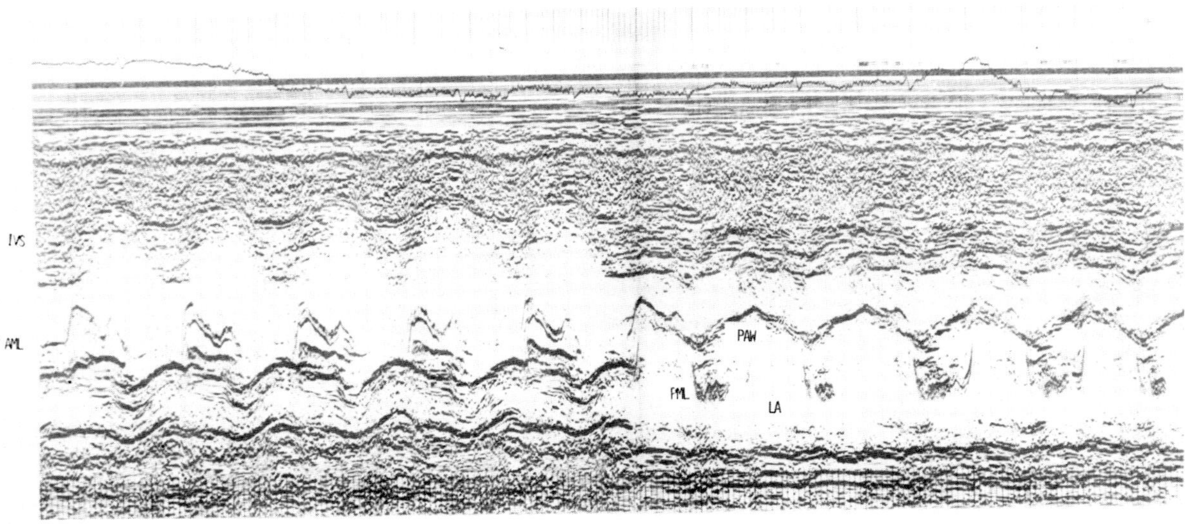

Figure 3-4

Echocardiographic scan of a 62-year-old patient with a pansystolic murmur and a fever. The scan is from the left ventricle at the level of the mitral valve to the left atrium at the level of the aortic root. Note the systolic echoes in the left atrium.

3-4.1. The echoes noted in the left atrium of this patient are most likely caused by:

A. Left atrial thrombus
B. Posterior mitral leaflet and/or vegetations
C. Mitral annular calcification
D. Atrial myxoma

will move much more rapidly than the posterior wall.

It must be emphasized that the mitral valve should be viewed not only as an anatomic structure but also as a physiologic reflector of events occuring on either side of the valves; that is, in the left atrium and left ventricle. Differences in atrial rhythm, such as atrial fibrillation, atrial flutter, or complete heart block, will produce their own distinct patterns of valve motion (Figure 3-7). Similarly, the E-F slope may be diminished not only by factors such as calcification that stiffen the mitral leaflets, but also by factors such as hypertrophy that decrease the compliance of the left ventricle. Other specific patterns of mitral valve motion have been reported to reflect elevated abnormal left ventricular diastolic pressure, including a relatively low-amplitude, rounded, early opening phase of the valve (D-E slope)[11] or a notch or interruption in the closure of the valve following atrial systole (A-C slope).

The degree of excursion of the mitral leaflets during diastole reflects flow across the mitral valve. In situations where trans-mitral valve flow is reduced, the excursion is diminished. Conversely, in situations where there is torrential trans-mitral valve diastolic flow, as in mitral regurgitation, the diastolic excursion is generally increased. Another measurement involving the mitral valve that may reflect left ventricular function is the distance from the E point (i.e., the peak of the early opening phase of mitral valve flow) to the ventricular septum. In normal people, this distance is less than 5.5 mm (Figure 1-11). Increases in this distance usually reflect a reduced ejection fraction, suggesting systolic decompensation of the left ventricle.[12,13]

Figure 3-8

M-mode echocardiogram showing diastolic fluttering of the anterior mitral leaflet.

3-8.1. The most likely cause of this abnormality is:

A. Flail anterior mitral leaflet
B. Flail posterior mitral leaflet
C. Mitral stenosis
D. Aortic valve insufficiency

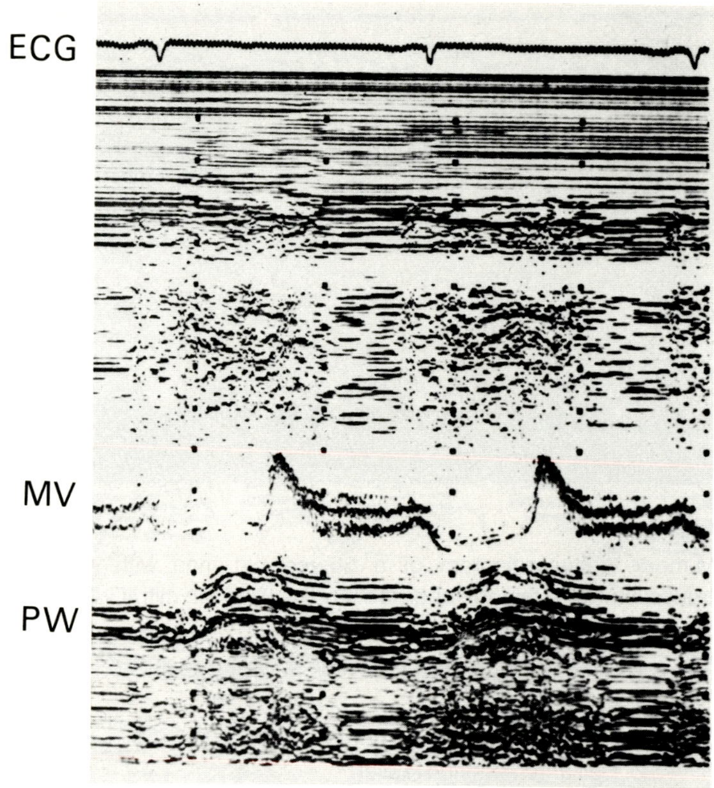

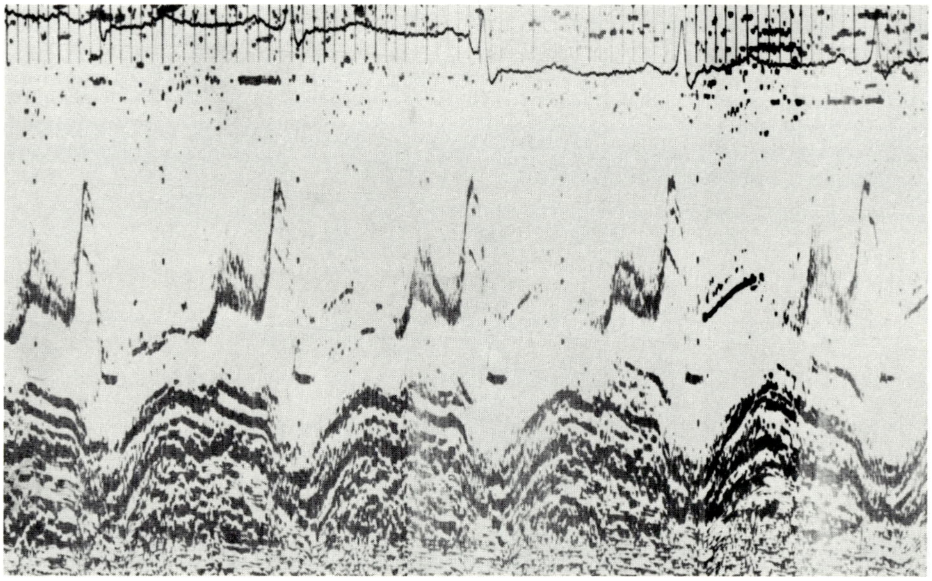

Figure 3-9

Echocardiogram of the anterior mitral leaflet in a patient with a diastolic murmur.

3-9.1. The abnormality noted in this mitral valve echocardiogram is:

A. Increased E–F slope
B. Large a-wave
C. Diastolic vibration or flutter of the anterior mitral leaflet
D. Flail anterior mitral leaflet

Aortic insufficiency is diagnosed echocardiographically when the *mitral* valve exhibits fine fluttering during diastole (Figure 3-8). The fluttering is the echocardiographic correlate of aortic regurgitant blood impinging upon the anterior mitral leaflet during diastole (Figure 3-9). Although the anterior mitral leaflet usually exhibits this phenomenon, the posterior leaflet, the ventricular septum, and left ventricular posterior wall may also exhibit fine oscillations during diastole. It is imperative to know the frequency-response characteristics of the ultrasound instrument utilized, since different instruments vary in their propensity for displaying fine mitral diastolic oscillations in normal subjects. Furthermore, this fine fluttering is commonly missed in mitral stenosis, since the calcified valve may not exhibit these oscillations.[14] Premature closure of the mitral valve (i.e., a mitral C point occurring before the onset of the QRS complex) has proved to be an important sign of acute severe aortic insufficiency.

REFERENCES

1. Cope GD, Kisslo JA, Johnson ML, Behar VS: A reassessment of the echocardiogram in mitral stenosis. Circulation 52:664-676, 1975
2. Driscoll DJ, Gutgesell HP, McNamara DG: Echocardiographic features of congenital mitral stenosis. Am J Cardiol 42:259-266, 1978
3. Fisher ML, Parisi AF, Plotnick GD, Defelice CE, Carliner NH, Fortuin NJ: Assessment of severity of mitral stenosis by echocardiographic leaflet separation. Arch Intern Med 139:102-106, 1979
4. Inoh T, Nakai K, Fukuzaki H, Hashimoto K, Asada S: Evaluation of mitral valvular lesion of mitral stenosis by M-mode echocardiography, with special reference to the indication for commissurotomy. Kobe J Med Sci 26:127-136, 1980
5. Nichol PM, Gilbert BW, Kisslo JA: Two-dimensional echocardiographic assessment of mitral stenosis. Circulation 55:120-128, 1977
6. Martin RP, Rakowski H, Kleiman JH, Beaver W, London E, Popp RL: Reliability and reproducibility of two-dimensional echocardiographic measurement of the stenotic mitral valve orifice area. Am J Cardiol 43:560-568, 1979
7. Umeda T, Kuwako K, Machii K: M-mode and cross-sectional echocardiographic evaluation of rheumatic mitral valve disease. Jpn Circ J 43:297-304, 1979
8. Mintz GS, Kotler MN, Segal BL, Parry WR: Two-dimensional echocardiographic recognition of ruptured chordae tendineae. Circulation 57:244-250, 1978
9. Mintz GS, Kotler MN, Parry WR, Segal GL: Statistical comparison of M-mode and two-dimensional echocardiographic diagnosis of flail mitral leaflets. Am J Cardiol 45:253-259, 1980
10. Child JS, Skorton DJ, Taylor RD, Krivokapich J, Abbasi AS, Wong M, et al: M-mode and cross-sectional echocardiographic features of flail posterior mitral leaflets. Am J Cardiol 44:1383-1390, 1979
11. Jugdutt BI, Lee SJ, McFarlane D: Non-invasive assessment of left ventricular function from the mitral valve echogram. Relation of final anterior mitral leaflet closing velocity to peak DP/DT and aortic velocity. Circulation 58:861-871, 1978
12. Stewart JA, Morin FR, Winsberg F: Malapposition of the mitral valve: A two-dimensional echocardiographic sign of left ventricular dysfunction. Radiology 130:399-402, 1979
13. Lew W, Henning H, Schelbert H, Karliner JS: Assessment of mitral valve E point-septal separation as an index of left ventricular performance in patients with acute and previous myocardial infarction. Am J Cardiol 41:836-845, 1978
14. D'Cruz I, Cohen HC, Prabhu R, Ayabe T, Glick G: Flutter of left ventricular structures in patients with aortic regurgitation, with special reference to associated mitral stenosis. Am Heart J 92:684-691, 1976

ADDITIONAL ILLUSTRATIONS AND EXERCISES

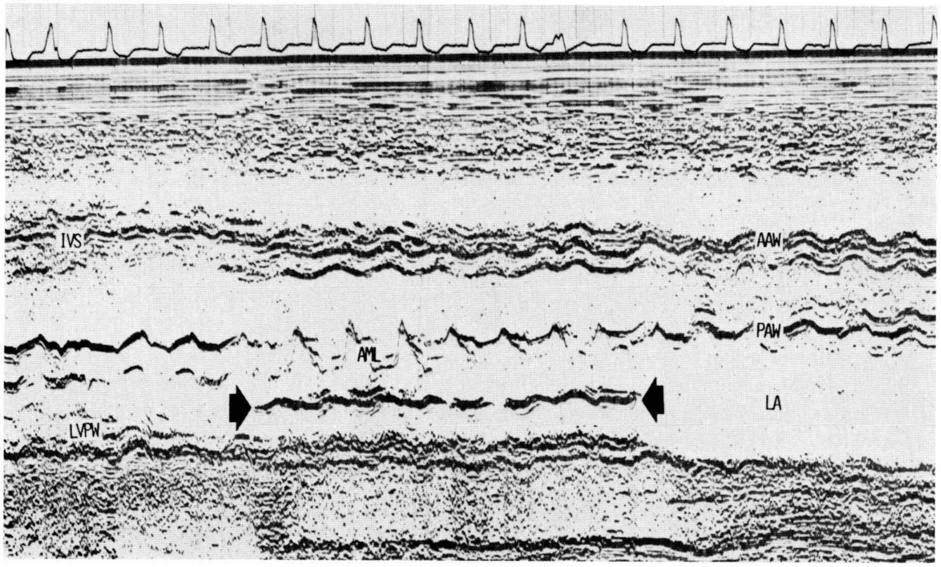

Figure 3-10

Slow-speed echocardiographic scan from the left ventricle at the level of the chordae tendineae, through the anterior mitral leaflet, and into the aortic root. Note thickening of the chordae tendineae anterior to the posterior wall.

3-10.1. The abnormality between the arrows is:

A. Flail posterior mitral leaflet
B. Flail anterior mitral leaflet
C. Mitral stenosis
D. Mitral annular calcification

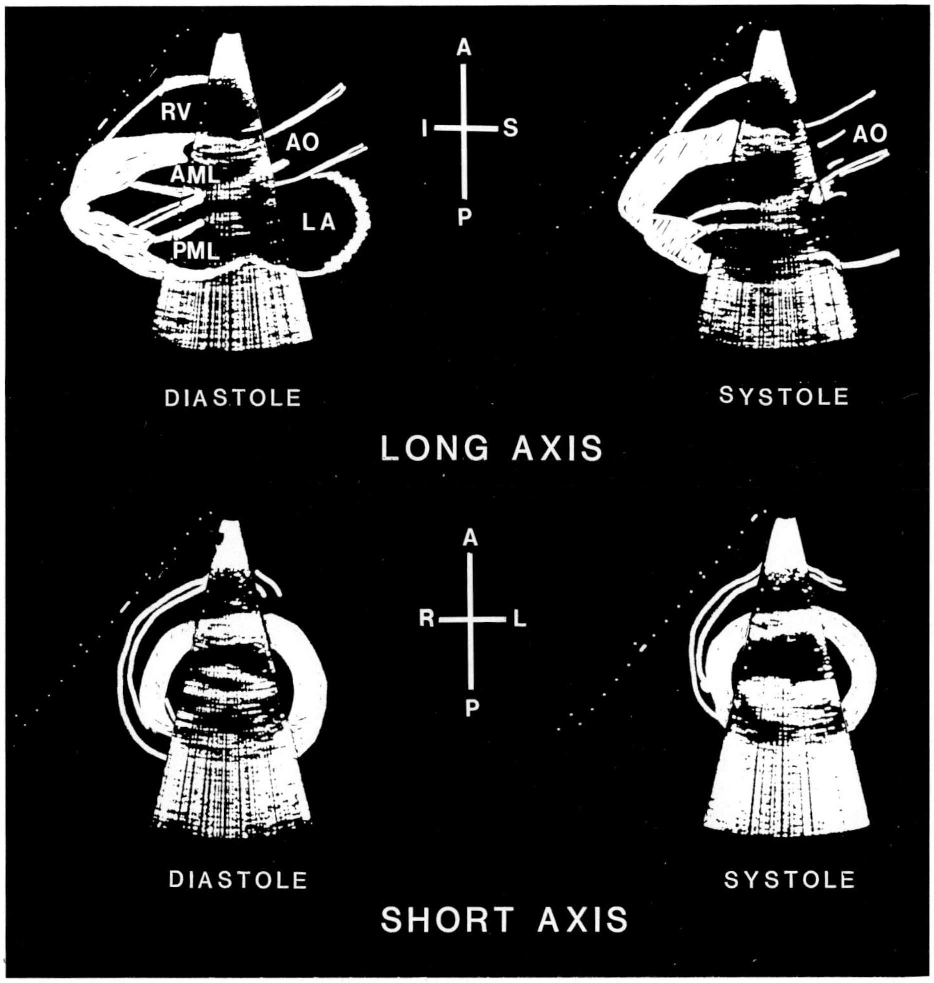

Figure 3-11

Two-dimensional 30° mechanical scan of the mitral valve in long axis and short axis during diastole and systole. Note the thickening of the anterior and posterior leaflets in diastole and the neutral position of the posterior leaflet in both diastole and systole. In short axis, the mitral orifice is seen in diastole.

3-11.1. In calculating the mitral valve area, which of the following statements are correct?

A. The mitral valve orifice is best measured in short axis at the most inferior portion of the mitral leaflets where the anterior and posterior mitral leaflets are seen.

B. The mitral valve orifice is best measured in short axis at the body or midpoint of the anterior mitral leaflets.

C. The mitral valve orifice is best measured in long axis.

D. The mitral valve orifice is best calculated with the receiver or coarse gain set high in order to image both leaflets well.

E. The mitral valve orifice is best measured with the receiver gain or coarse gain set low to just image the mitral orifice and to prevent blooming.

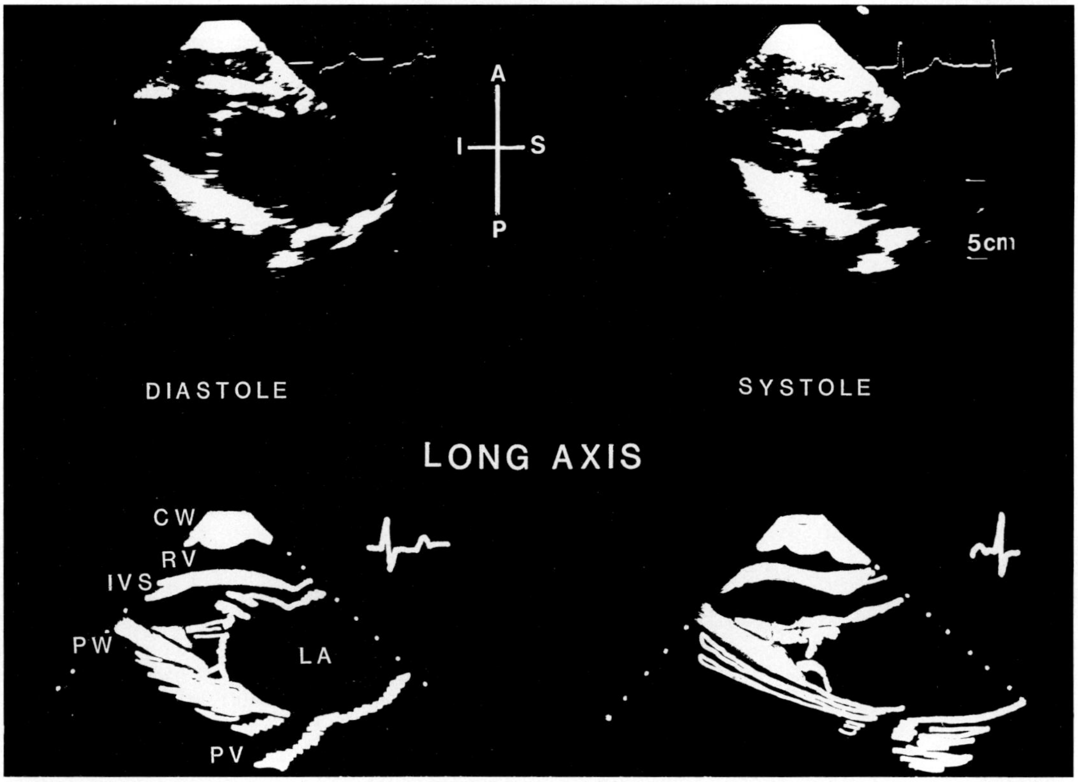

Figure 3-12

Two-dimensional 90° echocardiogram, in long axis in diastole and systole, of a patient with moderate mitral– stenosis without mitral annular calcification. The lines to the right of the display indicate 5 cm. Note the enlarged left atrium, the angulation of the anterior mitral leaflet during diastole, and the neutral position of the posterior mitral valve. During systole, there is complete coaptation of the anterior and posterior mitral leaflets.

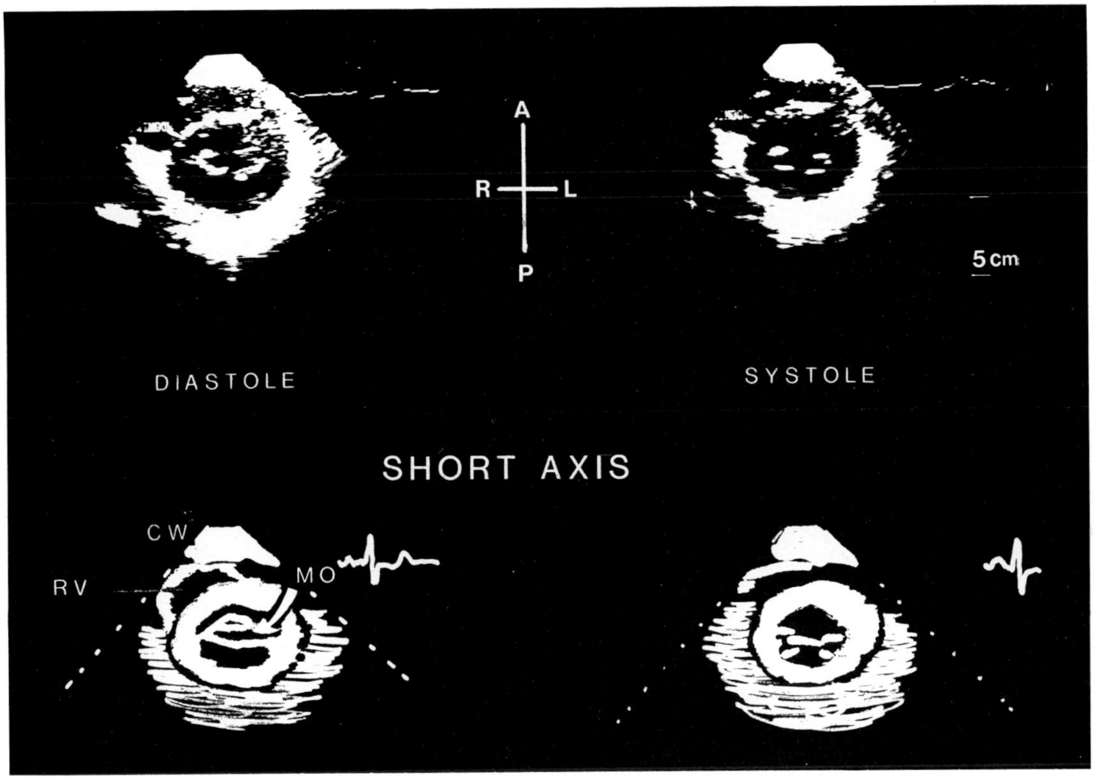

Figure 3-13

Two-dimensional 90° echocardiogram in short axis of the patient in Figure 3-12. Note the reduced mitral orifice during diastole. The calculated mitral orifice by echocardiogram was 1.5 cm^2. Note the thickened chordae tendineae, which appear as four dense lines during systole.

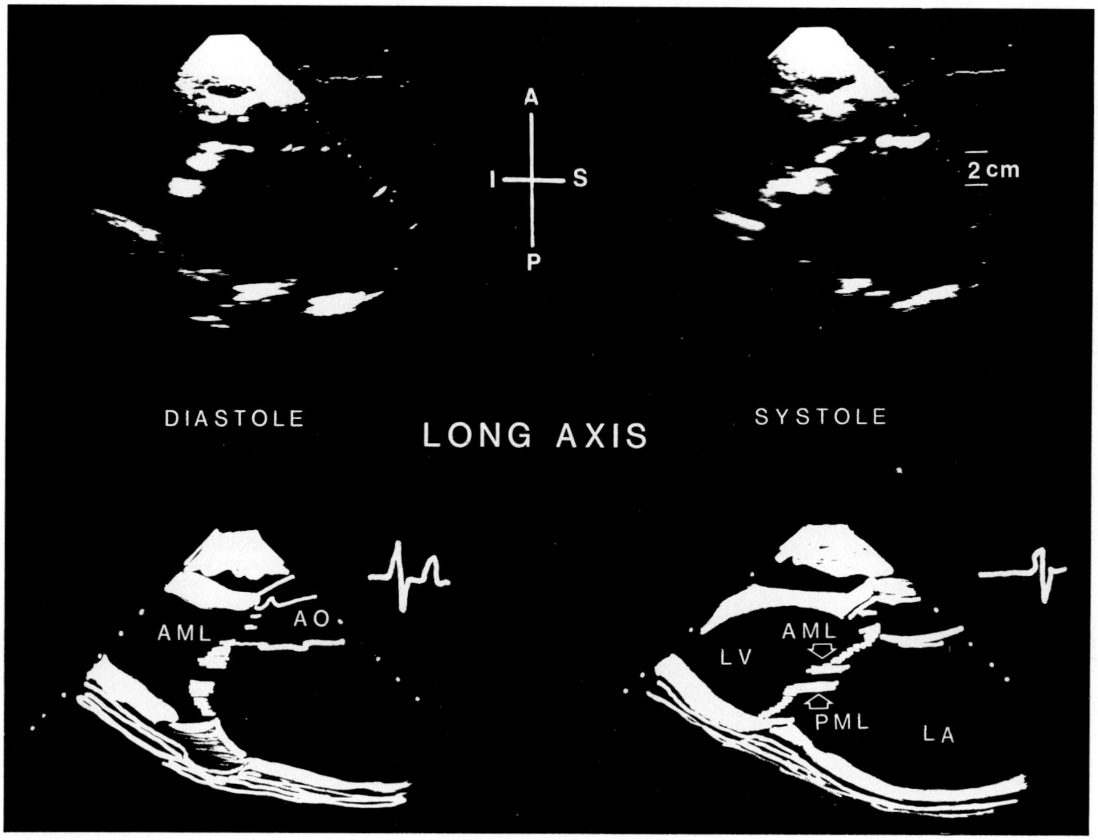

Figure 3-14

Two-dimensional 90° echocardiogram, in long axis in diastole and systole, of a patient with severe mitral stenosis and mitral annular calcification. The lines to the right indicate 2 cm. Note the enlarged left atrium, the angulation of the anterior mitral leaflet during diastole, and the neutral position of the posterior mitral leaflet. Note also that, during systole, the anterior and posterior leaflets do not coapt completely; this incomplete systolic coaptation was associated with mitral regurgitation.

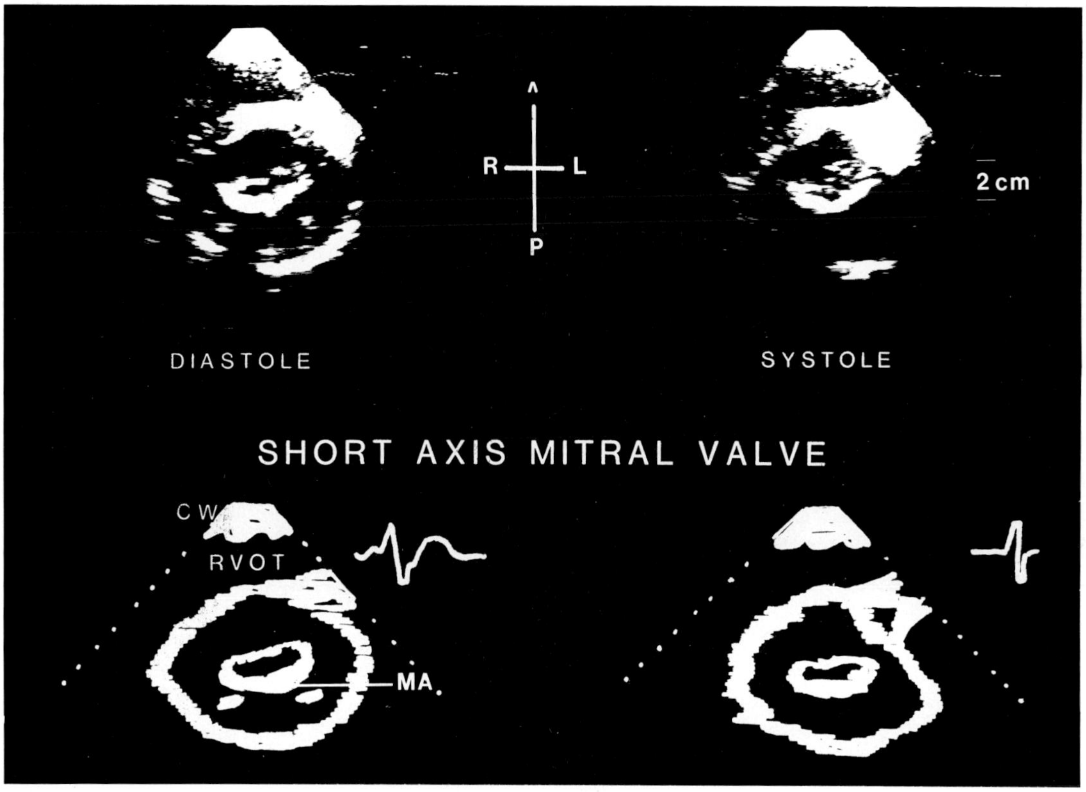

Figure 3-15

Two-dimensional 90° echocardiogram in short axis of the patient in Figure 3-14. Note the thickened anterior and posterior mitral leaflets and the reduction in mitral valve orifice size. The calculated mitral valve orifice in this patient was 0.9 cm^2. The heavy, dense line below the mitral orifice is a calcified mitral annulus.

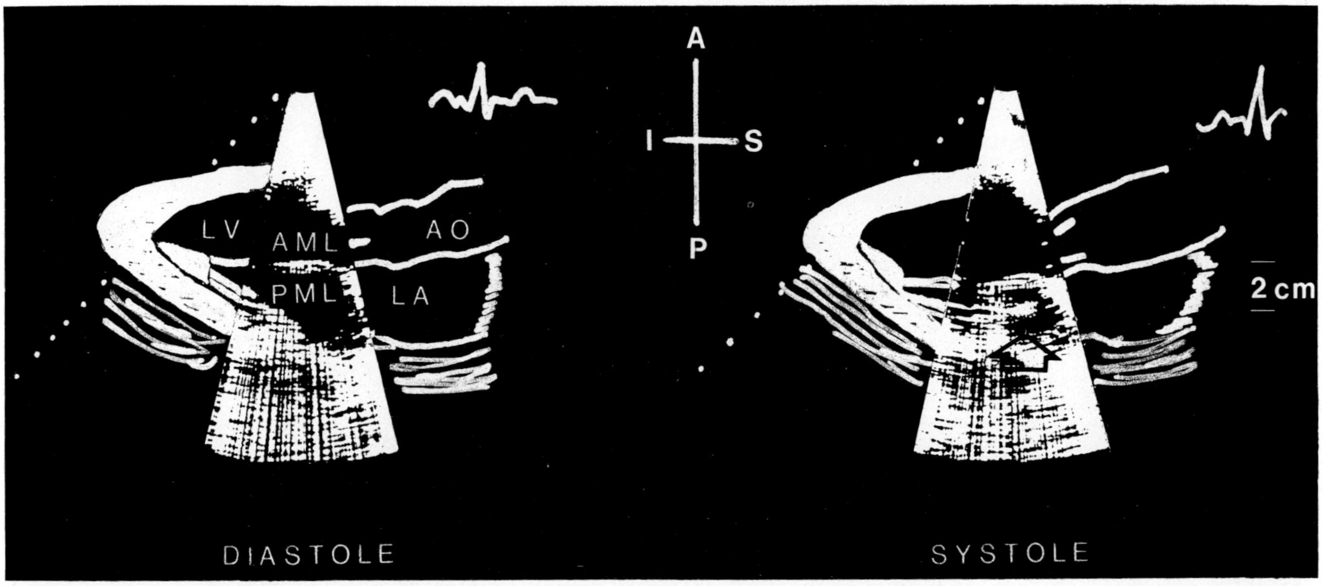

Figure 3-16

Two-dimensional 30° echocardiogram in long axis of left ventricle of a 72-year-old white woman with acute onset of mitral regurgitation and flail posterior mitral leaflet. Note the anterior mitral leaflet and the posterior mitral leaflet during diastole. Note also that, during systole, a portion of the posterior mitral leaflet is seen in the left atrium (open arrow). The left ventricle is at the upper limits of normal. The left atrial size is normal.

3-16.1. Which of the following statements are true in relation to the flail posterior mitral leaflet?

A. Flail mitral leaflet can be caused by ruptured chordae tendineae.

B. A flail mitral leaflet is diagnosed on M-mode or two-dimensional echocardiography whenever a portion of the leaflet is seen to move erractically in the left atrium during systole.

C. Flail mitral leaflet is *occasionally* associated with mitral regurgitation.

D. Flail mitral leaflet always causes enlargement of the left atrium.

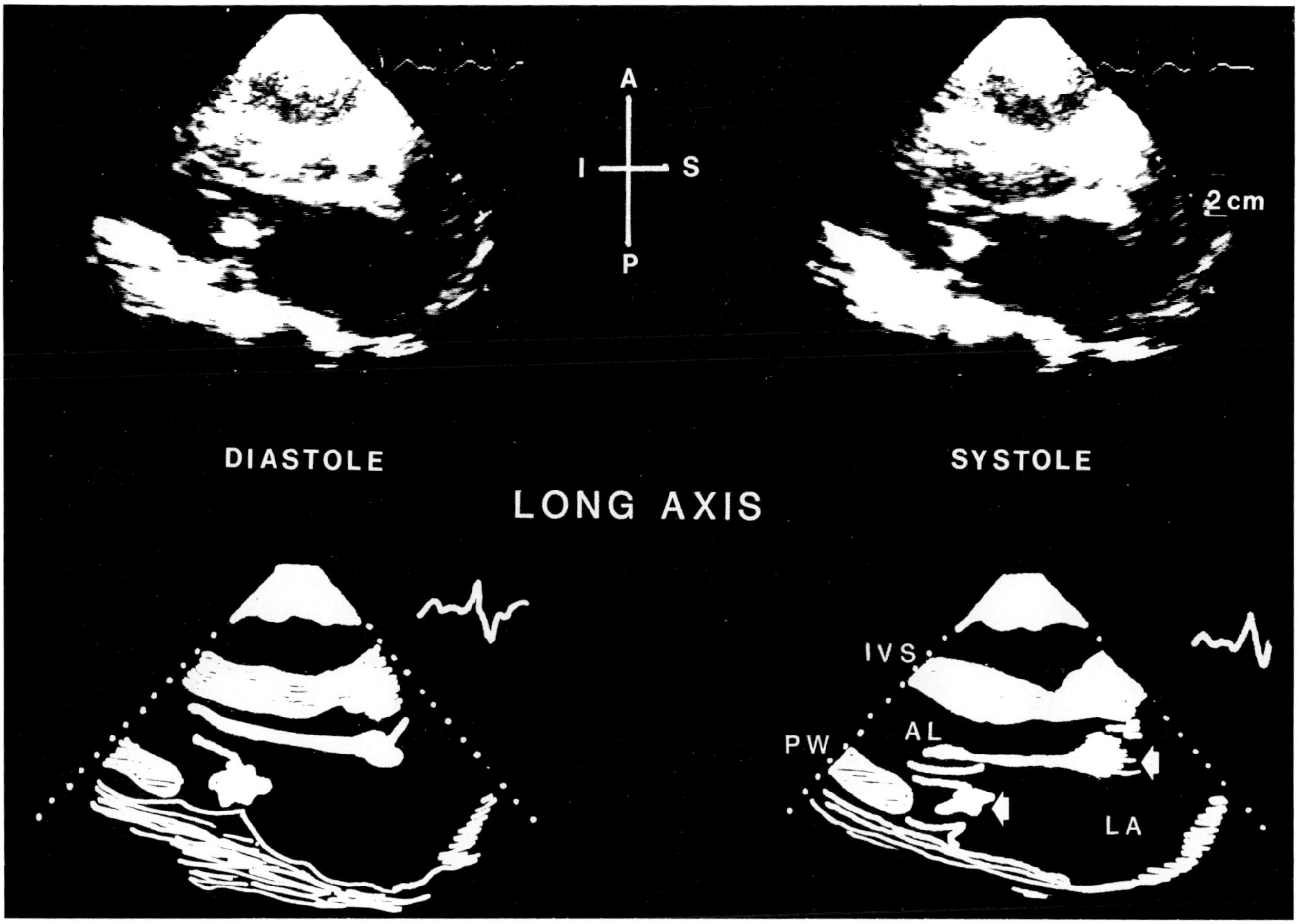

Figure 3-17

Two-dimensional 90° echocardiogram in long axis of a 78-year-old woman with a murmur and mitral regurgitation. Note the heavy, dense echoes in the anterior and posterior mitral annulus (white arrows). Lines to the right of the figure represent 2 cm. In this patient, calcification also extends into the aortic annulus. Left atrial size measures 5.0 cm.

3-17.1. As to mitral annular calcification, which of the following statements are true?

A. Mitral annular calcification is usually associated with mitral valve obstruction.

B. Mitral annular calcification is usually associated with mitral regurgitation.

C. Mitral annular calcification is commonly seen in young patients with mitral regurgitation.

D. Mitral annular calcification is frequently associated with calcification of the aortic valve annulus and aorta.

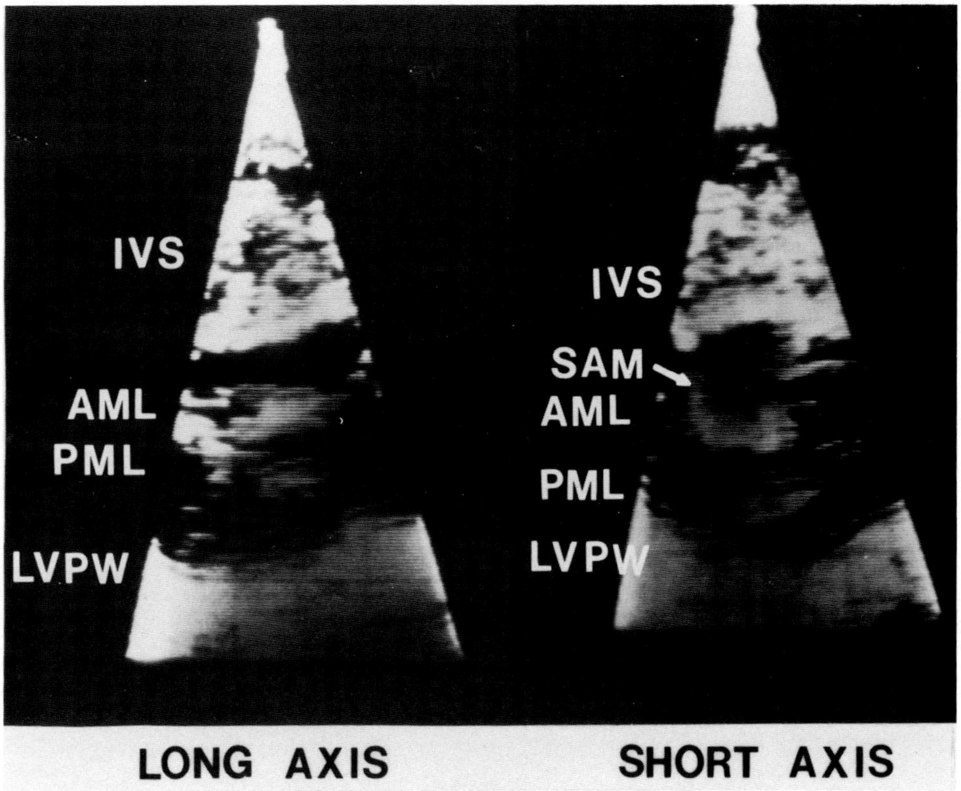

Figure 3-18

Two-dimensional 30° echocardiogram, in long and in short axis during systole, of a 28-year-old man with hypertrophic obstructive cardiomyopathy. Note the asymmetrically thickened septum (IVS), the systolic anterior motion of the mitral valve (SAM), and the proximity of the latter to the septum during systole.

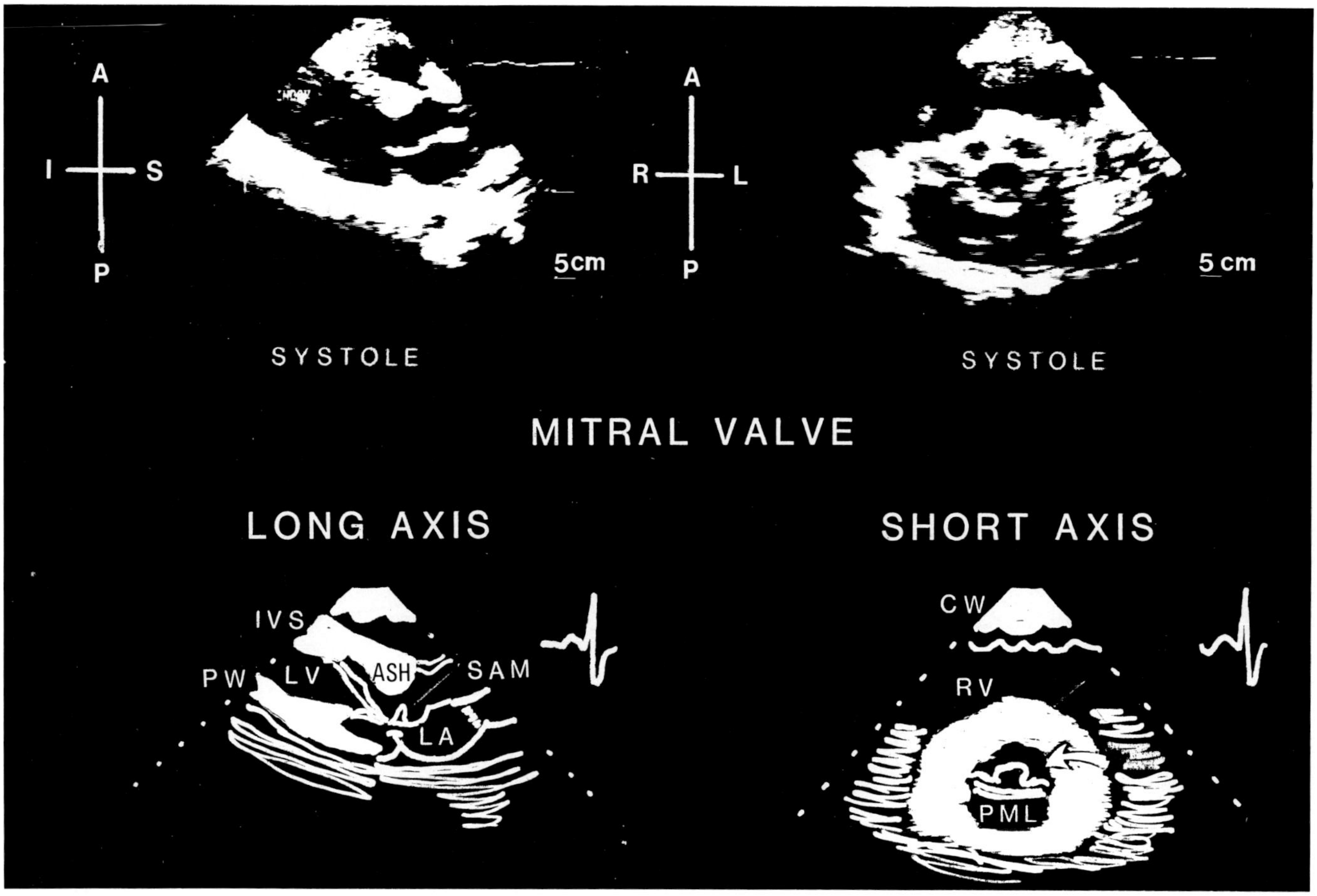

Figure 3-19

Phased-array 90° echocardiogram, in long and short axis during systole, of a 37-year-old man with hypertrophic obstructive cardiomyopathy. Note that, in systole, a light intervening echo is seen just anterior to the anterior mitral leaflet (SAM). In the short-axis view taken at the mitral valve, systolic anterior motion is noted as an outpocketing of the anterior leaflet in systole. Note the asymmetrical septal hypertrophy (ASH).

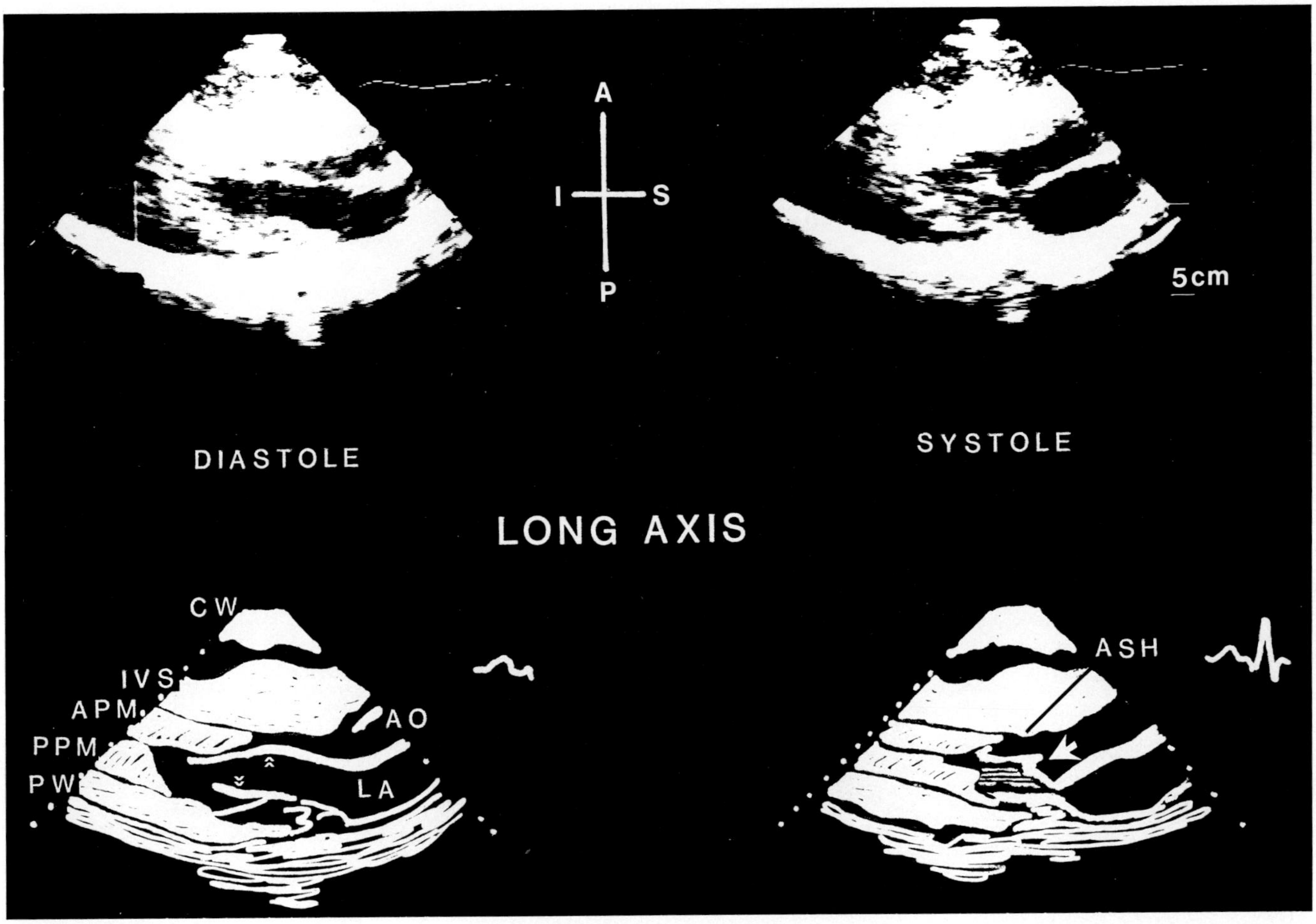

Figure 3-20

Phased-array 90° echocardiogram, in long axis during diastole and systole, of a 49-year-old man with hypertrophic obstructive cardiomyopathy. Note the thickened anterior (ˆ) and posterior (ˇ) mitral leaflets during diastole. During systole, the systolic anterior motion of the mitral valve and chordae tendineae (large white arrow) are seen. Note asymmetrical septal hypertrophy with hypertrophied anterior and posterior papillary muscles.

3-20.1. With respect to hypertrophic cardiomyopathy, the following statements are correct:

A. Systolic anterior motion can occur in the anterior mitral leaflet and chordae tendineae.
B. Systolic anterior motion occurs only in the anterior mitral leaflet.
C. Systolic anterior motion occurs both in the anterior and posterior mitral leaflets.
D. The finding of systolic anterior motion with asymmetrical septal hypertrophy generally implies an obstruction to the left ventricular outflow.

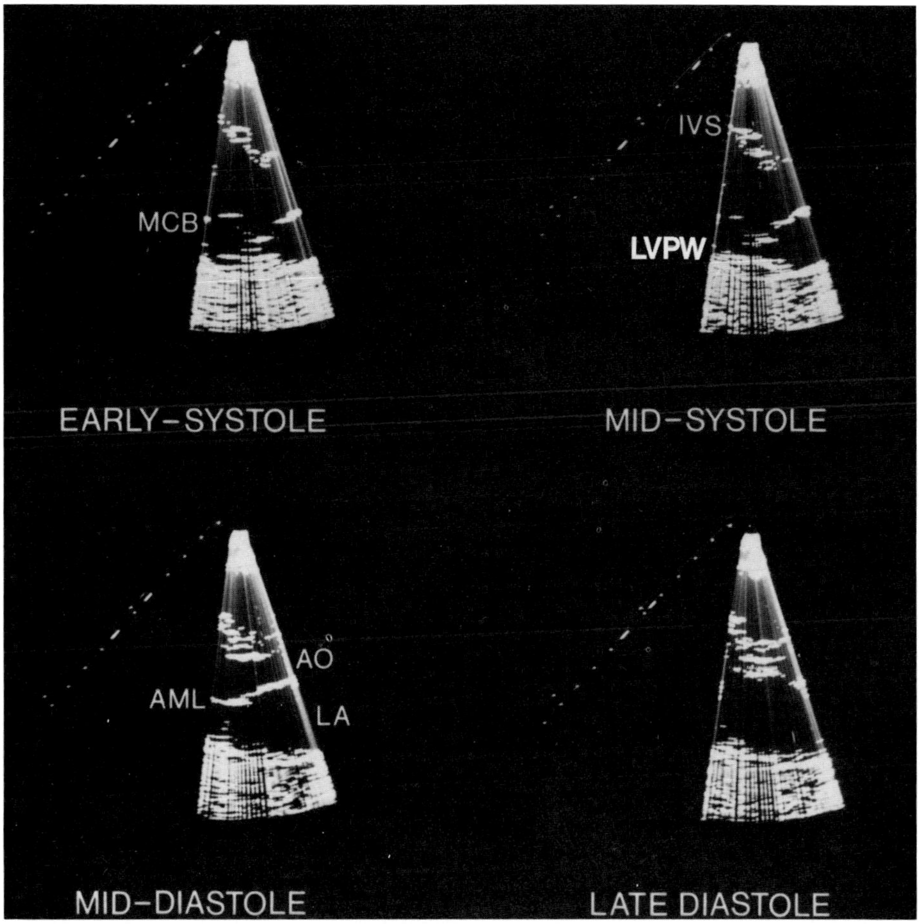

Figure 3-21

Mechanical 30° two-dimensional echocardiogram in long axis of a 27-year-old male patient with a form of systolic anterior motion of the chordae tendineae described as mitral chordal buckling (MCB). Note that during early and mid systole there is buckling of the mitral chordal apparatus anteriorly into the left ventricular outflow tract. This form of systolic anterior motion occurs without asymmetrical septal hypertrophy and left ventricular outflow tract obstruction.

3-21.1. Mitral chordal buckling can be seen in:

A. Normal patients
B. Mitral valve stenosis
C. Mitral valve prolapse
D. Aortic stenosis

James V. Talano

4

Mitral Valve Prolapse

M-MODE ECHOCARDIOGRAPHY

The clinical syndrome of mitral valve prolapse with its classic midsystolic click and mid- to late-systolic murmur is well known, as are the frequently associated findings of cardiac arrhythmias, nonspecific electrocardiographic abnormalities, and a complex of clinical symptoms, including chest pain. The M-mode echocardiographic picture of mitral valve prolapse is fairly characteristic. Normally, with the onset of systole, the mitral leaflets come into apposition or coapt (C-point); they then move slowly to a more anterior position (upsloping C–D line) until, at the beginning of the next diastole, they open. When mitral valve prolapse is present, one or both mitral leaflets are seen to move posteriorly, usually in midsystole, and to remain there until the end of systole — at which time they move anteriorly (Figure 4-1).

In some instances the two leaflets may move either parallel to the anterior chest wall (flat C–D slope) or only slightly posteriorly (negative C–D slope) before a more abrupt midsystolic posterior movement is seen (Figure 4-2).[1-3] In others there may be holosystolic mitral valve prolapse. Occasionally, the mitral leaflets are seen to move anteriorly in early systole and then posteriorly in mid and late systole (Figure 4-4). This initial anterior movement should not be confused with the abnormal mitral valve movement seen in idiopathic hypertrophic subaortic stenosis. In the latter, termed *systolic anterior motion,* a portion of the anterior mitral leaflet moves anteriorly after the onset of systole, and the leaflet remains anterior and adjacent to the interventricular septum throughout midsystole — returning to a more posterior position before the end of systole. In addition to these echocardiographic differences, the absence of the other features of idiopathic hypertrophic subaortic stenosis from mitral valve prolapse further helps to distinguish the two conditions. When early anterior movement of the mitral valve is a result of mitral valve prolapse, the mitral leaflets are seen to move into the left atrium in systole, against the posterior left atrial wall; this systolic anterior motion is due to a "kinking" of the large anterior leaflet into the left ventricular outflow tract.

In patients with **myxomatous** degeneration of the mitral valve (frequently associated with mitral valve prolapse), the leaflets may appear thickened, and multiple echoes may be seen during systole[4] (Figures 4-2 and 4-3). In the presence of pericardial effusion, mitral valve motion is distorted due to posterior movement of the entire heart in the pericardial space, giving the appearance of

CLINICAL SYMPTOMS

Clinical symptoms of chest pain, palpitations, neurological symptoms and dyspnea differ in patient groups with the various types. Patients in type 0 are generally asymptomatic. Symptoms appear more frequently in type 2 and type 3 patients but are not helpful in distinguishing these patients from type 1. The most prevalent symptom is atypical chest pain, which is experienced uncommonly in type 0 and type 1 patients but occurs in about half of type 2 and type 3 patients.[4-9]

CLINICAL AUSCULTATORY FEATURES

When clinical auscultatory features are compared to types of coaptations, nonejection clicks and apical mid- to late-systolic or holosystolic murmurs are most characteristic of the type 2 and 3 patterns. Nonejection clicks are present in none of the normals (type 0) and in only 10 percent of type 1 patients, whereas they are found in 60 percent of type 2 and 75 percent of type 3 patients. Similarly, apical systolic murmurs are present infrequently in type 0 and type 1 patients (5 percent and 30 percent, respectively) but are found in 80 percent of type 2 and 75 percent of type 3 patients.[9]

COMPARISON OF M-MODE FINDINGS WITH TWO-DIMENSIONAL MITRAL COAPTATION PATTERNS

When M-mode echocardiographic patterns of mitral valve prolapse (i.e., mid-, late-, or holosystolic prolapse) are evaluated in each of the four types and those of types 1, 2, and 3 are compared with normals (type 0), most patients in type 1 (80 percent) have no M-mode echocardiographic pattern of mitral valve prolapse. In contrast, two thirds of type 2 patients have an M-mode pattern of holosystolic mitral valve prolapse and one fifth have a pattern of mid- or late-systolic mitral valve prolapse. In only a few type 2 patients does the M-mode echocardiogram fail to reveal a pattern of mitral valve prolapse. In type 3 patients, mid- or late-systolic prolapse is found in 90 percent on M-mode echocardiography. Thus, type 2 coaptation is characterized by holosystolic mitral valve prolapse, whereas type 3 coaptation is characterized by mid- to late-systolic mitral prolapse. When type 0 and type 1 patients are compared with type 2 and type 3 patients, 90 percent of type 0 and type 1 patients—as opposed to only 8 percent of types 2 and 3—have a normal pattern on M-mode echocardiography.[9]

Using the long-axis parasternal view of mitral coaptation, several findings of abnormal mitral annular motion are noted in type 2 and type 3 patients. Mitral annular excursion is more prominent in types 2 and 3 than in types 0 and 1. An exaggerated **caudad** anterior movement of the mitral annulus is noted during systole in type 2 and type 3 patients and is not seen in type 0 or in type 1 patients. When measured by M-mode echocardiography, mitral annular excursion is significantly greater in types 2 and 3 than in types 0 and 1.[9]

To summarize, patients with type 2 or 3 mitral coaptation pattern as evidenced by two-dimensional echocardiography appear to have the auscultatory and M-mode echocardiographic features of Barlow's syndrome. Abnormal, exaggerated mitral annular excursion as determined by two-dimensional echocardiography appears to be characteristic of mitral valve prolapse. Type 2 pattern on two-dimensional echocardiography is characterized by holosystolic mitral valve prolapse on M-mode and appears to be due predominantly to anterior mitral leaflet prolapse. Patients with type 3 pattern on two-dimensional echocardiography are characterized by mid- to late-systolic mitral valve prolapse on M-mode. This pattern is characterized by late-systolic prolapse of the posterior mitral leaflet with undershooting of the anterior mitral leaflet. Type 1 pattern on two-dimensional echocardiography is characterized by few ausculatory or M-mode echocardiographic features of mitral valve prolapse and, as such, should be considered a varient of normal.

ASSOCIATED FINDINGS

Several recent studies have found a pathophysiologic correlation between mitral valve prolapse and dysfunction of the **autonomic nervous system.**[10] Increased **catecholamine excretion** has been found in patients with mitral valve prolapse, indicating that **hyperadrenergic** states may be responsible for several of the clinical symptoms and cardiac and echocardiographic findings associated with this disorder. The autonomic dysfunction may, in part, be responsible for the increased incidence of atrial and ventricular dysrhythmia. Perhaps an autonomic imbalance may be responsible for the association of QT prolongation on ECG with a propensity toward ventricular fibrillation.[11]

Several studies have confirmed the association of transient ischemic episodes, abnormality of vision, and strokes with mitral valve prolapse.[12,13] Cerebral angiography was performed in the patients studied, and cerebral emboli were demonstrated.[13] Several post-mortem studies in these patients have shown small platelet thrombi attached to the posterior mitral leaflet and posterior left atrial wall.[13,14] Cerebral lesions also have been found in these patients, indicating small platelet thromboemboli.

REFERENCES

1. Dillon JC, Haine DL, Chang S, Feigenbaum H: Use of echocardiography in patients with prolapsed mitral valve. Circulation 43:503-507, 1971
2. Popp R, Brown O, Silverman J, Harrison D: Echocardiographic abnormalities in the mitral valve prolapse syndrome. Circulation 49:428-433, 1974
3. Sahn DJ, Wood J, Allen H, Peoples W, Goldberg S: Echocardiographic spectrum of mitral valve motion in children with and without mitral valve prolapse: The nature of false-positive diagnosis. Am J Cardiol 39:422-431, 1977
4. Liedtke A, Babb JD, DeJoseph RL: Mitral valve echoes in patients with mitral valve prolapse syndrome. Am Heart J 97:286-290, 1979
5. Markiewicz W, London E; and Popp RL: Effect of transducer placement on echocardiographic mitral valve motion. Am Heart J, 96:555-556, 1978
6. Gilbert BW, Schatz RA, VonRamm DT, Behar VS, Kisslo JA: Mitral valve prolapse: Two-dimensional echocardiographic and angiographic correlation. Circulation 54:716-723, 1976
7. Cohen MV: Real-time sector scan study of the mitral valve prolapse syndrome. Br Heart J 40:964-972, 1978
8. Inoh T, Maeda K, Oda A: Diagnosis and classification of the mitral valve prolapse by the ultrasoundcardiotomography and the evaluation of the M-mode technic. Jpn Circ J 43:305-312, 1979
9. Talano JV, Gardin JM, Stephanides L: Mitral coaptation patterns in mitral valve prolapse. Am Heart J (in press).

10. Greenwald JG: Autonomic dysfunction in women with mitral valve prolapse. Circulation 60:910-913, 1979
11. Forbes RB, Morton GH: Ventricular fibrillation in a patient with unsuspected mitral valve prolapse and a prolonged Q - T interval. Can Anaesth Soc J 26:424-427, 1979
12. Saffro R, Talano JV: Transient ischemic attack associated with mitral systolic clicks. Arch Intern Med 139:693-694, 1979
13. Watson RT: TIA, stroke, and mitral valve prolapse. Neurology 29:886-889, 1979
14. Barnett HJ, Boughner DR, Taylor DW: Further evidence relating mitral valve prolapse to cerebral ischemic events. N. Engl J Med 302:139-149, 1980

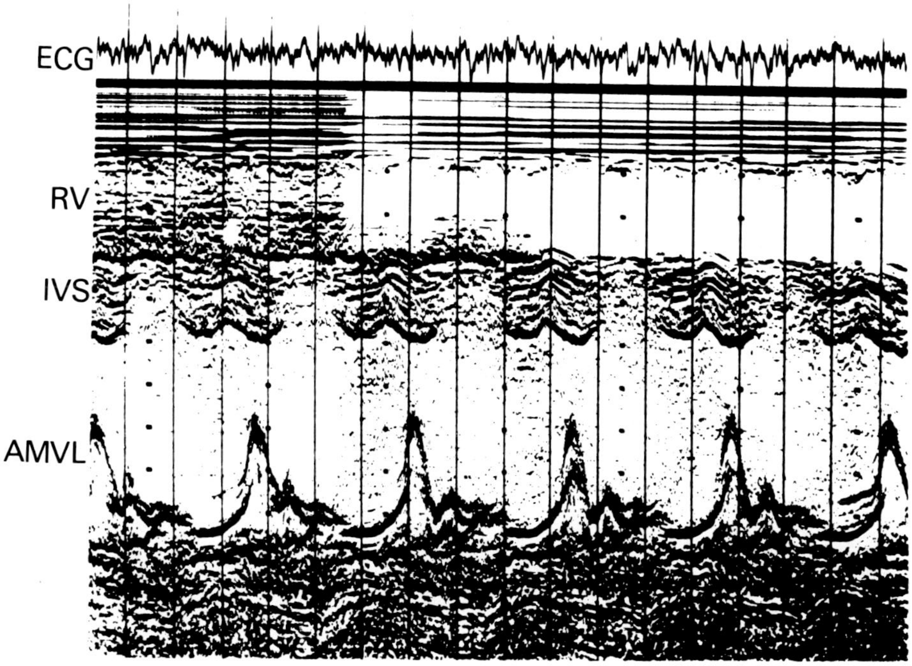

Figure 4-6

M-mode echocardiogram of a young female who presents with a history of palpitations, a diastolic decrescendo murmur at the fourth left interspace, and a systolic click at the left ventricular apex.

4-6.1. The findings of this echocardiogram are consistent with:

A. Late systolic prolapse of the mitral valve
B. Diastolic fluttering of the anterior mitral leaflet
C. Premature closure of the mitral valve
D. Holosystolic mitral valve prolapse

4-6.2. The M-mode echocardiogram is likely to indicate the presence of:

A. Aortic regurgitation with mitral valve prolapse
B. Mitral stenosis with mitral valve prolapse
C. Aortic stenosis and mitral valve prolapse
D. Ventricular septal defect and mitral valve prolapse

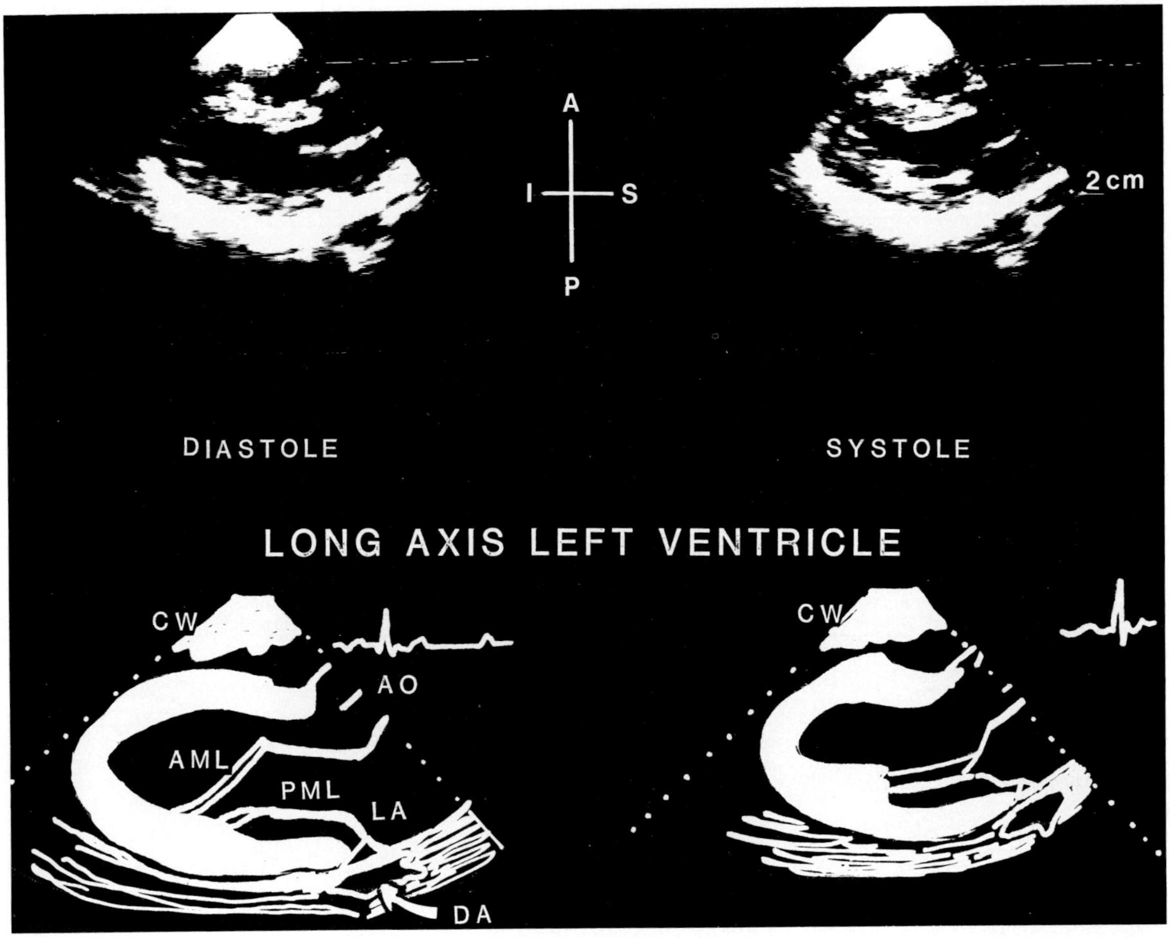

Figure 4-7

Two-dimensional echocardiograms in long axis of the left ventricle during diastole and systole. Note the type 0 coaptation of the anterior mitral and posterior mitral leaflets during systole: coaptation of the mitral valve occurs well within the left ventricular cavity.

4-7.1. This pattern of mitral coaptation is found frequently in which of the following situations:

A. Normal
B. Symptoms of chest pain and dizzyness
C. Midsystolic clicks and murmurs
D. Patients with idiopathic hypertrophic subaortic stenosis

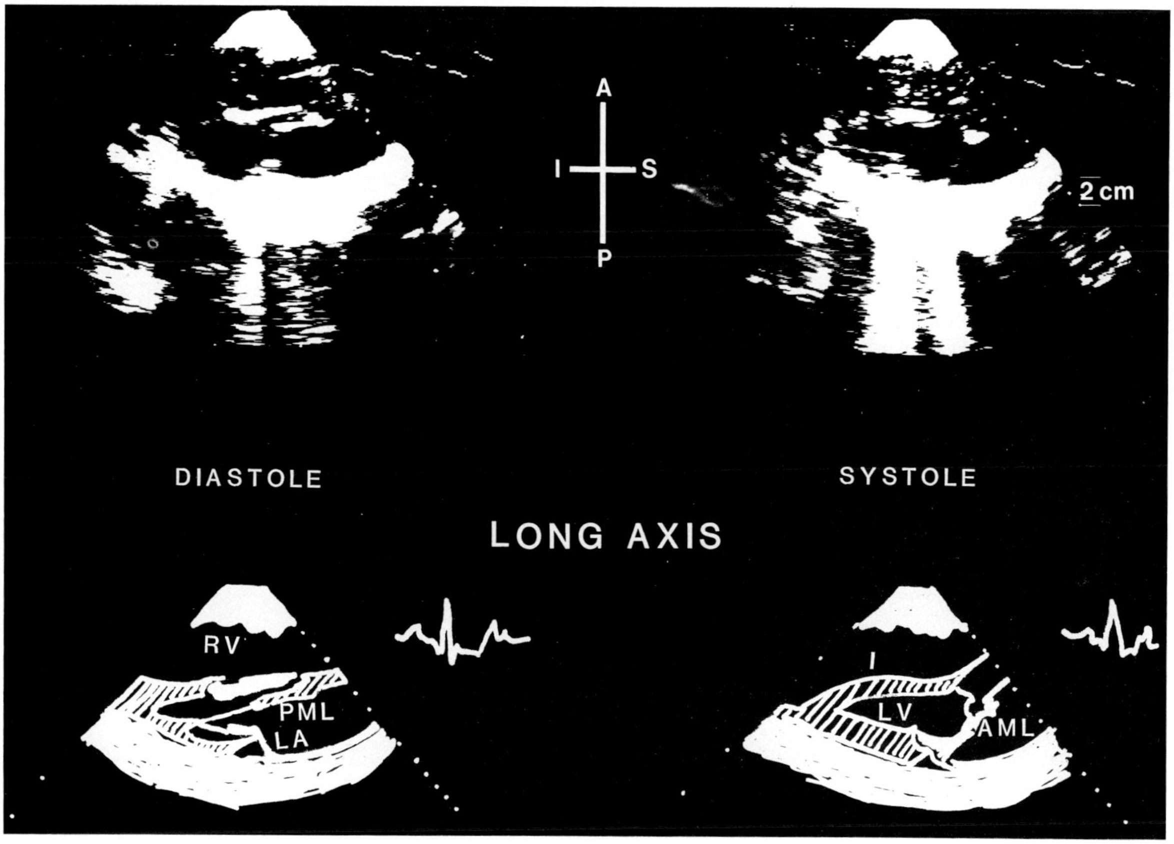

Figure 4-8

Two-dimensional echocardiograms in long axis of the left ventricle during diastole and systole of a patient with type 2 mitral coaptation. Note the prolapse of the anterior mitral leaflet well into the left atrium. The anterior leaflet bows well into the left atrium, almost touching the posterior left atrial wall. This patient also had a secundum atrial septal defect. (Note micro-bubbles in the right ventricle during systole.)

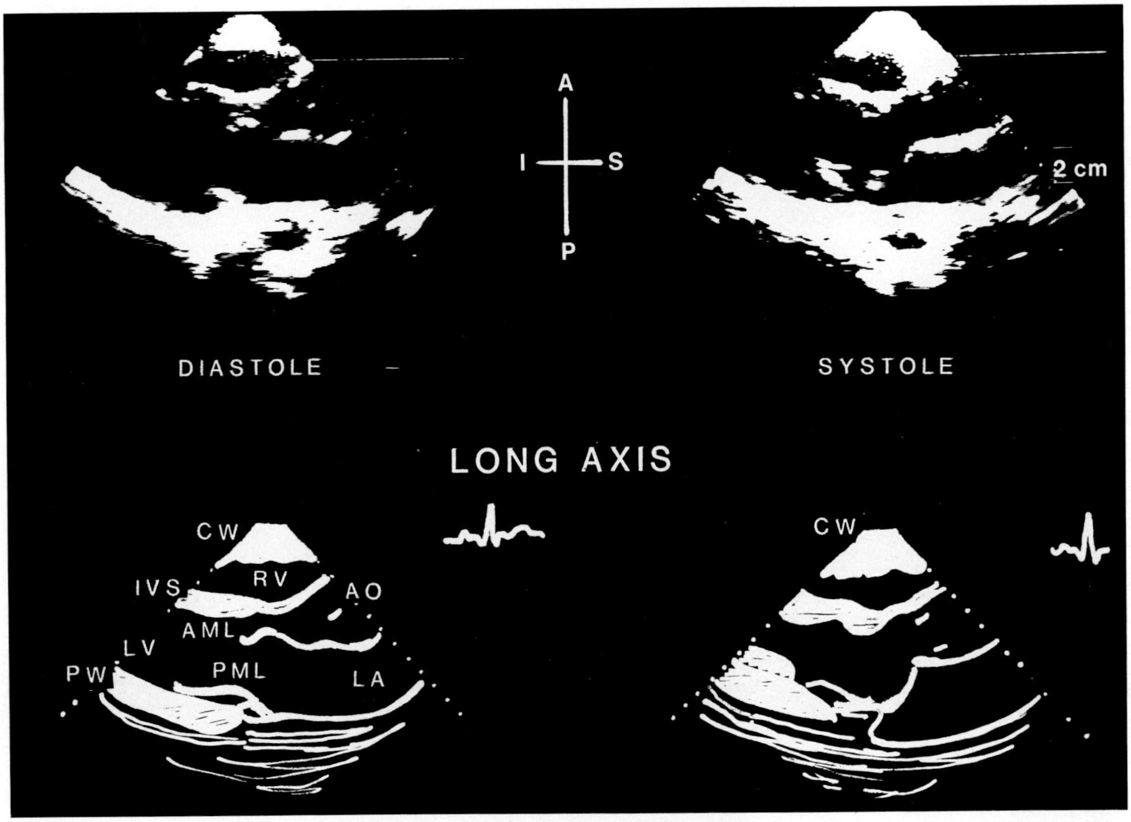

Figure 4-9

Two-dimensional echocardiograms in long axis of the left ventricle during diastole and systole of a patient with type 2 coaptation pattern. Note the cephalad bowing of the anterior mitral leaflet into the left atrium.

4-9.1. Type 2 pattern of mitral coaptation is seen frequently with which of the following:

A. Normals
B. M-mode late-systolic prolapse
C. Congenital heart disease
D. M-mode holosystolic prolapse

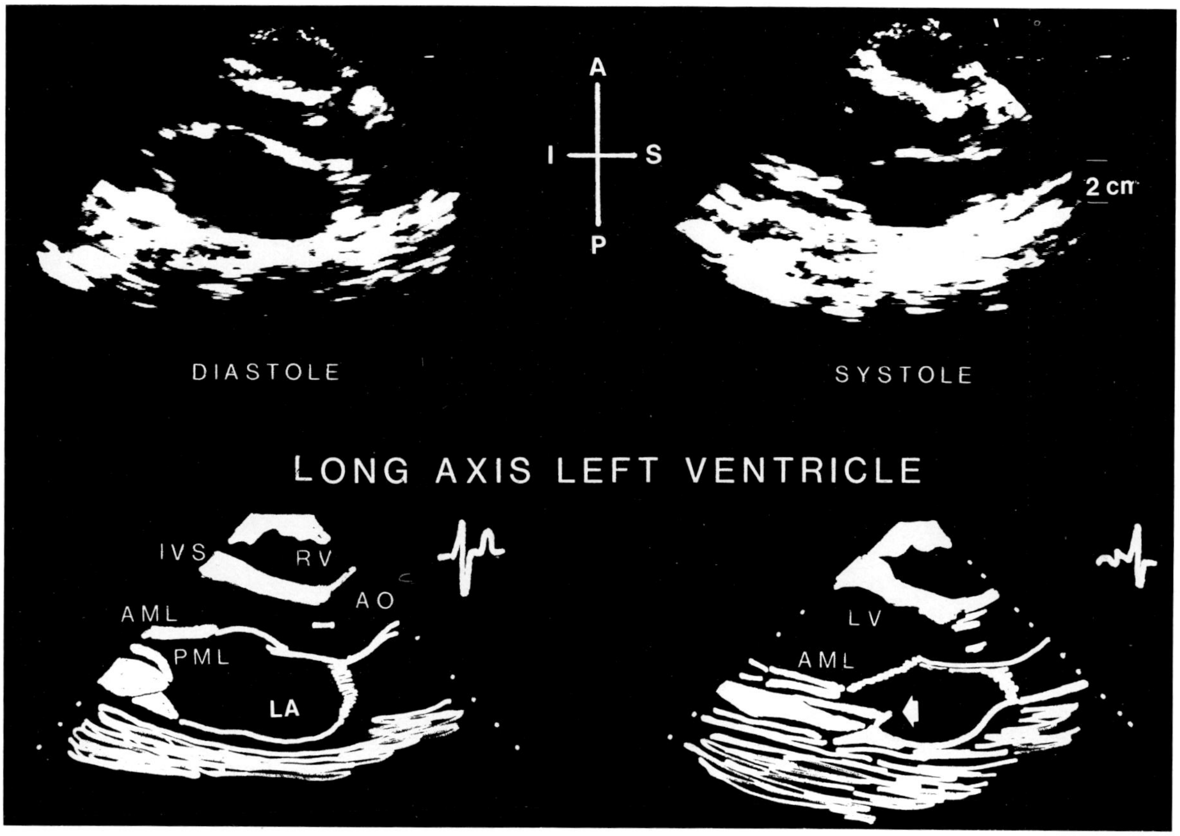

Figure 4-10

Two-dimensional echocardiograms in long axis of the ventricle during diastole and systole in a patient with type 3 coaptation. During early systole the posterior mitral leaflet was seen to coapt with the anterior mitral leaflet in the left ventricle. However, the posterior mitral leaflet moves cephalad into the left atrium during late systole (arrow).

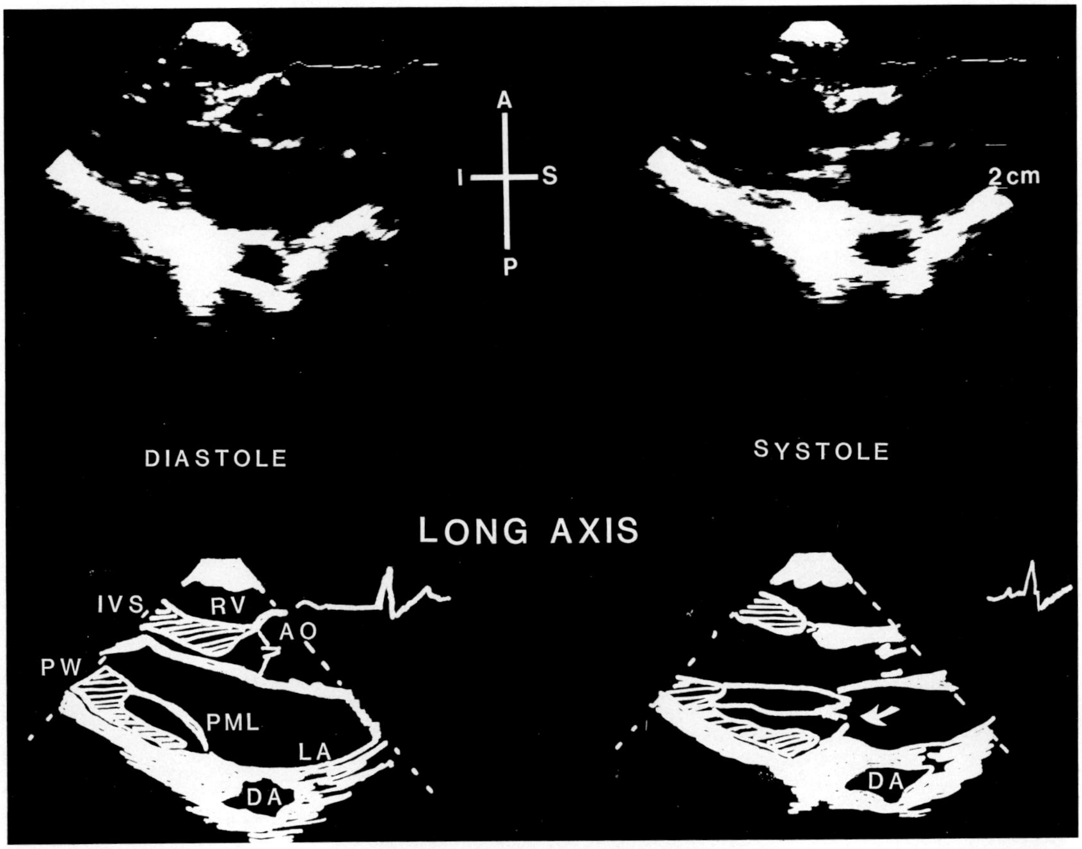

Figure 4-11

Two-dimensional echocardiograms in long axis of the left ventricle in a patient with type 3 coaptation. Note that during systole the anterior and posterior mitral leaflets move cephalad into the left atrium.

4-11.1 Type 3 coaptation pattern is seen frequently with which of the following:

A. Normals
B. Late-systolic prolapse on M-mode
C. Holosystolic prolapse on M-mode
D. Midsystolic clicks and late-systolic murmur
E. Congenital heart lesions

William R. Jacobs

5

Diseases of the Aorta and Great Vessels

Echocardiography is very useful in the examination of the aortic root and the left ventricular outflow tract. When the M-mode transducer is tilted superiorly from the mitral valve toward the aortic root, the continuity of the mitral valve and aorta can be seen. The anterior mitral leaflet is continuous with the posterior aortic wall, and the interventricular septum is continuous with the anterior aortic wall. The structure anterior to the aortic root is the right ventricular outflow tract, and the structure posterior to the aortic root is the left atrium. During systole the aortic root swings anteriorly and posteriorly and, then, in a more complex diastolic motion, moves posteriorly again (Figure 5-1). During diastole, the tips of the coapted aortic cusps (right aortic cusp, anteriorly; noncoronary cusp, posteriorly) can be seen in the middle of the aortic root. When left ventricular pressure exceeds the aortic diastolic pressure, the aortic cusps open rapidly, remaining about the same distance apart during systole, and then snap closed, forming a box-like pattern (Figure 5-2 A and 5-2 B). Since the aortic root moves anteriorly during systole, this box-like pattern is drawn into a parallelogram. A fairly wide ultrasonic beam crosses the circular aortic root, striking the aortic wall at many points along its curvature; the multiple reflected echoes that result give the impression that the aortic root is much thicker than it really is.

AORTIC ROOT

The simplest aortic abnormality demonstrable by M-mode echocardiography is **aortic root** dilatation. With aortic root dilatation, the walls of the aortic root maintain their normal parallel motion but are simply farther apart when measured from the anterior edge of the anterior wall echo to the anterior edge of the posterior aortic wall echo. In the dilated aortic root, in contrast to the normal, the aortic cusps do not impinge against the walls of the aorta in the open position. When the aortic root is greatly dilated, it may even be possible to image the aortic root from the right parasternal position.[1] In aortic dissection, the inner lining **(intima)** peels away from the thickened outer layer **(externa)** of the aortic root. The dissected aortic wall may appear as double lines (the two layers) separated by several millimeters. In aortic dissection, aortic cusp motion is seen between the inner lines which represent the intima, or inner lining of the aortic root.[2,3]

Figure 5-3

M-mode echocardiogram of the aortic root and aortic valve of a 58-year-old male with a murmur of aortic regurgitation.

5-3.1. The abnormality noted in the aortic cusp is:

A. Vegetation on cardiac leaflet
B. Aortic root dilatation
C. Sinus of Valsalva aneurysm
D. Eccentric closure of aortic valve

5-3.2. The most likely diagnosis in this patient is:

A. Aortic valve endocarditis
B. Sinus of Valsalva aneurysm
C. Aortic root dissection
D. Congenital bicuspid aortic valve

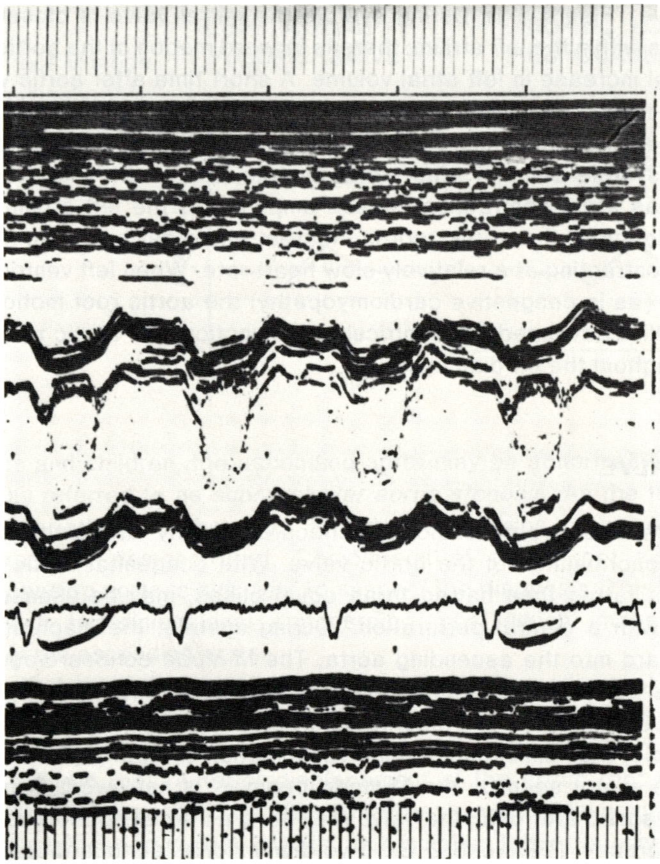

accumulate on the aortic cusps; this gives the cusps a thickened appearance, even though their motion usually remains normal. Vegetations appear as laminar or granular thickening of the cusps, which otherwise appear normal (Figure 5-2 G). These vegetations may be lifted up out of the ultrasonic beam when the aortic cusps open in systole. Thus they are often most prominent during diastole. When vegetations of the aortic valve destroy the substance of the cusp itself, one or more of the aortic cusps may become flail. When this occurs, blood may regurgitate into the left ventricle during diastole, causing diastolic vibrations of the flail aortic cusp (Figure 5-2 F). (Figure 5-4) Diastolic vibrations of the aortic cusp, like systolic vibrations of a mitral leaflet, are always abnormal and often are due to a flail cusp or endocarditis (Figure 5-2 F).[5] When the M-mode beam is tilted down into the left ventricular outflow tract, the flail aortic cusp or vegetations may be seen during diastole as a vigorously vibrating structure located in the left ventricular outflow tract between the septum and the anterior mitral leaflet.[6]

In other causes of aortic regurgitation, the aortic echocardiogram may not be as dramatically abnormal. In general, the aortic valve in aortic regurgitation may appear normal, or bicuspid (Figure 5-3) or the aortic root may be dilated. In the past it was thought that the M-mode appearance of a diastolic separation between the two aortic cusps indicated aortic regurgitation; this, however, has not proven to be correct in all cases. Diastolic cusp separation on two-dimensional echocardiography may, however, prove more useful in diagnosing aortic regurgitation. Perhaps the most common appearance of the aortic cusps in older adults with aortic regurgitation is that the cusps are thickened, and perhaps calcified, but have fair to good cusp motion. Aortic regurgitation is best detected by finding high-frequency or rapid diastolic vibrations of the anterior mitral leaflet; this, unfortunately, does not occur in every case (Figure 5-5).

In addition to demonstrating abnormalities of aortic cusp structure, echocardiography may be useful in demonstrating abnormal patterns of aortic cusp motion. During systole, the aortic cusps may demonstrate high-frequency systolic vibration (Figure 5-2 E); this high-frequency vibration is normal — in distinct contrast to diastolic aortic cusp vibration, which is always abnormal (Figure 5-4). The most interesting aortic cusp motion abnormalities are those which result from subvalvular left ventricular outflow obstruction. Perhaps the best known of these abnormalities is the left ventricular outflow tract obstruction that occurs in idiopathic hypertrophic subaortic stenosis (IHSS); in this abnormality, the left ventricular outflow tract is momentarily obstructed during systole by contact between the anterior mitral leaflet edge and the interventricular septum (systolic anterior motion of the anterior mitral leaflet). This results in partial mid-systolic closure of the aortic cusp(s) (Figure 5-2 D). Although this abnormal aortic cusp motion pattern is very sensitive when present, it is not very common in IHSS.

In **discrete subaortic stenosis,** there is a fibrous narrowing or discrete membrane in the left ventricular outflow tract below the aortic valve. The aortic cusps open quickly, then immediately begin to close, (early aortic cusp notching) and then vibrate and slowly reopen for the duration of systole (Figure 5-2 H). This unusual aortic cusp motion is yet unexplained but apparently relates to turbulence generated in the aortic root during systole.[7,8]

Since the aortic cusps are separated by the action of the left ventricle, it is not surprising that severe left ventricular dysfunction may cause abnormal aortic cusp motion. With severe impairment of left ventricular function, as in advanced congestive cardiomyopathy, the aortic cusps open late after the onset of QRS and appear to separate gradually, inscribing a curved line rather than the usual brisk, straight, opening motion (Figure 5-2 I). The cusps may open less far and may

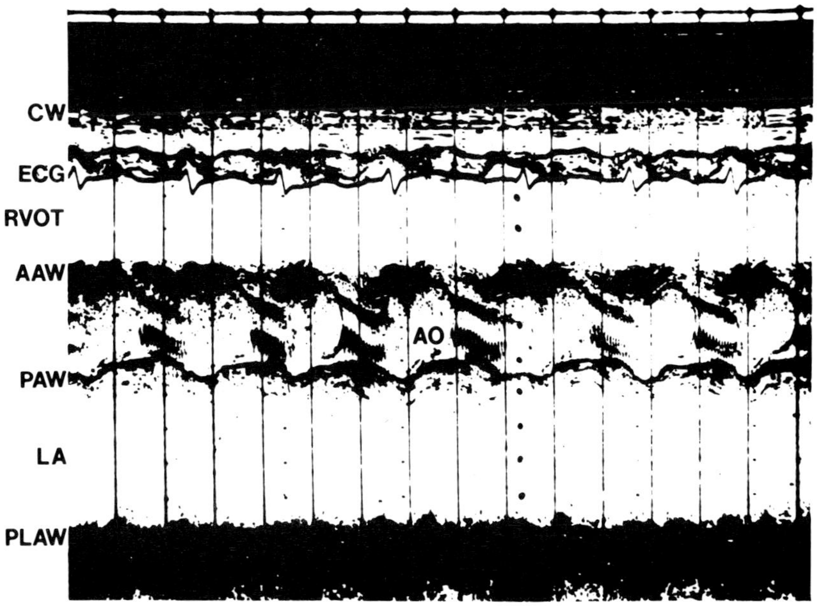

Figure 5-4

M-mode echocardiogram taken at the level of the aortic valve (PLAW, posterior left aortic wall).

5-4.1. The abnormality noted in the aortic leaflet in diastole is:

A. Ruptured noncoronary cusp
B. Aortic valve obstruction
C. Aortic root dissection
D. Sinus of Valsalva aneurysm

5-4.2. The size of the left atrium is:

A. Normal
B. Abnormal

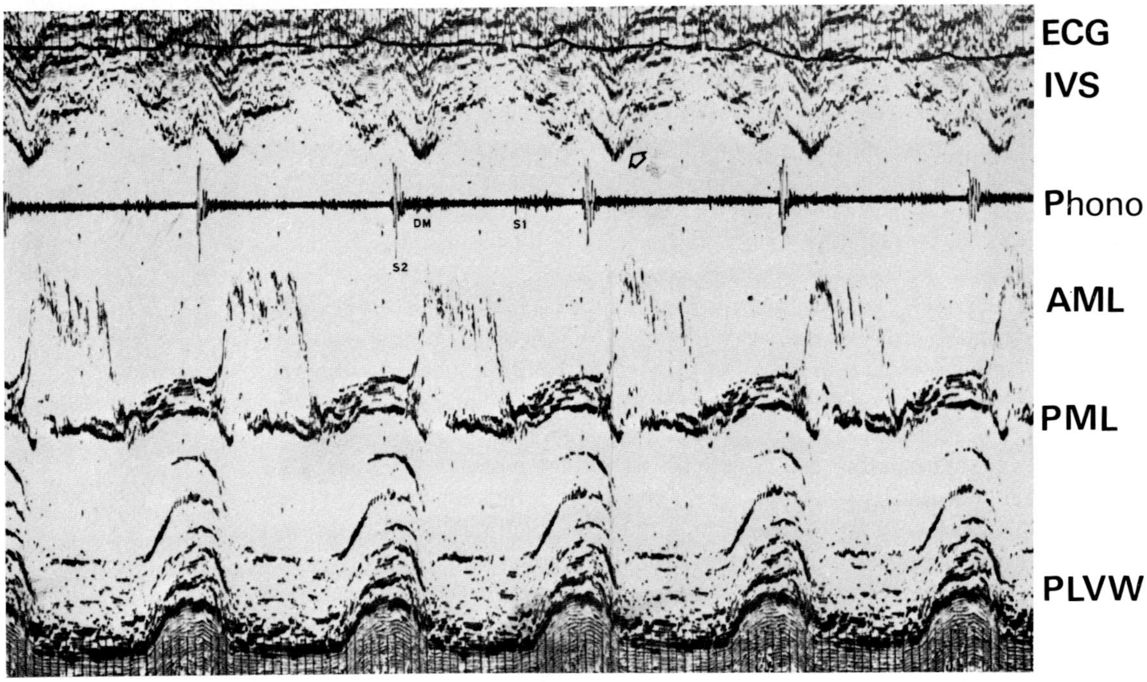

Figure 5-5

M-mode echocardiogram of the left ventricle at the level of the anterior and posterior mitral leaflet. A phonocardiogram is recorded showing a diastolic descresendo murmur (DM). The first heart sound (S1) and the second heart sound (S2) are noted. Note diastolic fluttering of the anterior mitral leaflet as well as that of the interventricular septum (open arrow). (PLVW, posterior left ventricular wall.)

5-5.1. The aortic valve abnormality associated with this echocardiogram is most likely:

A. Aortic stenosis
B. Bicuspid aortic valve
C. Sinus of Valsalva aneurysm
D. Idiopathic hypertrophic subaortic stenosis

gradually drift together during systole, rendering the entire pattern of aortic cusp motion more rounded and briefer than in the normal heart (Figure 5-2 I). In cases of very severe aortic insufficiency, the aortic cusps may actually open prematurely — before the onset of QRS (Figure 5-2 L).

REFERENCES

1. D'Cruz IA, Jain DP, Hirsch L, Levinsky R, Cohen HC, Glick G: Echocardiographic diagnosis of dilatation of the ascending aorta. Radiology 129:465-469, 1978
2. DeMaria AN, Bommer W, Neumann A, Weinert L, Bogren H, Mason DT: Identification and localization of aneurysms of the ascending aorta by cross-sectional echocardiography. Circulation 59:755-761, 1979
3. Hirschfeld DS, Rodriguez HJ, Schiller NB: Duplication of aortic wall seen by echocardiography. Br Heart J 38:843-850, 1976
4. Fowles RE, Martin RP, Abrams JM, Schapira JN, French JW, Popp RL: Two-dimensional echocardiographic features of bicuspid aortic valve. Chest 75:434-40, 1979
5. Krivokapich J, Child JS, Skorton DJ: Flail aortic valve leaflets: M-mode and two-dimensional echocardiographic manifestations. Am Heart J 99:425-437, 1980

6. Orita Y, Yamada A, Hirata T, Sese A, Tanaka S: Detection of flail aortic valve in bacterial endocarditis with real-time two-dimensional echocardiography: A case report. Jpn Heart J 21:141-148, 1980
7. Wilcox WD, Seward JB, Hagler DJ, Mair DD, Tajik AJ: Discrete subaortic stenosis: Two-dimensional echocardiographic features with angiographic and surgical correlation. Mayo Clin Proc 55:525-433, 1980
8. Berry TE, Aziz KU, Paul MH: Echocardiographic assessment of discrete subaortic stenosis in childhood. Am J Cardiol 43:957-961, 1979

ADDITIONAL ILLUSTRATIONS AND EXERCISES

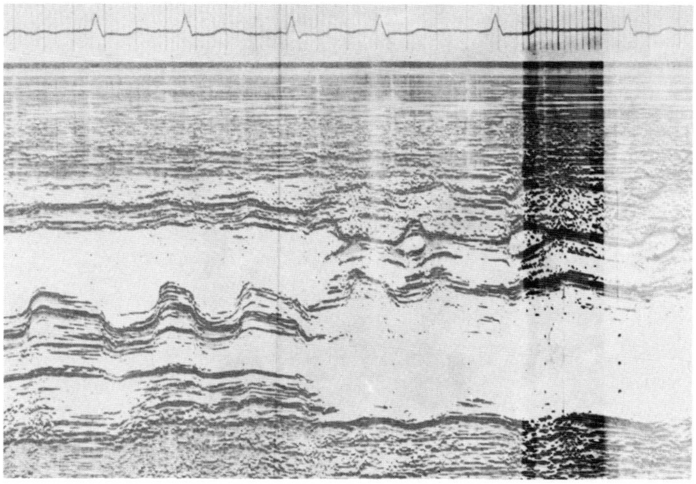

Figure 5–6

M-mode echocardiogram scan from the anterior mitral leaflet to the aortic valve. Note the heavy dense echoes originating from the anterior and posterior mitral leaflets. Also note the aortic opening at the level of the aortic root.

5-6.1. The mitral and aortic valve abnormalities noted are most likely due to:

A. Mitral valve prolapse and normal aortic valve
B. Mitral valve prolapse and congenital aortic stenosis
C. Idiopathic hypertrophic subaortic stenosis
D. Rheumatic mitral and aortic valve disease

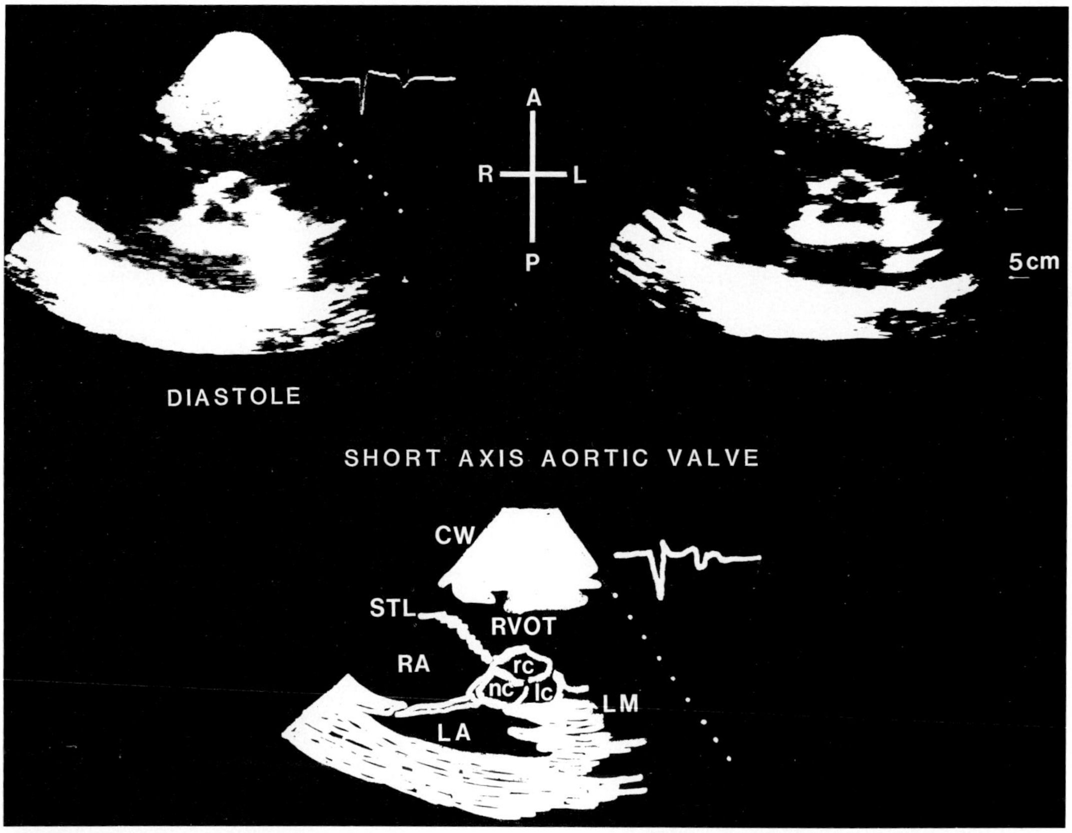

Figure 5-7

Two-dimensional echocardiogram in short axis of a normal aortic valve showing the three aortic valve cusps (rc, right cusp; nc, noncoronary cusp; lc, left cusp).

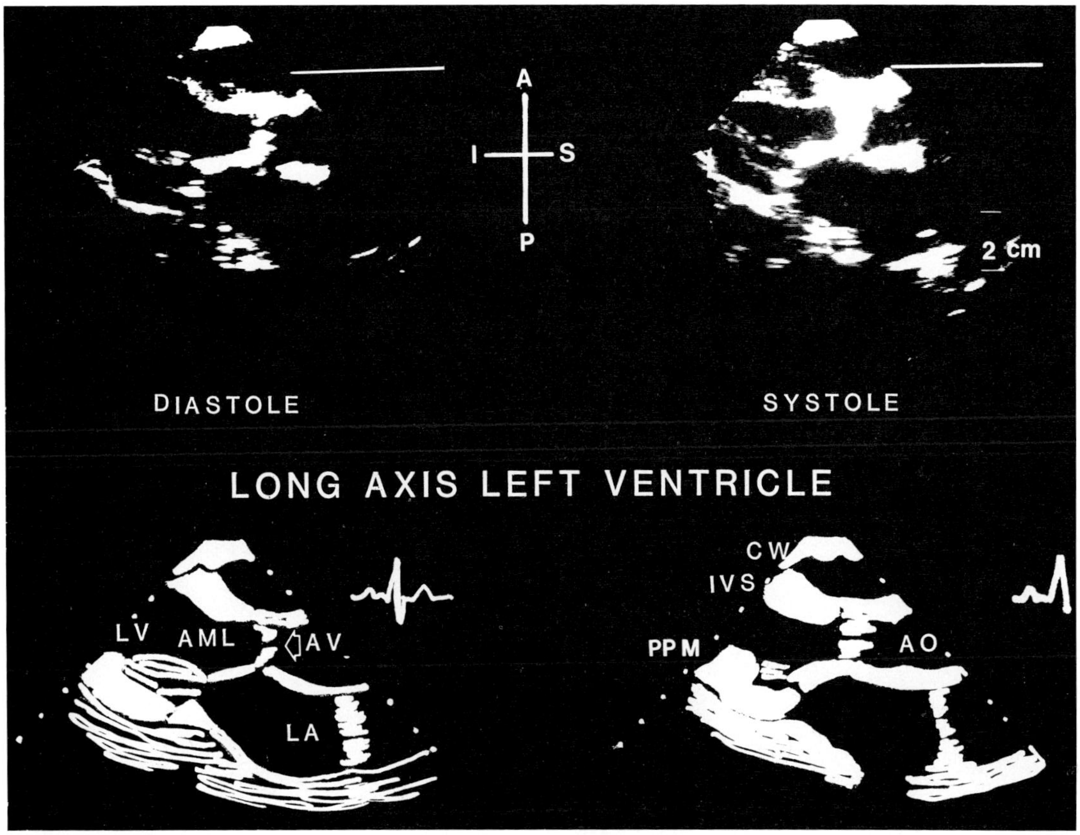

Figure 5-8

Long-axis two-dimensional echocardiogram of the left ventricular outflow tract and aortic valve during diastole and systole. Note the heavy dense echoes in the vicinity of the aortic valve. Note also the persistent separation of the aortic leaflets during diastole. During systole, separation of the aortic leaflets is only minimal: 0.6 cm (normal value exceeds 1.5 cm). Left ventricular hypertrophy was present.

5-8.1. The most likely diagnosis in this patient is:

- A. Aortic sclerosis
- B. Calcific aortic stenosis
- C. Subvalvular aortic stenosis
- D. Idiopathic hypertrophic subaortic stenosis

5-8.2. The severity of aortic stenosis can best be judged by which of the following parameters?

- A. Aortic leaflet separation by M-mode echocardiography
- B. Left ventricular hypertrophy by two-dimensional echocardiography
- C. Aortic leaflet separation by M-mode and left ventricular hypertrophy by two-dimensional echocardiography
- D. Aortic leaflet separation by Two-dimensional echocardiography and left ventricular hypertrophy by M-mode.

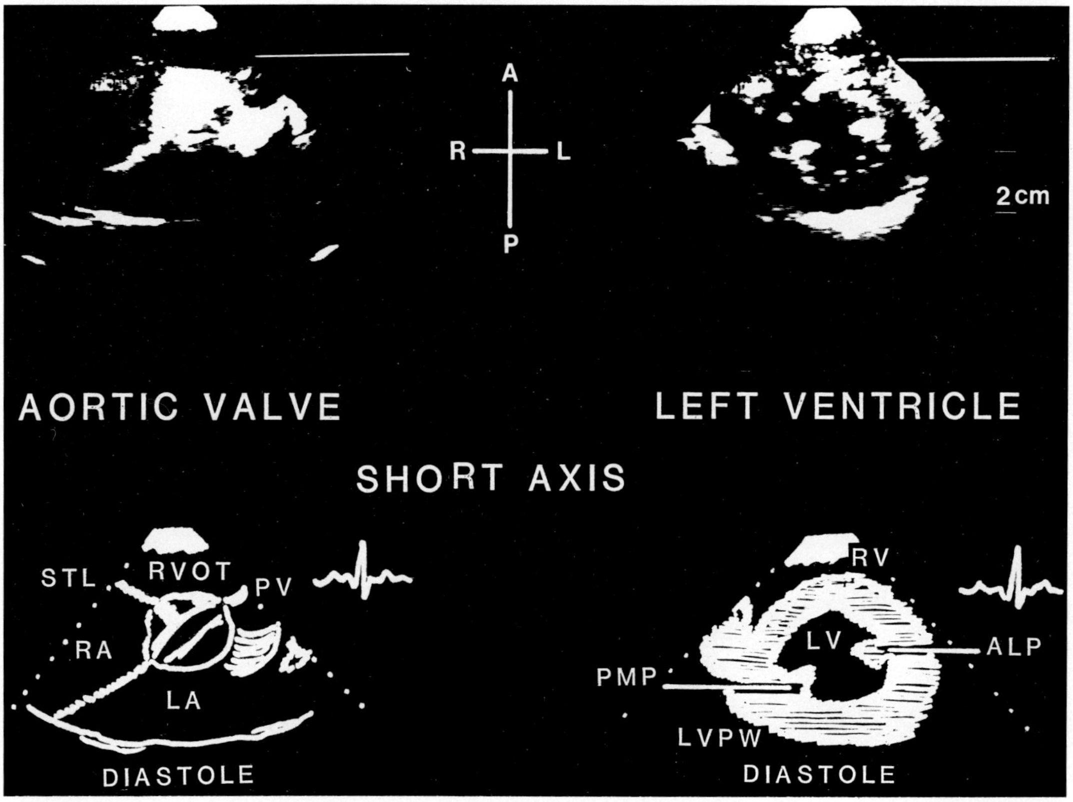

Figure 5-9

Two-dimensional echocardiogram of the aortic valve and left ventricle in short axis of a patient with congenital bicuspid aortic valve stenosis. Note two aortic leaflets which are heavily calcified in diastole. The short-axis view of the left ventricle is at the level of the papillary muscle in diastole. Note the concentric left ventricular hypertrophy. (Lines are 2.0 cm; PMP, posterior medial papillary muscle; ALP, anterior lateral papillary muscle.)

5-9.1. Concerning the echocardiographic diagnosis of aortic valve stenosis (i.e., a gradient across the aortic valve greater than 50 mm Hg), which of the following statements are true?

A. Persistent aortic cusp separation (diastole) of less than 1.0 cm is a good criterion.
B. The presence of concentric left ventricular hypertrophy makes aortic stenosis likely.
C. The absence of concentric left ventricular hypertrophy makes aortic stenosis unlikely.
D. Degree of aortic cusp separation in systole correlates well inversely with aortic valve gradient.

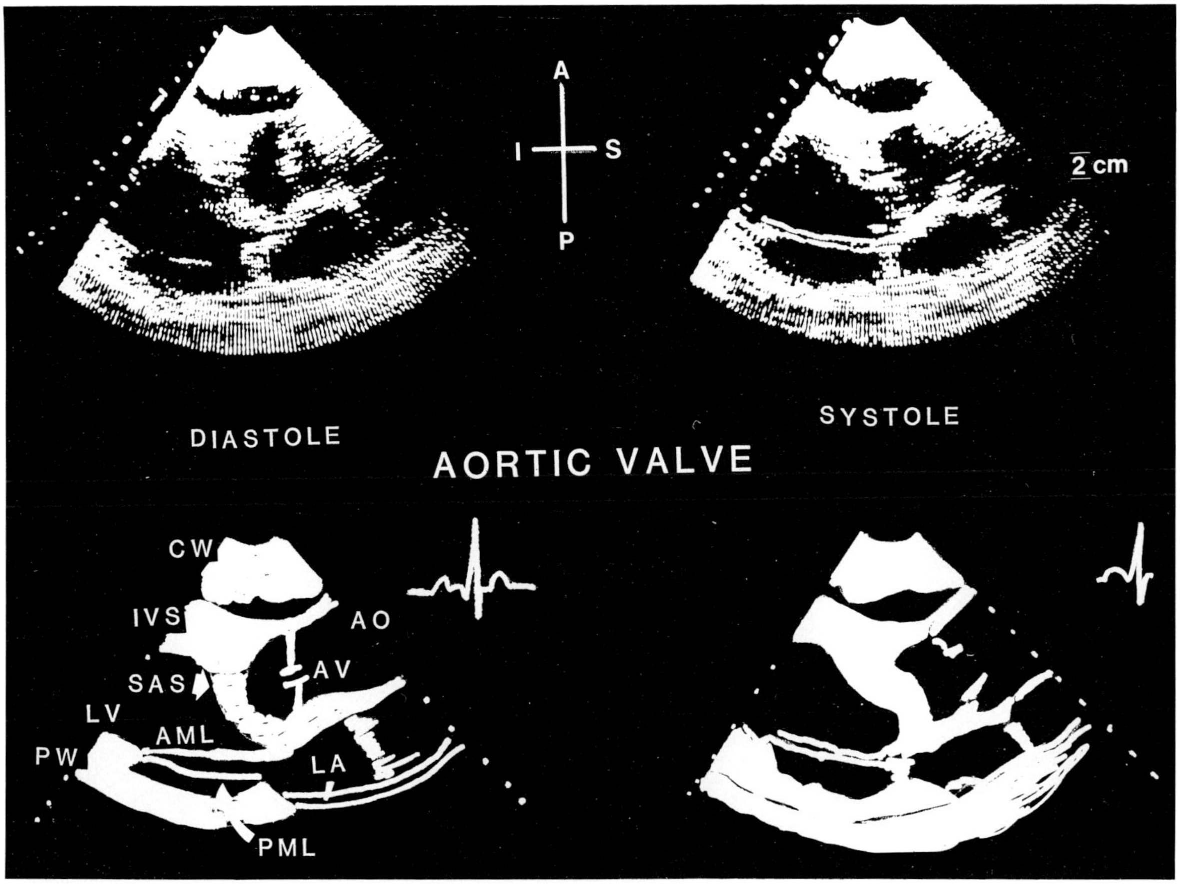

Figure 5-10

Two-dimensional long-axis view of the left ventricular outflow tract using a 87° mechanical scanner in a patient with congenital subaortic aortic stenosis. Note the aortic leaflets (AV) open normally during systole. However, below the aortic valve is a discrete membrane compatible with subaortic stenosis (SAS). Note the subaortic chamber below the aortic valve. At surgery, the subaortic membrane was due to an accessory aortic valve.

5-10.1. In discrete subaortic stenosis, the diagnosis can be made by each of the following echocardiographic signs *except:*

A. Demonstration of the subaortic membrane by two-dimensional echocardiography
B. Early systolic closure of the aortic valve by M-mode echocardiography
C. A narrowed left ventricular outflow tract when compared to the aortic root
D. Calcification and decreased opening of the aortic valve

5-10.2. In subaortic stenosis, the aortic valve opening which best describes the abnormality is:

A. Early-systolic notching of the aortic valve
B. Mid-systolic notching or closing of the aortic valve
C. Early-systolic notching with early preclosure of the valve accompanied by fluttering of the aortic valve leaflets
D. Mid-systolic notching with early closure and fluttering of the valve

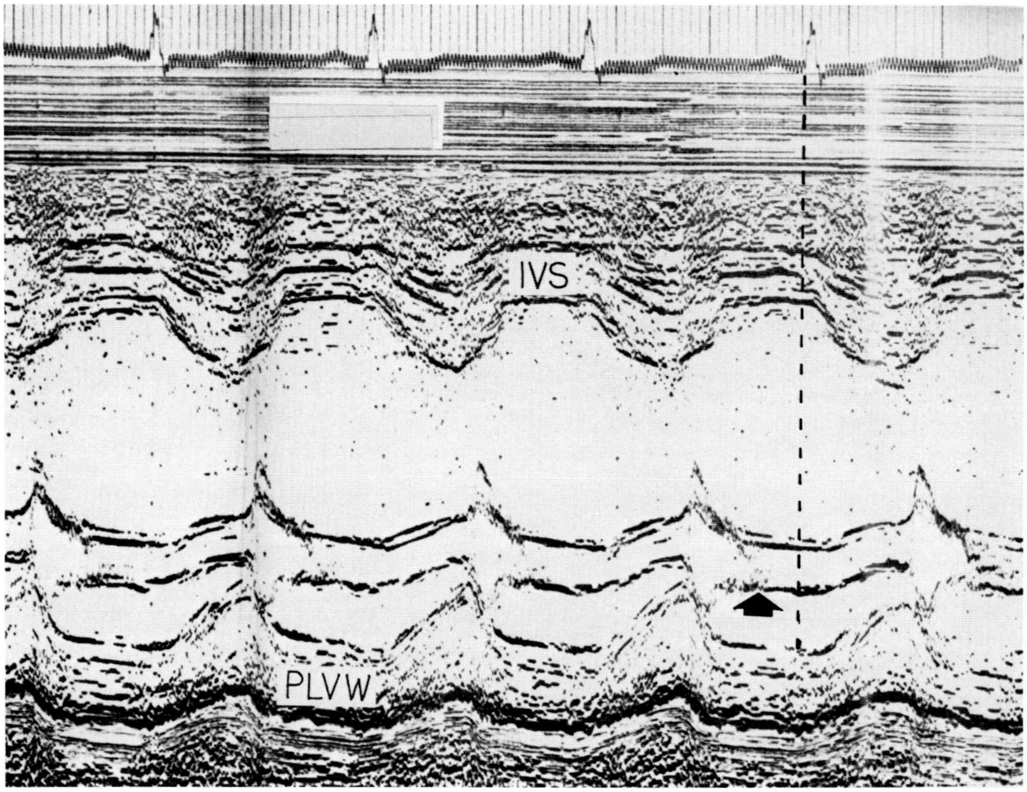

Figure 5-11

M-mode echocardiogram taken through the left ventricle at the level of the anterior and posterior mitral leaflet. Note the left ventricular enlargement (end-diastolic diameter, 6.2 cm) and increased motion of the interventricular septum and left ventricular posterior wall. Follow the anterior and posterior mitral leaflets to closure (arrow) and note the relationship of the mitral valve closure to the onset of the QRS complex.

5-11.1. The abnormality of the mitral valve is:

A. Decreased E–F slope of the anterior leaflet
B. Flail posterior mitral leaflet
C. Early mitral valve closure due to primary atrioventricular block
D. Early mitral valve closure due to severe aortic insufficiency

Ivan A. D'Cruz

6

Pericardial Effusion and Pericardial Disease

Diagnosis of the presence and size of pericardial effusions constitutes one of the most common and important applications of cardiac ultrasound in everyday clinical practice. The **specificity** and **sensitivity** of echocardiography is superior to other diagnostic methods for this purpose.[1]

In principle, the echocardiographic diasnosis is simple: it consists of the demonstration of an echo-free space between the left ventricular posterior wall and the subjacent pericardium. When a small pericardial effusion is present, a separation between the left ventricular posterior wall and the pericardium is seen in systole but not in diastole (Figure 6-1). As the amount of pericardial fluid increases, separation occurs in diastole as well; the larger the size of the effusion, the wider the echo-free space between the wall and the pericardium. When the patient is supine, pericardial fluid tends to pool in the most dependent part of the pericardial sac, behind the left ventricular posterior wall.

The appearance of an echo-free space anterior to the right ventricle may be noted in pericardial effusions of any size; however, anterior pericardial effusions often are not detectable in patients with only small fluid accumulations. In moderate or large pericardial effusion, the width of the anterior echo-free space generally is less than the posterior echo-free pericardial space. The quantity of anterior pericardial fluid tends to increase, however, when the patient sits up. The echocardiographic detection of pericardial effusions depends on the correct identification of the left ventricular posterior wall, **endocardium**, **epicardium**, and the **parietal pericardium** (Figure 6-1). This, in turn, is based upon (1) the proper adjustment of gain and reject ultrasound controls; (2) repeated scanning from the left ventricle to the left atrium, and (3) scanning at different levels of the left ventricle from base toward the apex.

There are many possible pitfalls in the diagnosis and estimation of size of pericardial effusions, all of which can be overcome by adequate experience and attention to scanning and recording techniques:[1-3]

- **Left pleural effusion,** which presents as echo-free space behind the heart, may be mistaken for pericardial effusions. Unlike pericardial effusion, however, pleural effusions may be seen to extend behind the left atrium as the ultrasound beam sweeps medially. Sometimes the pericardial-pleural membrane can be identified as a thin linear echo between the left ventricular

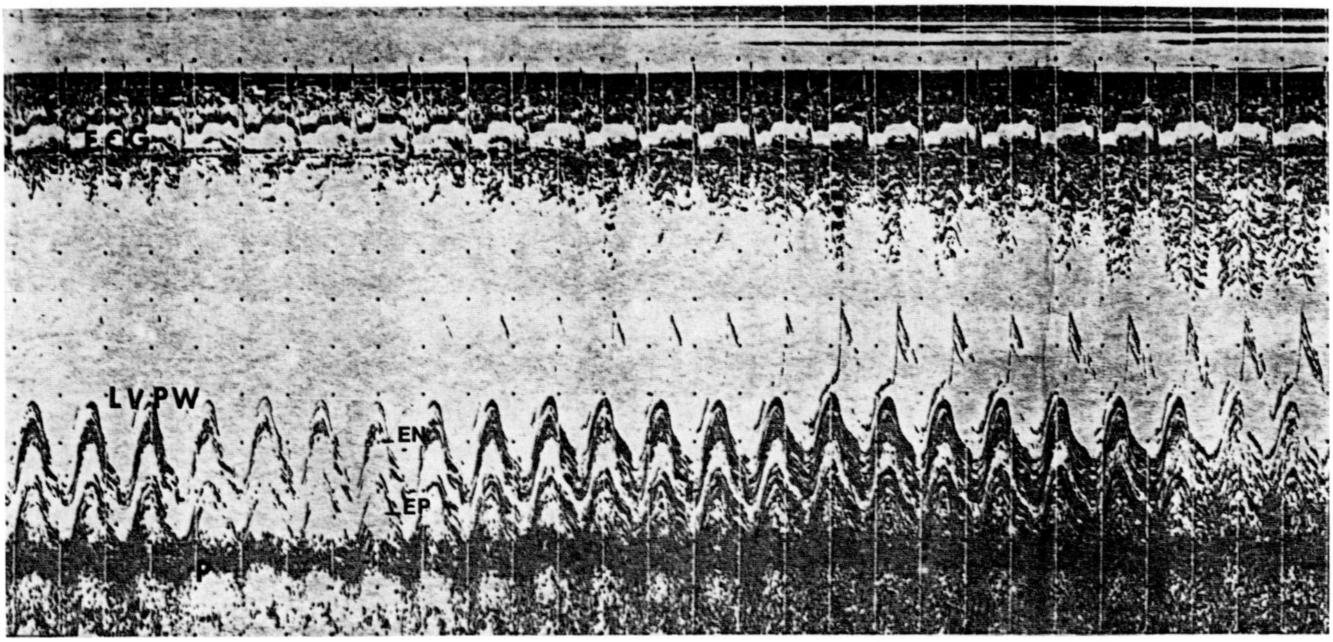

Figure 6-1

M-mode echocardiogram of a patient with a small pericardial effusion, demonstrating the role of the reject control. In the first three beats a small echo-free space representing pericardial fluid is seen between the left ventricular posterior wall and the pericardium in systole. This is the optimal setting. In the next four beats the reject was turned up too high so that the left ventricular posterior wall echoes were oversuppressed. In the succeeding few beats the reject setting is again at about the proper level so that the pericardial space is demonstrated. Thereafter (the last 10 beats) the reject was turned down so that the pericardial space was obscured by undersuppression of echoes in this region.

posterior wall and a wide posterior echo-free space (the pleural effusion); this is more likely to be identified if a small excess of pericardial fluid also is present. The *absence* of abnormal ventricular mobility (swinging heart) — in conjunction with a very wide posterior echo-free space — also favors the diagnosis of pleural effusion.

- A thickened pericardium or an organized pericardial exudate, the sequel of a previous episode of pericarditis, can present as a space of variable width behind the left ventricular posterior wall, mimicking a pericardial effusion (Figure 6-2). However, increasing the gain usually shows that this space is not echo-free but is filled with stratified or short linear-echos. Other differentiating features are that the width of thickened pericardium remains constant throughout systole and diastole and that it moves exactly parallel to the epicardium of the left ventricular posterior wall, being adherent to the latter (Figure 6-2).
- Mitral annular calcification or unusually prominent papillary muscle echoes can be mistaken for the left ventricular posterior wall, in which case the true width of the wall can be misdiagnosed as a pericardial effusion. Proper adjustments of gain and slow-speed scans from the left ventricle to the left atrium should avoid such errors.
- **Pericardial adhesions** or fluid loculation can cause disparities in the width of the echo-free space behind the left ventricular posterior wall at different

levels. Adhesions can also obliterate the pericardial space anteriorly, while permitting large quantities of fluid to accumulate posteriorly.[4]

- Varying the direction of the ultrasound beam can produce striking alterations in the echocardiograms of patients with pericardial effusions. Thus, large effusions can be associated with a narrow cardiac width and wide oscillations when the transducer is pointed caudally and laterally (leftward), but give a more "normal," less swinging appearance when the beam is swept up medially toward the base of the heart.[5,6]

A different type of diagnostic error can occur when anterior or posterior mediastinal masses that present as anterior or posterior echo-free space adjacent to the heart are mistaken for pericardial effusions. Anterior pericardial effusions also have been confused with prominent epicardial fat pads, hiatal hernia(s) through the foramen of Morgagni, and pericardial cysts, thymomas, and lymphomas. Posterior pericardial effusions have been mimicked by atypical left atrial enlargement, pericardial neoplasms, left ventricular pseudoaneurysms, malignant posterior mediastinal masses and mediastinal pancreatic pseudocysts, as well as by normal vascular channels such as the descending thoracic aorta and coronary sinus.

Most echocardiographers do not presume to assess the exact volume of pericardial fluid present in a particular patient, instead settling for an estimation of the size of the effusion: minimal, small, moderate (Figure 6-3), large, or very large (Figure 6-4).[4-7] This classification is based mainly on (1) the width of the posterior and anterior echo-free spaces, (2) in a small pericardial effusion, the difference between systolic and diastolic epicardial - pericardial separation, and (3) evidence of abnormal mobility or swinging of the heart as a whole, which suggests a large effusion.

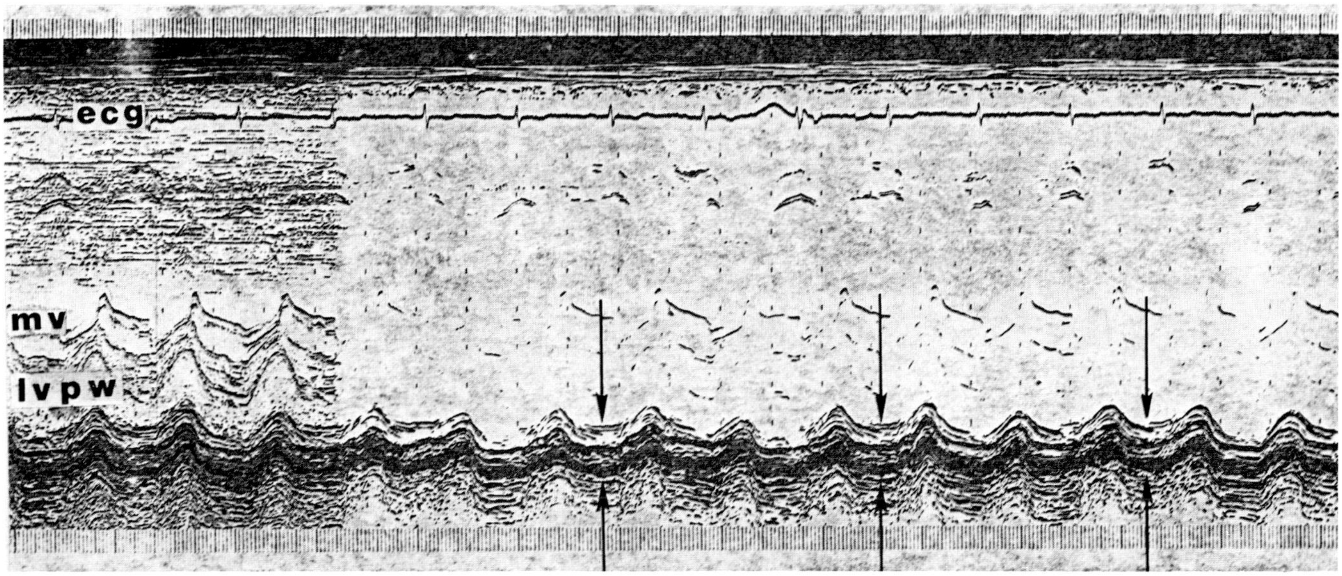

Figure 6-2

M-mode echocardiogram showing pericardial thickening from radiation for carcinoma of the breast. In the first three beats the left ventricular posterior wall is seen anterior to the thick sclerotic pericardium. As the reject control was abruptly turned up, echoes of the mitral valve and left ventricular posterior wall are suppressed, but those of the thick pericardium persist.

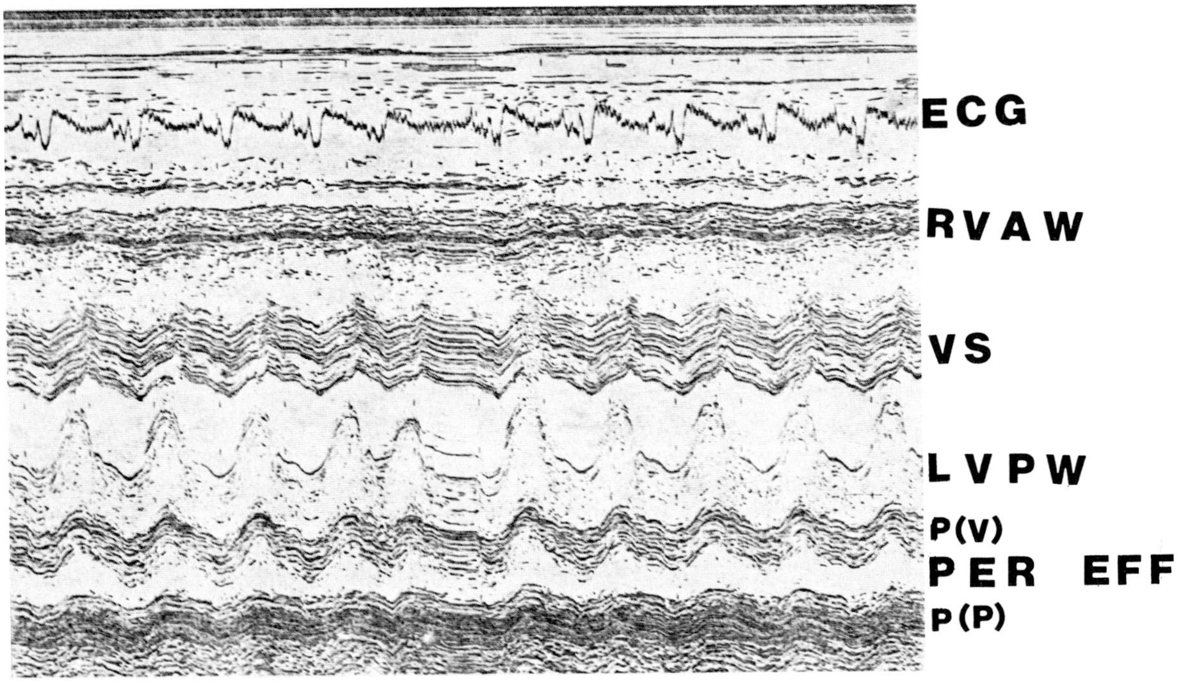

Figure 6-3
M-mode echocardiogram showing a posterior pericardial effusion (PER) of moderate size in a patient recovering from open heart surgery. The visceral pericardium, P(V), and the parietal pericardium, P(P), are both thickened.

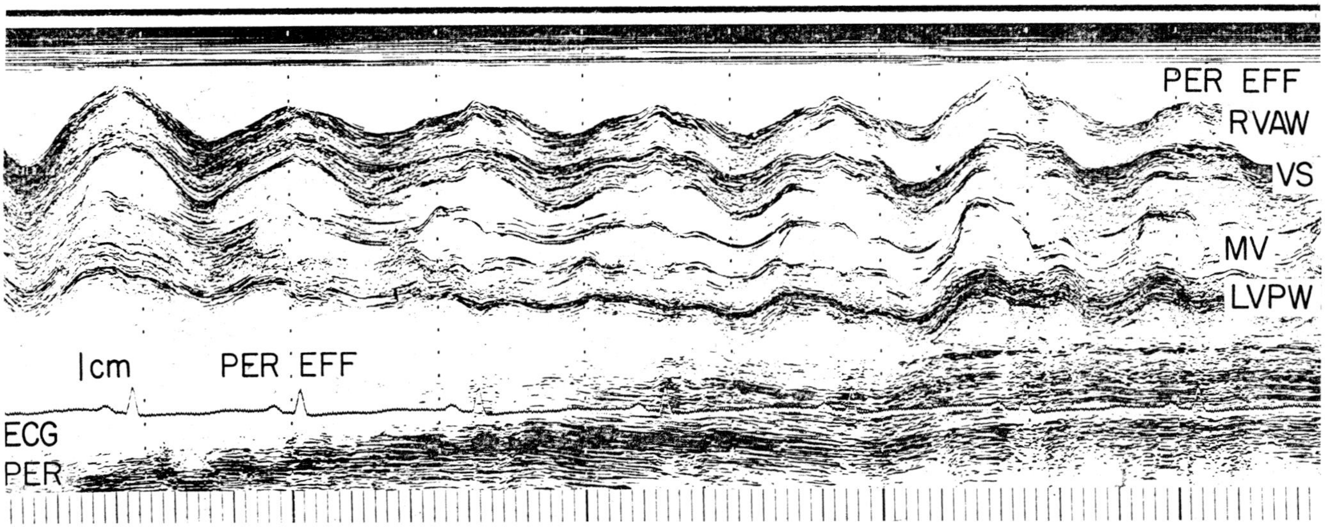

Figure 6-4
M-mode echocardiogram of a patient with a very large pericardial effusion, showing a wide echo-free space anterior as well as posterior to the heart, which "swings" in an abnormally mobile manner. The cardiac width appears wider toward the right of the figure than at the left as the ultrasound beam is scanned from the apex toward the base of the heart.

PERICARDIAL TAMPONADE

The principal echocardiographic manifestation of cardiac tamponade is a striking phasic variation in ventricular dimensions and/or mitral valve motion during respiration (the echo correlate of the **paradoxical pulse**). During inspiration the right ventricle increases, and the left ventricle decreases in size; concomitantly, the diastolic excursion (D-E) of the anterior mitral leaflet decreases and the mitral E-F slope diminishes.[8,9] During expiration the reverse changes occur. These findings are not entirely specific for pericardial tamponade, and have been described in occasional instances of acute pulmonary embolism, constrictive pericarditis, and chronic obstructive lung disease.[8,10] Schiller and Botvinick described narrowing of the right ventricle (to 7 mm or less) as a reliable sign of tamponade.[9] Vignola et al. called attention to a peculiar, early-systolic notching of the right ventricular wall motion found in patients with tamponade and not in those with other types of pericardial effusions.[11] Schilt et al. have recently called attention to a posterior diastolic motion of the right ventricular anterior wall observed in some patients with cardiac tamponade.[12] Although the sensitivity and specificity of these various echocardiographic signs of pericardial fluid are still being debated,[13] they have proved useful in the clinical management of patients with large pericardial effusions. Thus, their appearance de novo or their augmentation in serial tracings alerts the clinician to the possible presence, or imminence, of cardiac tamponade. The patient is then placed under more intense observation, and a decision to remove the pericardial effusion by **pericardiocentesis** or open drainage is rendered more likely.

Recently, it has become possible not only to recognize thickening and sclerosis of the parietal pericardium[14,15] but also to detect solid material within a pericardial effusion, such as layers of fibrin that organize blood or **exudate** from an infection.[15,16]

PERICARDIAL CONSTRICTION

The echocardiographic diagnosis of **constrictive pericarditis** is not as firmly based as that of pericardial fluid, because the abnormal findings in constriction are nonspecific and mostly inconsistent. When more than one of the following criteria occur in combination with a suitable clinical picture, however, pericardial constriction may be considered: (1) a marked degree of pericardial thickening;[15,16] (2) otherwise unexplained paradoxical septal motion;[17,18] (3) lack of normal gradual diastolic expansion of the left ventricle;[19] or (4) dense pericardial calcification.[15,16]

Serial echocardiograms to follow up the size of pericardial effusions are, of course, common practice in routine clinical cardiology.[15] It has not been sufficiently emphasized in the literature, however, that in selected cases of pericarditis with effusion (especially pyogenic pericarditis), serial echograms can reveal the transformation of an exudative pericarditis to dense pericardial fibrosis, often with a constrictive component. Similar changes may also be seen in blood within the pericardium following chest trauma.[20,21]

Two-dimensional echocardiography is not essential for confirming the diagnosis of pericardial effusion in most patients. However, in a few uncertain cases, it reveals a typical space behind the left ventricle, which widens in systole on real-time viewing (Figure 6-5).[22] Anterior and lateral fluid is also well seen on two-dimensional echo, as is the abnormal oscillatory cardiac mobility in large

Figure 6-5

Two-dimensional echocardiogram showing a pericardial effusion of small to moderate size. The left frame is in the short-axis view, the middle frame is in the long-axis view and the right frame is in a long axis near-apical (two-chamber) view. The posterior pericardial effusion is seen between the left ventricular posterior wall and pericardium.

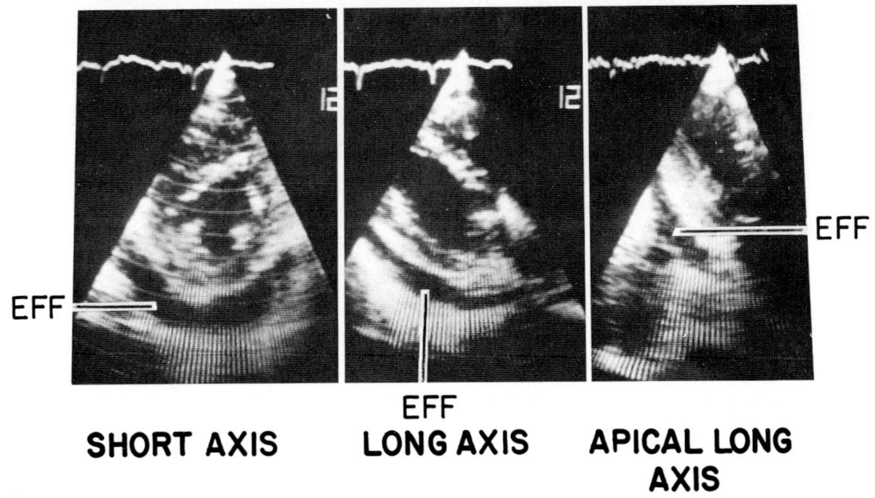

pericardial effusions.[23] An important advantage of two-dimensional echocardiography over M-mode technique is that the width of the pericardial space (separation between epicardium and parietal pericardium) can be visualized not only at basal and mid left ventricular levels but also at all other surfaces of the heart. This, in turn, provides a more complete picture of the size and distribution of the effusion and facilitates the choice of a suitable site for pericardiocentesis.[24] Extension of pericardial fluid into the oblique sinus behind the left atrium can be seen in patients

Figure 6-6

Two-dimensional echocardiogram showing a fairly large pericardial effusion posterior to the left ventricular posterior wall and even extending behind the left atrium in the two frames at right (arrows).

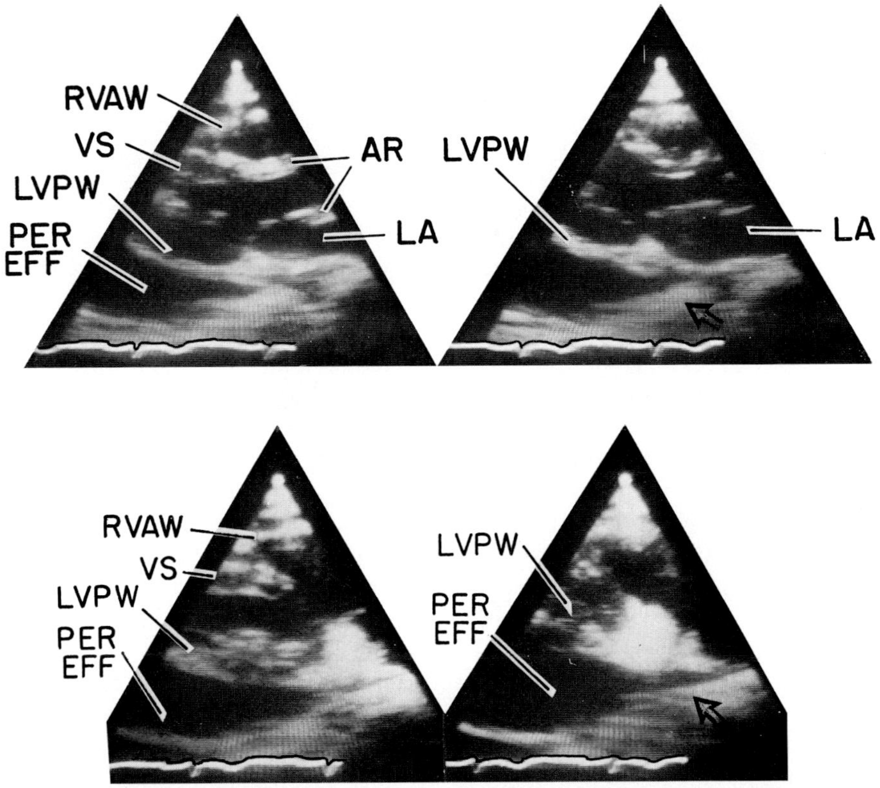

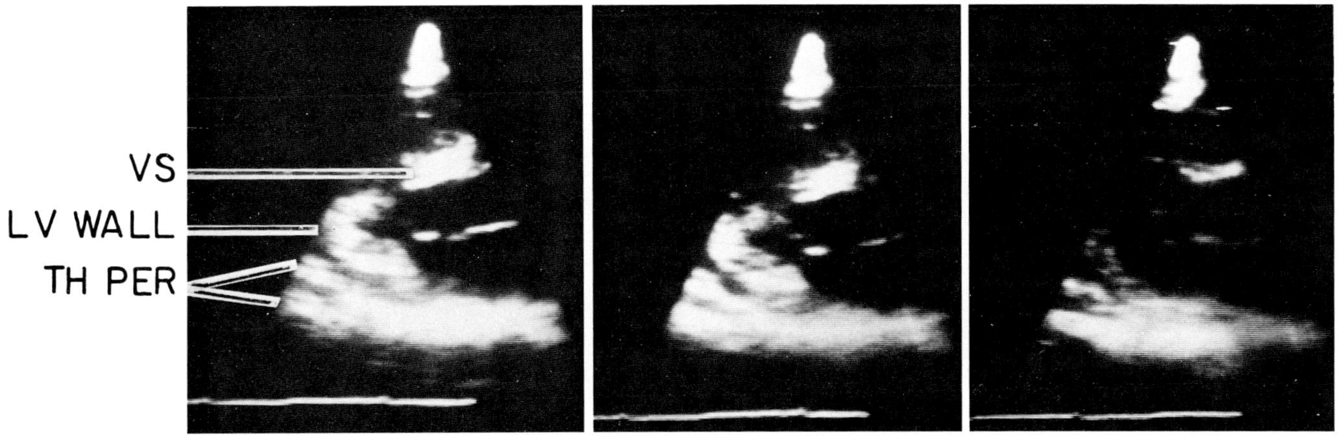

Figure 6-7

Two-dimensional echocardiogram in the long-axis view demonstrating dense, thick echoes from sclerotic thickened pericardium (TH PER). The left ventricular posterior wall and ventricular septum are seen in the first two frames, but have been suppressed in the third frame (right), whereas the thick pericardial echo persists.

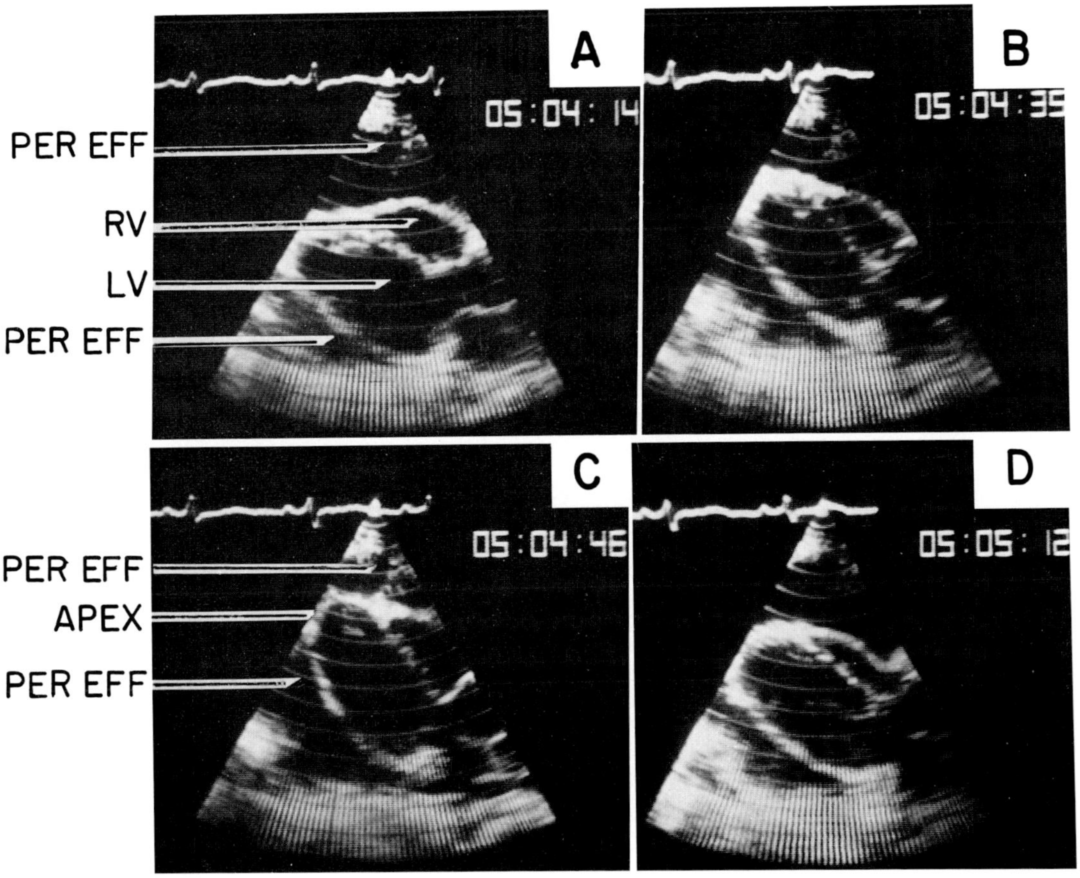

Figure 6-8

Two-dimensional echocardiogram in long axis of a patient with a large pericardial effusion secondary to pericardial metastasis of breast carcinoma. A–D are serial frames: B is 0.21 sec after A; C is 0.11 sec after B; D is 0.26 sec after C. The "swinging heart" motion results in a large-amplitude anterior motion of the ventricular apex from A to B and then C, followed by a posterior motion in D. Note that the ventricular positions in A and C are very different, even though they are taken at about the same time in the cardiac cycle (beginning of systole), because of the alternation of cardiac position from beat to beat. Electrical alternans is evident in the electrocardiogram.

Figure 6-9

Two-dimensional echocardiogram of a patient with a left pleural effusion (PL EFF). This patient had no pericardial effusion. In the long-axis view, the location of the small, circular echo-free space just posterior to the left atrium—representing the descending aorta (De Ao)—helps in differentiating pleural from pericardial effusions. The descending aorta lies in a plane anterior to that of a pleural effusion, whereas it would lie posterior to the plane of a pericardial effusion.

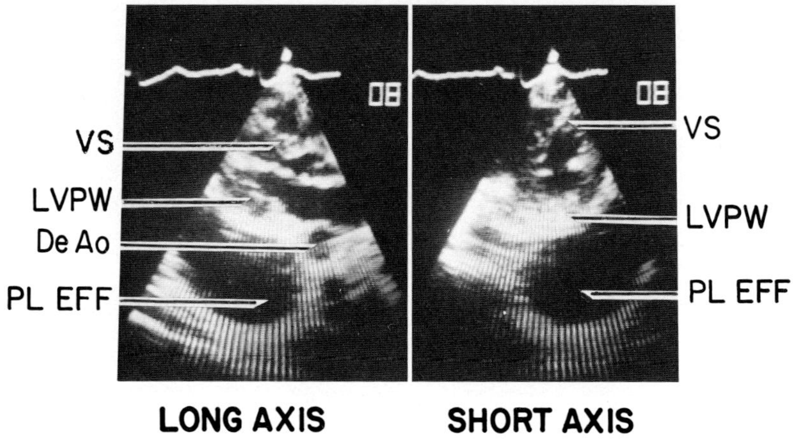

with large pericardial effusions (Figure 6-6). Fibrous thickening (Figure 6-7) or fibrinous bands or layers adhering to the epicardium or bridging the pericardial space between epicardium and pericardium are well seen on two-dimensional echocardiography — these fibrinous bands often exhibit an undulating or wavy motion due to currents set up in the pericardial fluid by cardiac motion.[25,26]

Another important advantage of the two-dimensional over M-mode technique is that it permits differentiation of nonpericardial echo-free spaces (anterior or posterior to the heart) from pericardial fluid. Two-dimensional echocardiography reveals that such extracardiac spaces have geometric shapes or anatomic relationships different from that of pericardial fluid accumulations. Thus, anterior pericardial effusions can usually be distinguished from anterior **mediastinal cysts, lymphomas,** or **hematomas,** and posterior pericardial effusions can be distinguished from echo-free spaces with contours characteristic of pleural effusions, descending aorta,[27] dilated coronary sinus, left ventricular pseudoaneurysm, or left atrial enlargement behind the left ventricle.[28]

In patients with large pericardial effusions, the large amplitude of ventricular motion, commonly known as the swinging heart appearance, is very typical and unmistakable (Figure 6-8). Cases have occasionally occurred in which two-dimensional echocardiography clinched the diagnosis of a large pericardial effusion when the M-mode findings were indistinct or equivocal.

The echocardiographer is often faced with the diagnostic task of deciding whether a large echo-free space behind the heart is a pericardial or pleural effusion. Though the M-mode tracing can usually be relied upon for this purpose, the two-dimensional echocardiogram may be of additonal help, especially if the descending aorta can be visualized (Figure 6-9).

REFERENCES

1. Jacobs WR, Talano JV, Loeb HS: Echocardiographic interpretation of pericardial effusion. Arch Intern Med 138:622-625, 1978
2. Walinsky P: Pitfalls in the diagnosis of pericaridal effusion. Cardiovascular Clin 9:11-15, 1978
3. Berger M, Bobak L, Jelveh M, Goldberg E: Pericardial effusion diagnosed by echocardiography: Clinical and electrocardiographic findings in 171 patients. Chest 74:174-179, 1978

4. Teichholz LE: Echocardiographic evaluation of pericardial diseases. Prog Cardiovasc Dis 21:133-140, 1978
5. Horowitz MS, Rossen R, Harrison DC: Echocardiographic diagnosis of pericardial disease. Am Heart J 97:420-427, 1979
6. Berger M, Bobak L, Jelveh M, Goldberg E: Pericardial effusion diagnosed by echocardiography: Clinical and electrocardiographic findings in 171 patients. Chest 74:174-179, 1978
7. Markiewicz W, Brik A, Brook G, Popp R: Pericardial rub in pericardiac effusion: Lack of correlation with amount of fluid. Chest 77:634-641, 1980
8. D'Cruz IA, Cohen HC, Prabhu R, Glick G: Diagnosis of cardiac tamponade by echocardiography: Changes in mitral valve motion and ventricular dimensions, with special reference to paradoxical pulse. Circulation 52:460-466, 1975
9. Schiller NB, Botvinick EH: Right ventricular compression as a sign of cardiac tamponade: An analysis of echocardiographic ventricular dimensions and their clinical implications. Circulation 56:774-781, 1977
10. Settle HP, Adolph RJ, Fowler NO: Echocardiographic study of cardiac tamponade. Circulation 56:951-958, 1977
11. Vignola PA, Pohost GM, Caufman GD, Myers GS: Correlation of echocardiographic and clinical findings in patients with pericardial effusion. Am J Cardiol 37:701-707, 1976
12. Schilt BF, Feigenbaum J, Weyman AE, Dillon JC: A new echocardiographic sign for cardiac tamponade, (abstract). Circulation 62 (suppl 3):100, 1980
13. Martins JB, Kerber RE: Can cardiac tamponade be diagnosed by echocardiography: Experimental studies. Circulation 60:737-742, 1979
14. Pate JW, Gardner HC, Norman RS: Diagnosis of pericardial effusion by echocardiography. Ann Surg 165:826-832, 1967
15. Allen JW, Harrison EC, Camp JC, Borseri A, Turnier E, Lau FYK: The role of serial echocardiography in the evaluation and differential diagnosis of pericardial disease. Am Heart J 93:560-566, 1977
16. Schnittger I, Bowden RE, Abrams J, Popp R: Echocardiography: Pericardial thickening and constrictive pericarditis. Am J Cardiol 42:388-395, 1978
17. Pool PE, Seagren SC, Abbasi AS, Charuzi Y, Kraus R: Echocardiographic manifestations of constrictive pericarditis: Abnormal septal motion. Chest 68:684-688, 1975
18. Candel-Riera J, Garcia del Castillo H, Permanyer-Miralda G, Soler-Soler J: Echocardiographic features of the interventricular septum in chronic contrictive pericarditis. Circulation 57:1154-1158, 1978
19. Feigenbaum H: Echocardiography. Philadelphia, Lea and Febiger, 1976
20. Cohen MV, Greenberg MA: Constrictive pericarditis: Early and late complication of cardiac surgery. Ann J Cardiol 43:657-661, 1979
21. Schwartz DJ, Thanavaro S, Kleiger RE, Krone RJ, Connors JP, Oliver C: Epicardial pacemaker complicated by cardiac tamponade and constrictive pericarditis. Chest 76:226-227, 1979
22. Martin RP, Rakowski H, French J, Popp RL: Localization of pericardial effusion with wide angle phased array echocardiography. Am J Cardiol 42:904-912, 1978
23. Matsuo H, Matsumoto M, Hamanaka Y, Ohara T, Senda S, Inoue M, Abe H: Rotational excursion of heart in massive pericardial effusion studied by phased-array echocardiography. Br Heart J 41:513-521, 1979
24. Friedman MJ, Sahn DJ, Haber K: Two-dimensional echocardiography and B-mode ultrasonography for the diagnosis of loculated pericardial effusion. Circulation 60:1644-1649, 1979
25. Chiaramida SA, Goldman MA, Zema MJ, Pizzarello RA, Goldberg HM: Echocardiographic identification of intrapericardial fibrous strands in acute pericarditis with pericardial effusion. Chest 77:85-89, 1980
26. Martin RP, Bowden R, Filly K, Popp FL: Intrapericardial abnormalities in patients with pericardial effusion: Findings by two-dimensional echocardiography. Circulation 61:568-572, 1980

27. Haaz WS, Mintz GS, Kotler MN, Parry W, Segal BL: Two-dimensional echocardiographic recognition of the descending thoracic aorta: Value in differentiating pericardial from pleural effusions. Am J Cardiol 46:739-743, 1980
28. Greene DA, Kleid JJ, Naidu S: Unusual echocardiographic manifestation of pericardial effusion. Am J Cardiol 39:112-119, 1977

ADDITIONAL ILLUSTRATIONS AND EXERCISES

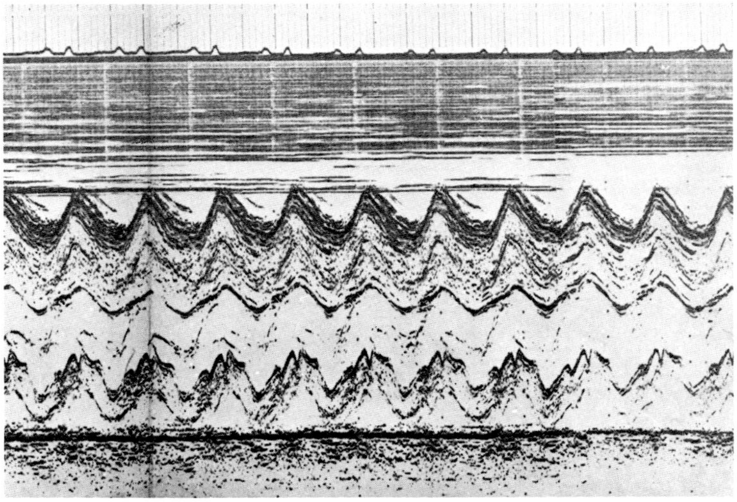

Figure 6-10

M-mode echocardiogram of the left ventricle at the atrial ventricular groove.

6-10.1. What would this patient's chest x-ray show?

A. Pericardial calcification
B. Cardiomegaly — enlarged cardiac silhouette
C. Left ventricular hypertrophy
D. Pulmonary venous congestion

6-10.2. What is the likely amount of pericardial effusion in this patient?

A. None
B. Minimal
C. Small
D. Large

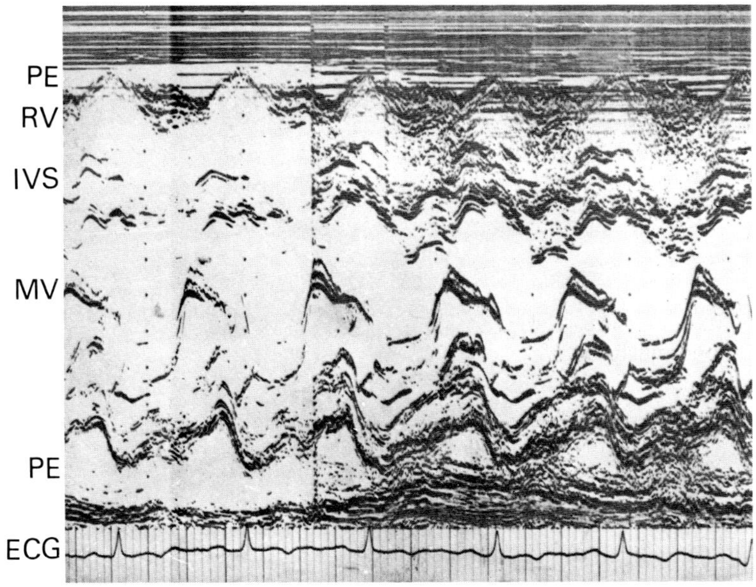

Figure 6-11

6-11.1. How large would you estimate the size of the pericardial effusion in this patient to be?

A. Small
B. Moderate
C. Large

6-11.2. What changes in the mitral valve are noted?

A. Mitral valve prolapse
B. Flail posterior mitral leaflet
C. Mitral valve pseudo-prolapse
D. Mitral stenosis

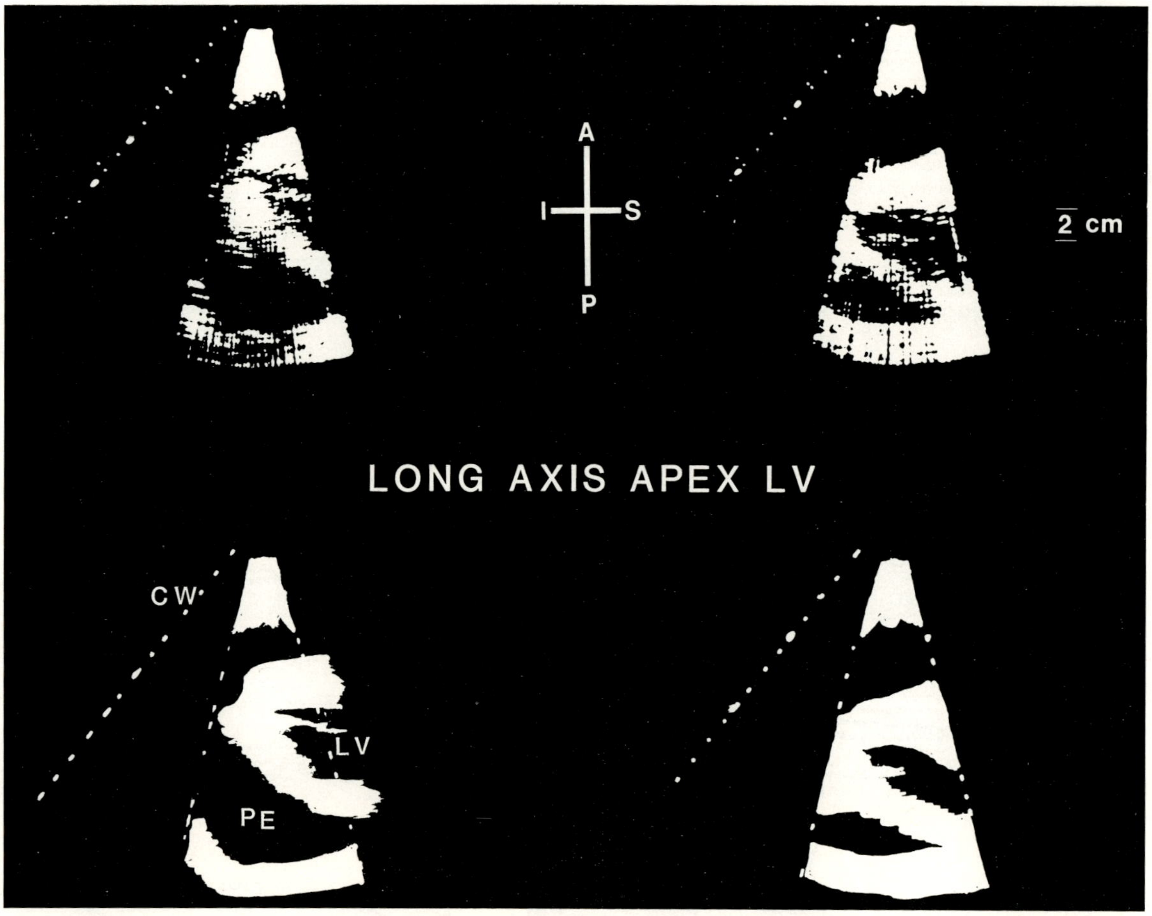

Figure 6-14

Two-dimensional 30° echocardiogram of a patient with a large pericardial effusion. The left and right panels are taken during two successive beats at the same time during the cardiac cycle. The transducer is stationary. Note the differences in position of the cardiac apex.

6-14.1. The following clinical findings are likely in this patient, *except* for:

A. Electrical alternans (alternating ECG height of the QRS on successive beats)
B. Cardiomegaly on chest x-ray
C. An enlarged left atrium
D. Acoustical alternans (alternation in the heart sounds on successive beats)

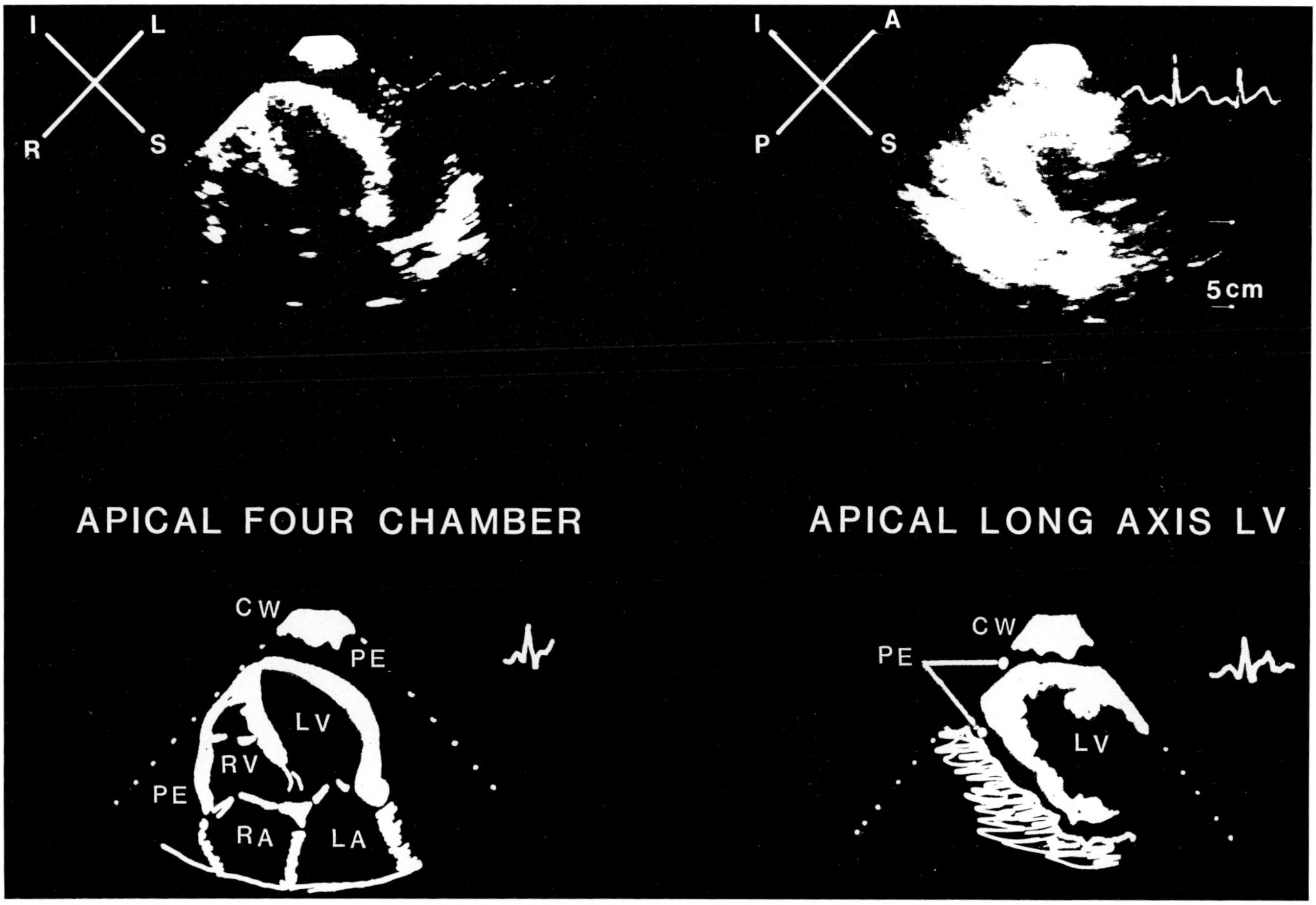

Figure 6-15

Phased-array 90° echocardiogram of a patient showing a malignant pericardial effusion in the apical four-chamber view and the apical long-axis two-chamber view. Note the continuity of the pericardial echo-free space extending even behind the left atrium.

6-15.1. From observation of this figure, which of the following statements are true?

A. A large pericardial effusion is present.
B. The effusion is loculated.
C. There is a large left pleural effusion.
D. A needle placed in the apical pericardial space should result in effective decompression of the pericardial effusion.

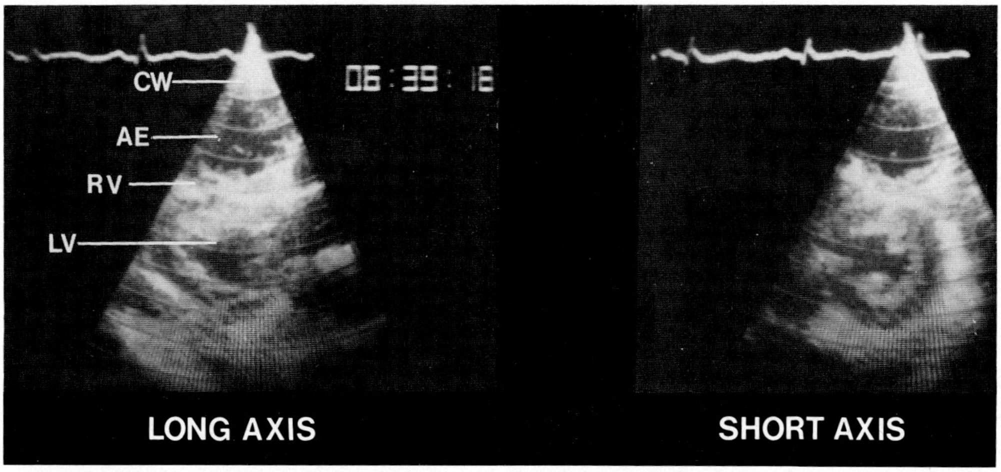

Figure 6-16

Ten-year-old boy with an anterior echo-free space (AE) seen on M-mode echocardiography. A two-dimensional echocardiogram is taken in the long-axis and short-axis views at the level of the mid left ventricle. Note the round structure (best seen in short axis) in the anterior echo-free space.

6-16.1. Anterior echo-free spaces can be the direct cause of which of the following?

A. Pericardial effusion
B. Mediastinal cysts
C. Prominent epicardial fat
D. Dilated coronary sinus
E. Hematomas

6-16.2. The most likely cause of the echo-free space as noted in this two-dimensional echocardiogram is:

A. Pericardial effusion
B. Mediastinal cysts
C. Prominent epicardial fat
D. Dilated coronary sinus
E. Hematomas

William R. Jacobs

7

Abnormalities of the Left Ventricle and Interventricular Septum

In M-mode echocardiography, left ventricular function is determined from two small areas of the interventricular septum and posterior left ventricular wall (Figure 7-1). Despite limitations resulting from sampling from these small areas of the left ventricle, M-mode echocardiography is still quite useful in identifying abnormalities of structure and function. With two-dimensional echocardiography, on the other hand, the entire left ventricle can be visualized. With improvements in technique and equipment, two-dimensional echocardiography promises to be a valuable tool in the evaluation of normal and abnormal ventricular function.[1,2] In addition, both M-mode and two-dimensional echocardiography are useful in measuring wall thickness and are capable of providing estimates of left ventricular mass.

To ensure accuracy and reproducibility, proper technique is critical. First it is necessary to select a location on the chest wall from which an M-mode echocardiogram produces the most consistent and accurate results. It has been found that the **standard interspace** provides the area from which the most reliable and reproducible measurements of left ventricular size are made. The standard interspace is defined as that intercostal space (interspace) from which the anterior mitral leaflet is imaged with slight medial angulation but without superior or inferior transducer angulation. After this interspace is found, the transducer is angulated inferiorly toward the left ventricular apex until the mitral leaflets are no longer seen and only the chordae tendineae are present between the two left ventricular endocardial surfaces. Internal landmarks such as the papillary muscles and the mitral valve are also used to determine correct imaging of the long-axis view in two-dimensional echocardiography.

Once correct transducer placement and beam direction are achieved instrument settings must be adjusted to provide maximum definition of the left ventricular endocardium in order to study left ventricular function by either M-mode or two-dimensional echocardiography. Smooth surfaces in and around the heart, such as the anterior mitral leaflet and the pericardium, are strong reflectors of ultrasound and are generally easy to image. Unfortunately, the trabeculated (ridged) lining of the left ventricle (endocardium) tends to scatter the ultrasonic beam, which makes it more difficult to demonstrate echocardiographically. The endocardium of the left ventricular posterior wall is particularly difficult to image, since it not only is trabeculated but also is relatively distant from the transducer.

Due to the endocardial trabeculation and nearby chordae tendineae, multiple echoes may be reflected from the left ventricular posterior wall. Indocyanine green dye studies have shown that the fastest-moving echo (that is, the one with the steepest upward slope during systole) is likely to be the endocardium.

Different echocardiographic instruments utilize different methods for providing increased amplification of distant echoes. Whichever instrument is used, it is usually necessary to use maximum amplification in demonstrating the left ventricular posterior wall endocardium—which, in normal patients, looks like a finely pencilled line. When a line near the posterior left ventricular wall appears to be dense — as if it were drawn with a felt-tip marking pencil—be cautious. Such a strongly reflected echo is rarely produced by normal endocardium and is more likely to be reflected from some other posterior echo-producing surface, such as the epicardial - pericardial interface.

The thickness of the lines produced by various intracardiac structures varies somewhat with the gain (amplification) settings of the instrument. When gain settings are increased, the line tends to thicken; the upper surface of the line stays at the same point and widening occurs posteriorly (downward). Consequently, to make gain-independent measurements, it is necessary to use the leading (upper) edge method. It is apparent that echocardiographic measurements must be precisely vertical. (For a discussion of echocardiographic measurements and techniques see Chapter 1.) Every echocardiogram should also contain an aorta-to-apex sweep recorded at a slow paper speed (25 mm/sec or less).

Most measurements of left ventricular structure and function assume that the normal left ventricular cavity is ovoid (egg-shaped or, in geometric terms, a prolate ellipsoid), with a length that is twice its width. If these configurational assumptions are correct, then a formula for determining the volume of such an ovoid structure can be simplified; the volume of the ventricle can be estimated by merely cubing the left ventricular minor-axis dimension obtained by M-mode

Figure 7-1

The portion of the left ventricle imaged by M-mode from the standard position. Note that the apex of the left ventricle is not imaged by this technique.

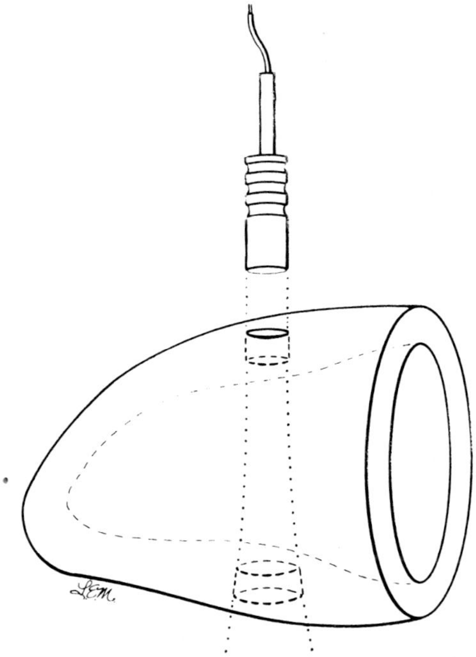

echocardiography as described in Chapter 1. It is assumed that in cross section the left ventricle is circular in shape and that all parts of the ventricle contract equally.

When the left ventricle enlarges, its cavity tends to become spherical. In that situation, the volume estimations made by cubing the width will be larger than the actual volume of the ventricle. An equation has been developed to correct for the assumption that the left ventricular length is twice its width:[1,2]

$$EDV = \left(\frac{7}{2.4 + EDD}\right)(EDD^3)$$

where EDV = left ventricular end-diastolic volume
EDD = left ventricular end-diastolic diameter, i.e., width

Coronary artery disease causes the cubed-width estimation of left ventricular volume to be inaccurate, especially in systole. In coronary artery disease, a segment of the ventricle may fail to contract or may even bulge during systole (dyskinesis).

A widely used measurement of left ventricular function is the ejection fraction, previously described. However, as distortion of the ventricle occurs in disease states, the assumptions used to calculate ejection fraction do not hold up and errors in estimation occur. In ventricles with an abnormal systolic or diastolic shape, the left ventricular ejection fraction may be more accurately estimated by determining **mitral E point – septal separation.** In normal ventricles, as the anterior mitral leaflet swings open, it approaches and often touches the septum at the E point (Figure 1-11). When left ventricular function is depressed, the anterior mitral leaflet does not swing as far anteriorly, and there is a separation of more than 5 mm between the E point of the mitral valve and the furthest posterior excursion of the interventricular septum. The mitral E point - septal separation is determined by drawing a horizontal line on the echocardiogram at the maximum posterior excursion of the left ventricular septal endocardium. A vertical measurement is then made from the E point of the mitral valve to this line. This is the mitral E point - septal separation, and it correlates well with the left ventricular ejection fraction, even though the echocardiographic beam may not pass through the abnormal segmental area of the left ventricle. Accordingly, in a ventricle with a large apical aneurysm, although the left ventricular dimensional in short axis may be normal by M-mode, the mitral E point - septal separation will usually be abnormal. Rheumatic mitral valve disease and aortic insufficiency both affect the free motion of the anterior mitral leaflet during diastole, and mitral E point - septal separation has not been considered as useful in these two conditions.

Quantitation of abnormalities of left ventricular size are made by examining the thickness and motion of the septum and posterior left ventricular wall and by measuring the end-diastolic and end-systolic dimensions. Perhaps the most common abnormality to be present is left ventricular dilatation, which can occur with increased **(hyperkinetic)** (Figure 7-2 B) or decreased **(hypokinetic)** (Figure 7-2 D) left ventricular wall motion. Increased thickness of the left ventcular walls **(hypertrophy)** occurs in conditions of elevated left ventricular systolic pressure **(pressure overload state)** (Figure 7-2 C). In idiopathic hypertophic subaortic stenosis, the septum is greatly thickened (asymmetrical septal hypertrophy) and moves little (hypokinetic or akinetic) (Figure 7-2 K).

The aorta and that portion of the interventricular septum near the anterior wall

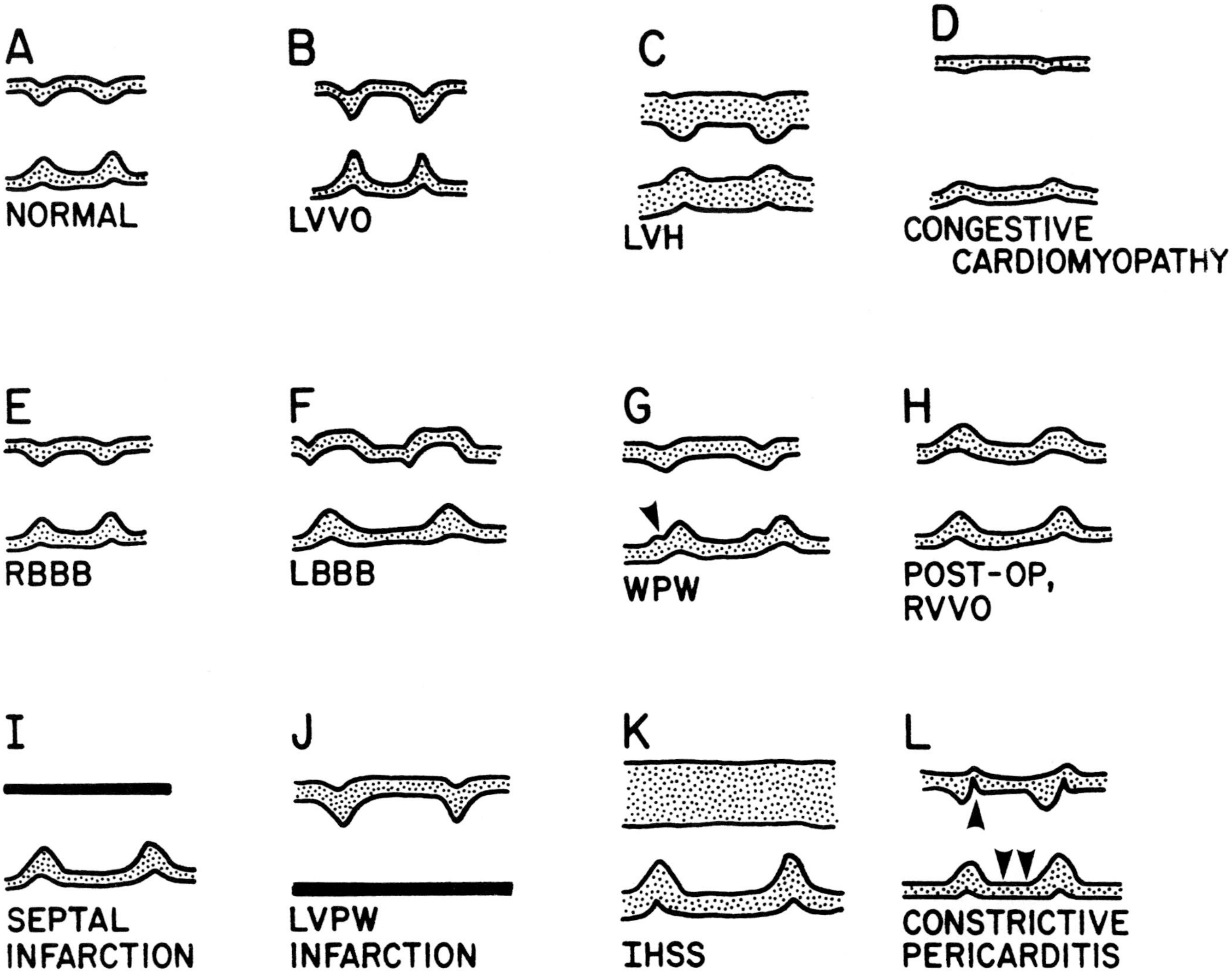

Figure 7-2

Various patterns of left ventricular wall motion by M-mode echocardiography. (LVVO, left ventricular volume overload; LVH, left ventricular hypertrophy; RBBB, right bundle branch block; LBBB, left bundle branch block; WPW, Wolff-Parkinson-White syndrome; IHHS, idiopathic hypertrophic subaortic stenosis.)

of the aorta move anteriorly during systole. A little further down from the aorta (caudad) toward the cardiac apex, septal motion disappears or is flat; the point at which this occurs is called the *hinge point.* On the apex side of this hinge point, anterior to the chordae tendineae, left ventricular septal motion is posterior during systole (Figure 7-2 A). In the normal left ventricle, then, a beam passing through the chordae tendineae from the standard interspace crosses the septum at a point where septal motion is posterior during systole (Figure 7-2 A). If the interventricular septum or posterior left ventricular wall has been replaced by scar tissue (a previous infarction) or suddenly lacks an adequate blood supply (acute myocardial ischemia or infarction), its motion will be impaired (Figure 7-2 I, J). Systolic thickening of that wall will be diminished as well.[3-6]

Since the interventricular septum is shared by both ventricles, right ventricular abnormalities may cause abnormal septal motion as well. In **right ventricular volume overload,** as occurs in atrial septal defect tricuspid and pulmonary regurgitation, the right ventricle has to pump a greater stroke volume than normal.[7] The motion of the interventricular septum then becomes reversed (paradoxical) and parallels the motion of the posterior left ventricular wall (Figure 7-2 H). One explanation for this abnormal motion is that the overdistended right ventricle indents the septum into the left ventricle during diastole; then, in systole the left ventricle assumes its normal circular configuration, and the septum moves back anteriorly into the right ventricle.[8]

After valvular or coronary bypass surgery, septal motion generally becomes **paradoxical** but returns to normal within a few months. Abnormalities of left ventricular depolarization, such as left bundle branch block and **Wolff – Parkinson – White syndrome,** may also affect wall motion (Figure 7-2 F, G).[9,10] Right bundle branch block, on the other hand, does not affect interventricular septal motion (Figure 7-2 E). In constrictive pericarditis, several abnormalities have been reported, including abnormal septal motion — sometimes with an early-diastolic notch (paradoxical septal motion) — and decreased (less than a millimeter) diastolic posterior wall motion (Figure 7-2 L).

In left ventricular volume overload (which can be caused by anemia, mitral regurgitation, aortic regurgitation, or atrioventricular fistula) the excursions of both the septum and the posterior wall are increased (hyperkinetic) (Figure 7-2 B), with increases in the excursion of the interventricular septum being especially prominent. In coronary heart disease, when either the septum or the posterior wall is damaged (infarcted)[3,5,11] the opposite wall of the heart often exhibits hyperkinetic motion (Figure 7-2 I, J). Left ventricular posterior wall motion may also be altered in the Wolff - Parkinson - White syndrome (Figure 7-2 G) or with posterior wall infarction (Figure 7-2 J).

The apex of the left ventricle is a blind spot for M-mode echocardiography. A left ventricular apical aneurysm may not be apparent, since wall motion nearer the mitral valve may still be normal. Since the entire left ventricle can usually be imaged in several planes by two-dimensional echocardiography, this technique is the most effective for demonstrating abnormalities in the *shape* of the left ventricle as well as segmental abnormalities such as scar formation and aneurysm. Areas of decreased (hypokinetic) or absent **(akinetic)** motion or even bulging **(dyskinetic)** may be seen, similar to left ventricular angiography. The left ventricular apex, being the segment farthest from the origin of the coronary arteries, is often involved in left ventricular aneurysm formation and is best seen with two-dimensional echocardiography. Apical aneurysms demonstrated by this technique are often seen to contain clots.[12]

REFERENCES

1. DeMaria AN, Neumann A, Schubart PJ, Lee G, Mason DT: Systematic correlation of cardial chamber size and ventricular performance determined with echocardiography and alterations in heart rate in normal patients. Am J Cardiol 43:1-9, 1979
2. Gueret P, Meerbaum S, Wyatt HL, Uchiyama T, Lang TW, Corday E: Two-dimensional echocardiographic quantitation of left ventricular volumes and ejection fraction: Importance of accounting for dyssynergy in short-axis reconstruction models. Circulation 62:1308-1318, 1980
3. Connetta DA, Christie LG, Wise DE, Myers RR, Conti CR: Echocardiographic analysis

of systolic and diastolic left ventricular wall motion in normal man. Chest 76:76-82, 1979

4. Weiner I, Meller J, Packer M, Herman MV, Teichholz LE: Prognostic value of echocardiographic evaluation of septal function in acute anteroseptal myocardial infarction. Am Heart J 97:726-732, 1979
5. Cody RJ, Salcedo EE, Phillips DF, Tarazi RC: M-mode echocardiography in anteroseptal myocardial infarction, lack of sensitivity. Chest 77:781-783, 1980
6. Barthelemy M: Two-dimensional echocardiography in acute myocardial infarction, letter. Intensive Care Med 5:203, 1979
7. Kerber RE, Dippel WF, Abbound FM: Abnormal motion of the interventricular septum in right ventricular volume overload. Circulation 48:86-96, 1973
8. St. John Sutton MG, Tajik AJ, Mercier LA, Seward JB, Giuliani ER, Ritman EL: Assessment of left ventricular function in secundum atrial septal deffect by computer analysis of the M-mode echocardiogram. Circulation 60:1082-1090, 1979
9. Abbasi AS, Eder LM, MacAlpin RN, Kattus AA: Paradoxical motion of interventricular septum in left bundle branch block. Circulation 49:423-427, 1977
10. Fuji J, Wantanabe H, Wanatabe T, Takahashi N, Ohta A, Kato K: M-mode and cross-sectional echocardiographic study of the left ventricular wall motions in complete left bundle-branch block. Br Heart J 42:255-260, 1979
11. Snider AR, Silverman NH, Schiller NB, Ports TA: Echocardiographic evaluation of ventricular septal aneurysms. Circulation 59:920-926, 1979
12. Lewin RF, Vidne B, Sclarovsky S, Agmon, J: Two-dimensional real-time echocardiographic detection of a left ventricular aneurysm associated with mobile pedunculated thrombi. Chest 77:704-706, 1980

ADDITIONAL ILLUSTRATIONS AND EXERCISES

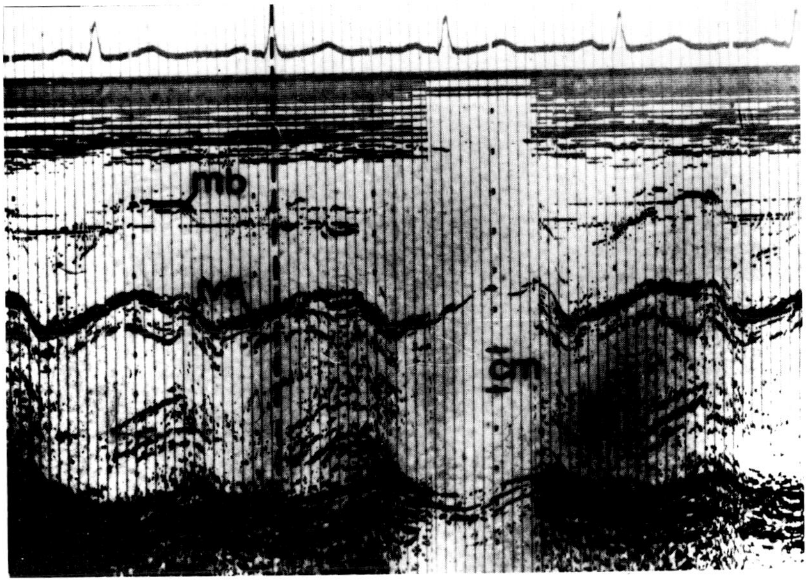

Figure 7-3

Echocardiogram taken from a patient with cardiomegaly and increased pulmonary blood flow seen on the chest x ray. Depth markers are 1.0 cm. The right ventricle is enlarged (mb, moderator band in the right ventricle).

7-3.1. Septal motion during systole is:

A. Normal
B. Abnormal, hypokinetic
C. Abnormal, paradoxical

7-3.2. Septal motion is compatible with:

A. Right ventricular volume overload
B. Complete left bundle branch block
C. Complete right bundle branch block
D. Normal variant

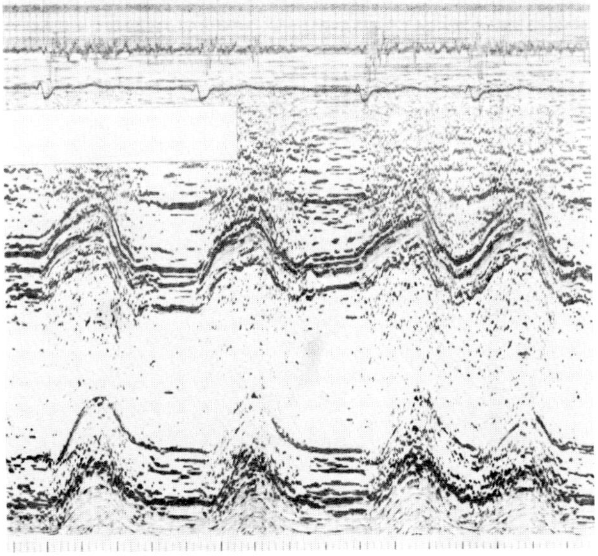

Figure 7-4

Echocardiogram taken from a middle-aged man who has undergone mitral valve replacement. He continues to have significant tricuspid regurgitation. The right ventricle is enlarged.

7-4.1. Which states contribute to the abnormality noted in the interventricular septum?

A. Paradoxical septal motion due to left bundle branch block
B. Paradoxical septal motion due to right ventricular volume overload
C. Paradoxical septal motion due to open heart surgery
D. Paradoxical septal motion due to an intraoperative anterior septal myocardial infarction

7-4.2. Other causes of paradoxical septal motion include:

A. Atrial septal defect
B. Pulmonic regurgitation
C. Anomalous pulmonary venous drainage
D. Aneurysm of the interventricular septum
E. All of the above

Figure 7-5

M-mode echocardiogram taken in a patient who has a history of supraventricular tachycardia. Note the arrows pointing to the left ventricular posterior endocardium.

7-5.1. The interventricular septal motion is:

A. Normal

B. Abnormal

7-5.2. The abnormality pointed out by the arrow on the left ventricular posterior wall is compatible with:

A. Wolff-Parkinson-White syndrome (preexcitation)

B. Posterior myocardial infarction

C. Left bundle branch block

D. Right bundle branch block

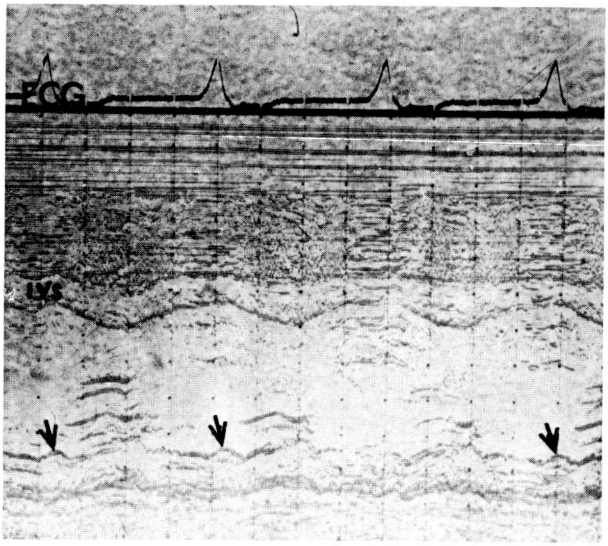

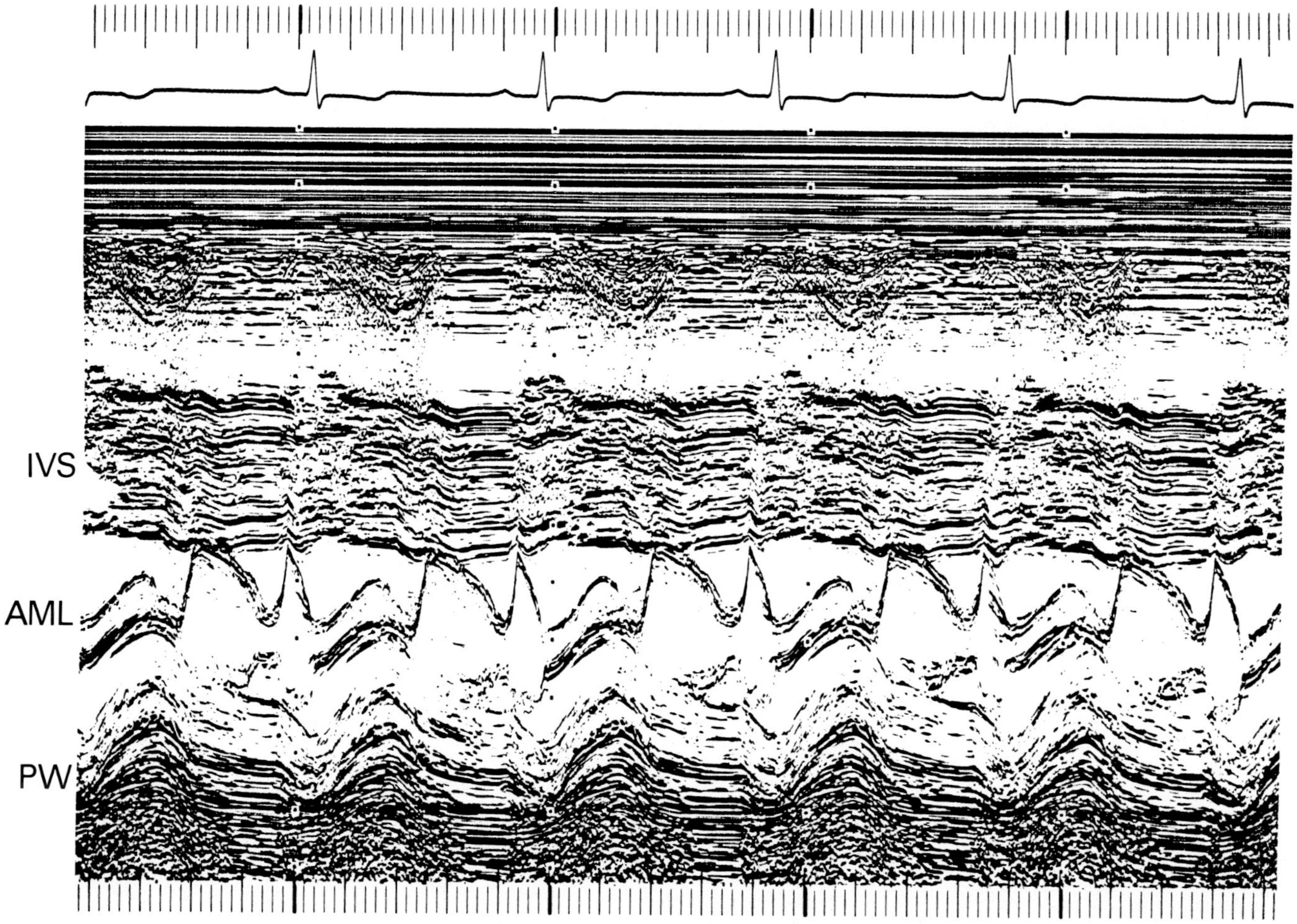

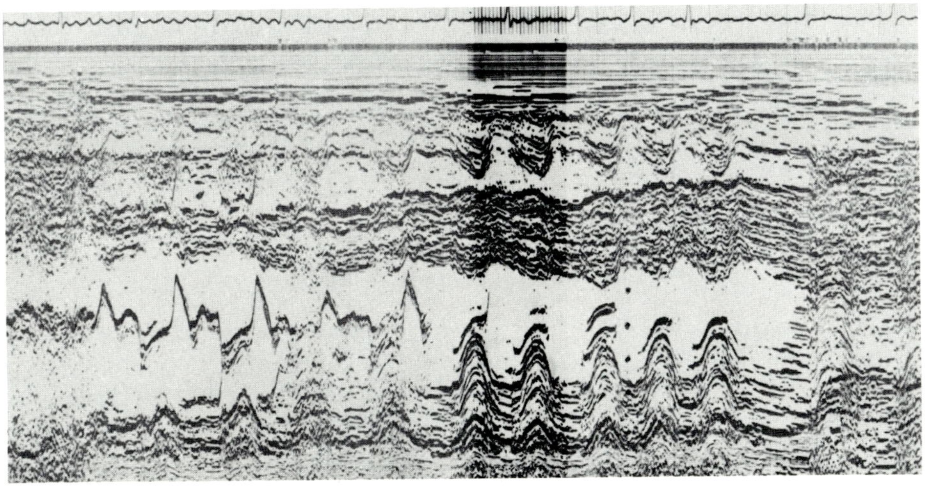

Figure 7-7

Echocardiogram taken of a 21-year-old male with normal blood pressure and no cardiac murmurs. The electrocardiogram is shown above, with the patient in atrial fibrillation. Depth markers are 1.0 cm.

7-7.1. The most likely diagnosis in this patient is:

A. A normal echocardiogram
B. Asymmetrical septal hypertrophy with obstruction (IHSS)
C. Hypertrophic nonobstructive cardiomyopathy
D. Anterior myocardial infarction

Figure 7-6

Echocardiogram taken at the level of the anterior and posterior mitral leaflet.

7-6.1. This echocardiogram demonstrates:

A. A thickened, calcified mitral valve
B. Thickened, flat (akinetic) septal motion
C. A diminished E–F slope of the mitral valve
D. Systolic anterior motion
E. Vegetations on the anterior leaflet of the mitral valve

7-6.2. The most likely diagnosis in this patient is:

A. Aortic valvular stenosis
B. Bacterial endocarditis with vegetations of the mitral valve
C. Idiopathic hypertrophic subaortic stenosis
D. Congestive cardiomyopathy
E. Flail anterior mitral leaflet

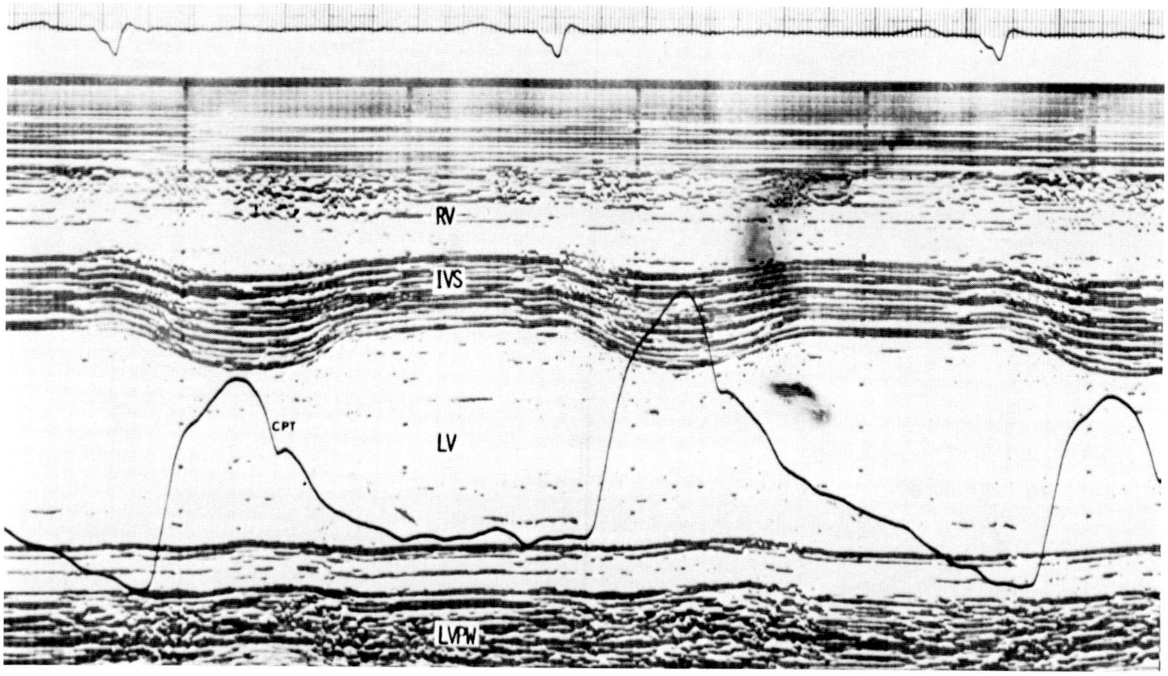

Figure 7-8

Echocardiogram taken at the level of the left ventricle on a patient who has recently presented with chest pain, diaphoresis, and shortness of breath. Depth markers are 1 cm. (CPT, carotid pulse tracing.)

7-8.1. The abnormalities seen in this tracing are:

A. Evidence of left ventricular hypertrophy
B. Decreased left ventricular posterior wall motion
C. Normal but exaggerated motion of the interventricular septum
D. Pericardial effusion

7-8.2. The most likely diagnosis on this patient is:

A. Anterior myocardial infarction
B. Posterior (inferior) myocardial infarction
C. Posterior pericardial effusion
D. Pericardial thickening

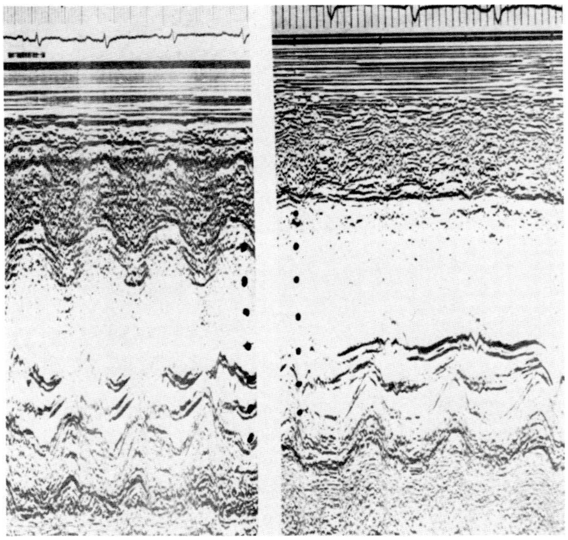

Figure 7-9

Two sequential left ventricular echocardiograms of a young black man with endocarditis and mitral and aortic regurgitation. The left panel was taken at the initial hospitalization; the right panel was taken when shock and pulmonary edema supervened.

7-9.1. The abnormalities noted in this echocardiogram are:

A. Left ventricular volume overload (left panel)
B. Right ventricular volume overload (right panel)
C. Akinetic septal motion (right panel)
D. Hypokinetic posterior wall (right panel)

7-9.2. The most likely cause of the change to the echocardiogram on the right in this patient is:

A. Ruptured chordae tendineae with mitral regurgitation
B. Flail aortic leaflet with severe aortic regurgitation
C. Septal myocardial infarction, probably secondary to a coronary embolus
D. Papillary muscle rupture

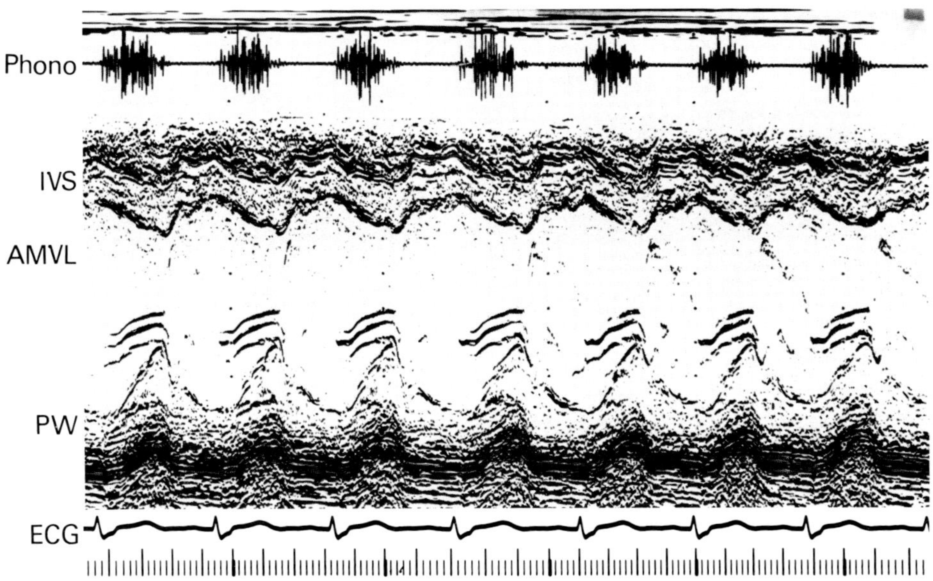

Figure 7-10

M-mode echocardiogram taken at the level of the left ventricle in a 39-year-old Oriental male with a loud pansystolic murmur since birth. His phonocardiogram is shown at high-frequency settings at the fourth left intercostal space. Only a portion of the anterior mitral valve leaflet is seen. Note the enlargement of the left ventricle and the vigorous contraction of the interventricular septum and left ventricular posterior wall. Left atrial size was 3.4 cm, which was normal.

7-10.1 The left ventricular changes noted in this patient are most likely caused by:

A. Prolonged systemic hypertension with left ventricular hypertrophy
B. Ventricular septal defect with left ventricular volume overload
C. Aortic stenosis with left ventricular pressure overload
D. Hypertrophic obstructive cardiomyopathy (IHSS)

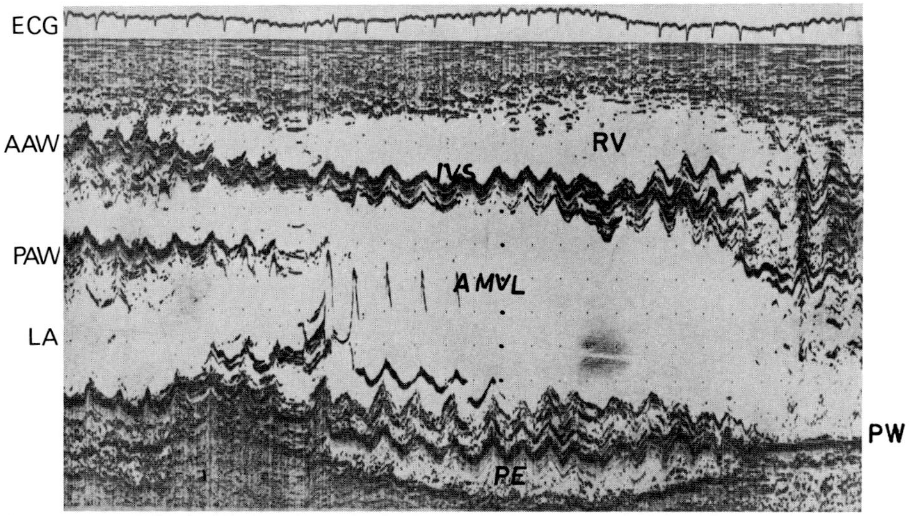

Figure 7-11

M-mode echocardiographic slow-speed scan of a patient who presents with cardiomegaly, atrial fibrillation, and a gallop rhythm.

7-11.1. The abnormalities noted in this echocardiogram include:

A. Marked left ventricular enlargement
B. Marked left atrial enlargement
C. Increased E point–septal separation compatible with diminished ejection fraction
D. Localized posterior pericardial effusion
E. Posterior basilar infarction

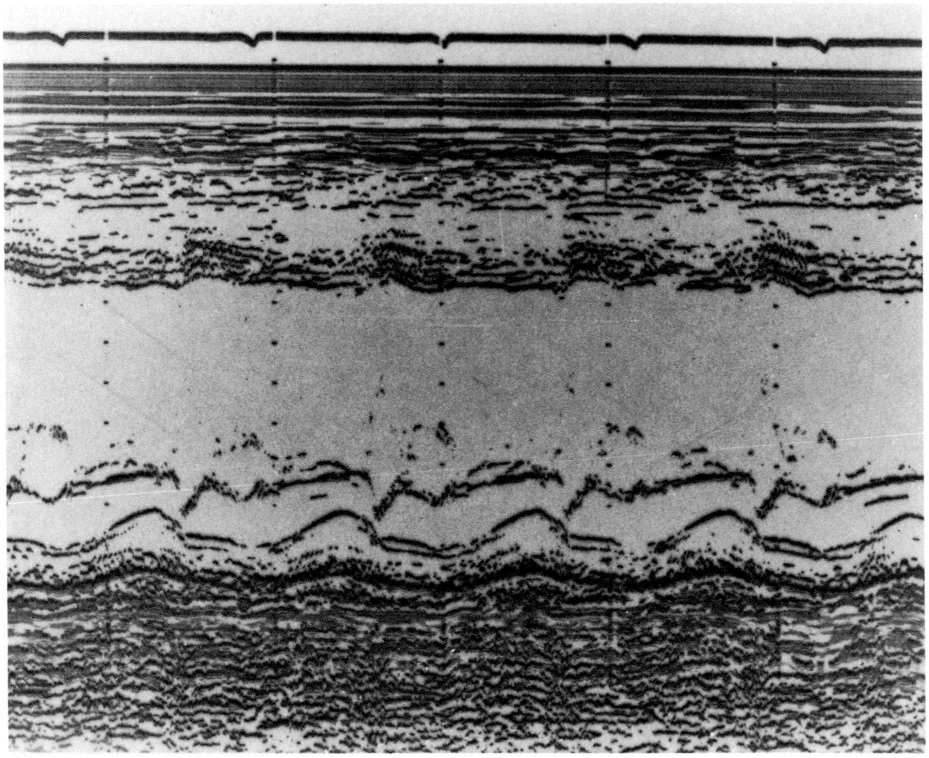

Figure 7-12

Echocardiogram taken in a patient who presents with congestive heart failure.

7-12.1. The interventricular septal motion is:

A. Normal
B. Abnormal
C. Unimportant
D. Indistinguishable
E. None of the above

7-12.2. Septal thickening during systole is:

A. Normal
B. Absent
C. Unimportant
D. Indistinguishable

7-12.3. The correct diagnosis in this patient is most likely:

A. Previous anterior septal myocardial infarction
B. An atrial septal defect
C. Mitral stenosis
D. Complete left bundle branch block
E. None of the above

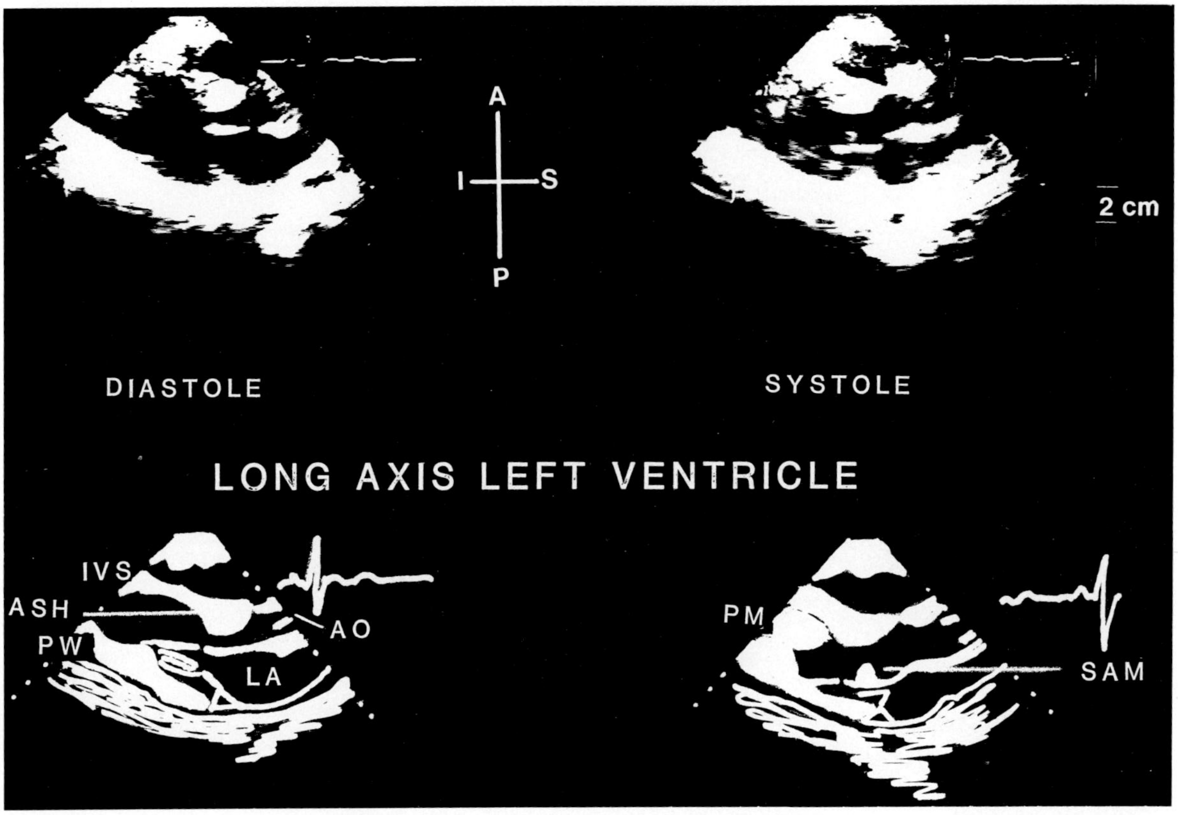

Figure 7-13

Phased-array 90° two-dimensional echocardiogram of a patient with idiopathic hypertrophic subaortic stenosis with asymmetrical septal hypertrophy (ASH). Note the localized thickened septum (ASH). During systole there is systolic anterior motion of the mitral valve (SAM). The patient had left ventricular outflow tract obstruction. Depth lines are 2 cm.

7-13.1. An M-mode echocardiogram taken at the thickened portion of the septum (ASH) might show which of the following?

A. A thickened hypokinetic or akinetic septum
B. A diminished E–F slope of the anterior mitral leaflet
C. Systolic anterior motion of the posterior leaflet
D. Thickened aortic valve with a diminished aortic opening

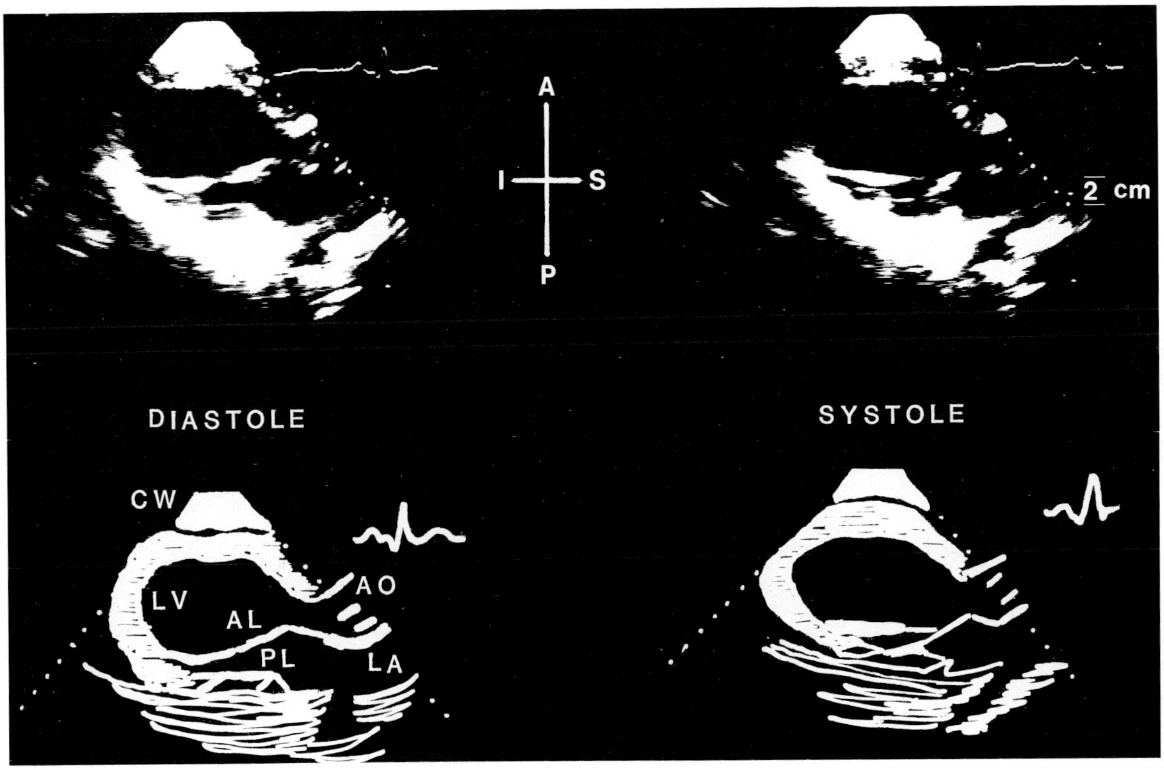

Figure 7-14

Phased-array 90° echocardiogram of a patient with a congestive cardiomyopathy and recurrent ventricular tachycardia. Note the large left ventricle during systole and diastole with diffuse left ventricular hypokinesis. Note the increased distance (5.0 cm) in diastole of the anterior mitral leaflet to the septum (E point – septal separation). The ejection fraction was 13 percent. (AL, anterior mitral leaflet; PL, posterior mitral leaflet.)

7-14.1. An M-mode echocardiogram taken of this patient would be expected to show all of the following, *except:*

A. Left ventricular enlargement
B. Wide diastolic excursion of the anterior mitral leaflet
C. Hypokinesis of the septum and left ventricular posterior wall
D. An apical aneurysm
E. Increased mitral E point – septal separation

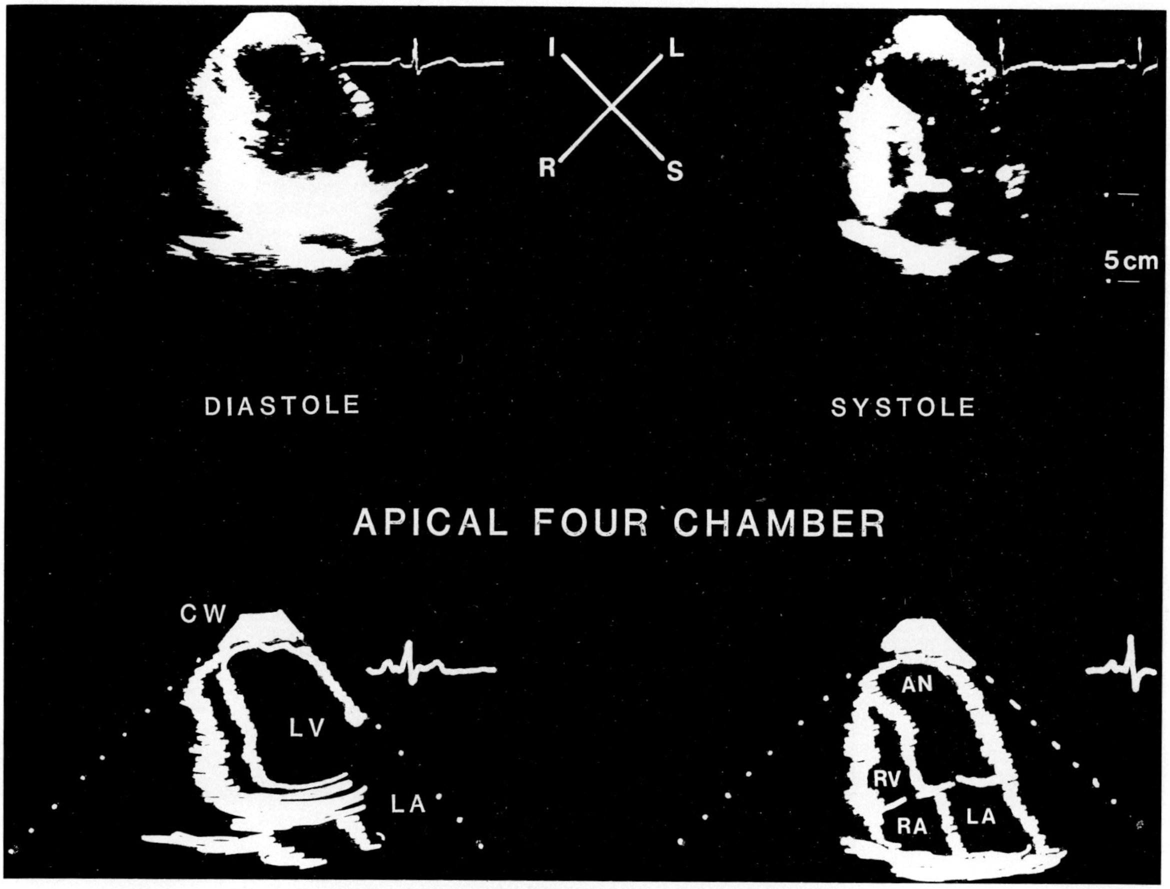

Figure 7-15

Phased array 90° two-dimensional echocardiogram of a patient with an extensive anterior apical infarction noted in an apical four-chamber view during diastole and systole. Note the prominent left ventricular apical aneurysm (AN) best seen during systole with paradoxical motion of the apical septal segment.

7-15.1. An M-mode echocardiogram taken in the standard position of this patient would be expected to show which of the following:

A. Paradoxical septal motion
B. An apical aneurysm
C. Left ventricular enlargement
D. Dyskinesis of the left ventricular apex
E. Increased mitral E point–septal separation

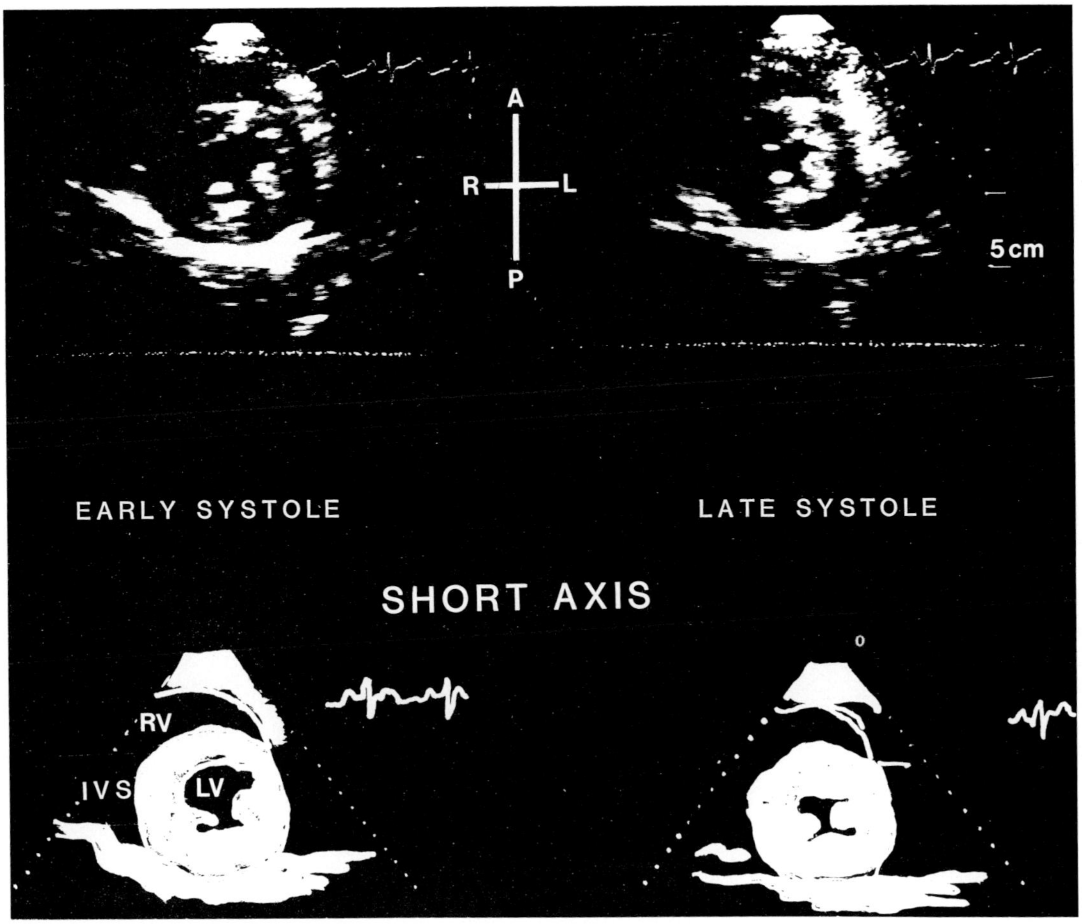

Figure 7-16

Phased-array 90° two-dimensional echocardiogram of a patient with systemic lupus erythematosus and severe hypertension taken in short-axis view. Note the concentric left ventricular hypertrophy and prominent anterior lateral and posterior medial papillary muscle.

7-16.1. An M-mode echocardiogram taken in this patient at the standard position of the ventricle would be expected to show:

A. Left ventricular enlargement
B. Thickened septum but normal posterior wall thickness
C. Thickened septum and posterior walls
D. Systolic anterior motion of the mitral valve

Carl L. Tommaso

8

Tricuspid and Pulmonic Valves

TRICUSPID VALVE

The tricuspid valve may be difficult to visualize, particularly in normal patients. It is usually detected by first finding the mitral valve echo and then directing the transducer medially. The tricuspid valve, as the name implies, is a trileaflet valve; it lies between the right atrium and right ventricle. Occasionally only one leaflet of the valve — usually the septal leaflet — is recorded moving in diastole; it is seen to move in a "W"-shaped pattern similar to that of the posterior mitral leaflet, on the right ventricular side of the septum. The anterior tricuspid leaflet, which resembles the anterior mitral leaflet, frequently can be recorded as well, with careful scanning of the right heart. As the right ventricle increases in size, recording of the valve becomes easier, and often two leaflets are recorded. The valve at this time appears similar in configuration to the mitral valve. The changes in this configuration during disease states and hemodynamic changes are thus very similar to those observed in the echocardiographic recording of the mitral valve in these conditions.

Tricuspid stenosis may be detected in the M-mode echocardiogram as a reduced D-E excursion and diminished tricuspid E-F slope. The degree of calcification of the tricuspid valve is much less than that of the mitral valve; the valve may take on the appearance of only fibrosis or thickening of the leaflets (Figure 8-1).

Ebstein's anomaly of the tricuspid valve is a condition in which the valve is attached in an abnormally low (caudad) position in the right ventricle.[1] The initial clue often is a simultaneous recording of the tricuspid and the mitral valves at the same position. The simultaneous recording is helpful because it demonstrates the delayed closure of the tricuspid valve which, in this condition, closes 50 msec after the mitral valve. Reduced diastolic slope (E-F) and increased amplitude of the tricuspid valve echos are other diagnostic features.

Tricuspid valve prolapse may also be readily diagnosed in the tricuspid valve echocardiogram. It may be seen as a posterior systolic motion of the valve's anterior leaflet. Isolated tricuspid valve prolapse is very rare; usually the valve prolapses in association with prolapse of mitral valve (Figure 8-2).

The presence of **pulmonic valve regurgitation** also can be detected from the motion of the tricuspid valve. When regurgitation of the pulmonic valve is present, the anterior tricuspid valve leaflet will be seen to vibrate, at a medium frequency, during diastole. The tricuspid valve echocardiogram also can reflect

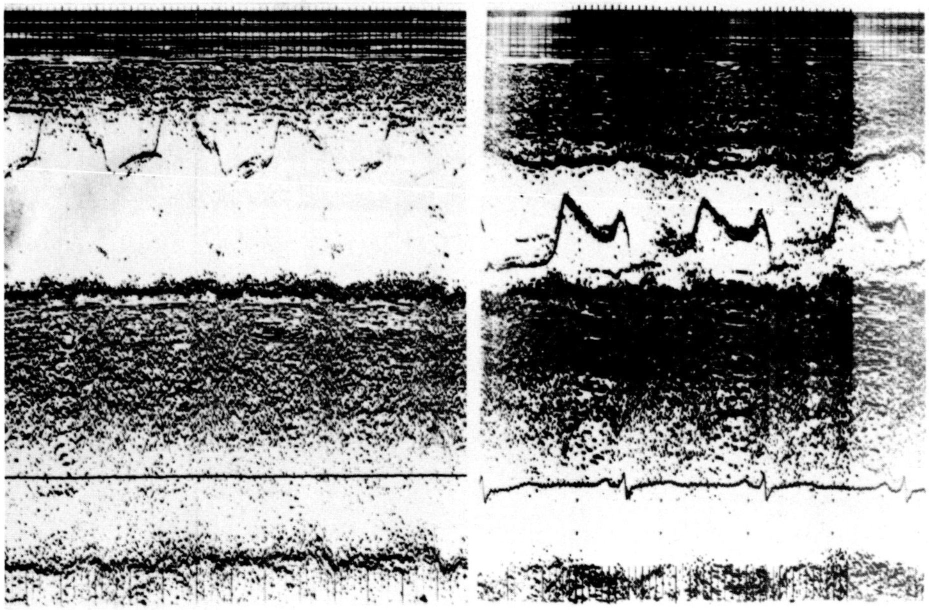

Figure 8-1

M-mode echocardiogram taken at the level of the tricuspid valve (left panel) and mitral valve (right panel) in a 17-year-old girl who presented with a diastolic murmur at the fourth left interspace. To some observers, the murmur increased with inspiration.

8-1.1. The tricuspid valve demonstrates which of the following:

A. Decreased D–E excursion
B. Decreased E–F slope
C. Thickened anterior tricuspid leaflet
D. Loss of normal a-wave

8-1.2. The most likely diagnosis of this patient is:

A. Congenital tricuspid valve stenosis
B. Congenital mitral valve stenosis
C. Primary pulmonary hypertension
D. Ebstein's anomaly of the tricuspid valve

diastolic pressure changes in the right ventricle — just as the mitral valve recording reflects changes in diastolic left ventricular pressure. Hence, interrupted closure (during the A–C slope) of the tricuspid valve may be found in patients with elevated right ventricular end-diastolic pressures (Figure 8-3). In addition, the filling velocity of the right ventricle is reflected in the E–F slope of the tricuspid valve, and cardiac states such as pulmonary hypertension that reduce this velocity will diminish the E–F slope. Care must be taken that such states are not confused with tricuspid stenosis.

Using two-dimensional echocardiography, the tricuspid valve can be visualized from the long-axis view from either the left or right parasternal locations (Figure 8-4), in the short-axis view at the aortic valve in the left parasternal position, or simultaneously with the mitral valve from the apical four-chamber position. Tricuspid stenosis is best seen in long axis, where fusion and incomplete opening of the leaflets may be noted. Right atrial enlargement may also be noted from this view. The long-axis view is helpful also in the evaluation of tricuspid valve prolapse, in which portions of any or all of the leaflets may be seen to move

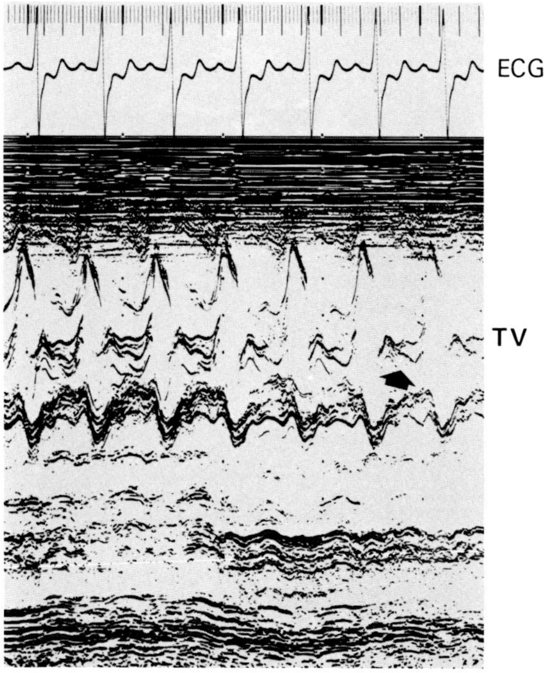

Figure 8-2

M-mode echocardiogram of the anterior and septal leaflets of the tricuspid valve. Note the diastolic motion of the tricuspid valve (arrow).

8-2.1. What is suggested by this echocardiogram of the tricuspid valve?

A. Pulmonic insufficiency
B. Tricuspid valve vegetation
C. Tricuspid valve prolapse
D. Tricuspid stenosis

cephalad into the right atrium during systole (Figure 8-5). The apical four-chamber view also may be useful when tricuspid prolapse is suspected.[2]

Ebstein's anomaly is best evaluated using the apical four-chamber view. Simultaneous visualization of the tricuspid and mitral valves permits their sites of attachment and the length and the relative closure of the tricuspid leaflets to be seen and the diagnosis ascertained.[1] **Tricuspid regurgitation** is best detected with two-dimensional echocardiography using peripheral vein injections; on injection of a dextrose solution, regurgitation of small air bubbles **(microcavitation)** within the hepatic veins and inferior vena cava is observed (not seen in normals) (Figure 8-6). Similar to shunt detection, this method is safe, reproducible, and sensitive for tricuspid regurgitation.[3]

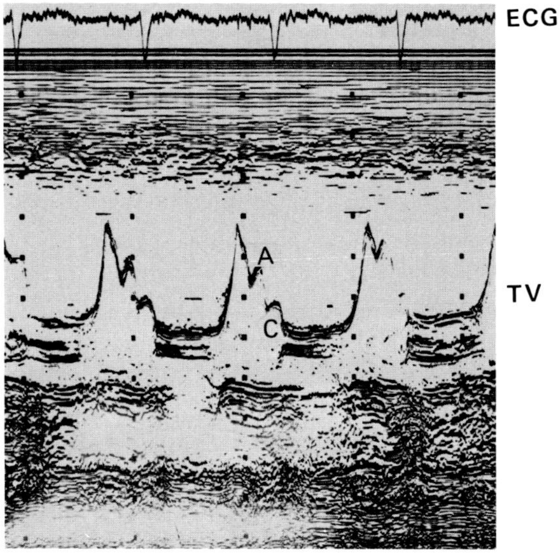

Figure 8-3

M-mode echocardiogram of the anterior and septal leaflets of the tricuspid valve in a patient with chest pain and dyspnea. Note the A–C slope of the anterior tricuspid leaflet.

8-3.1. What abnormality is noted here?

A. Ebstein's anomaly
B. Primum atrial septal defect
C. Interrupted tricuspid valve closure
D. Pulmonic insufficiency

8-3.2. The most likely cause is:

A. Pulmonic valve regurgitation
B. Pulmonic valve stenosis
C. Elevated right ventricular end-diastolic pressure
D. Tricuspid stenosis

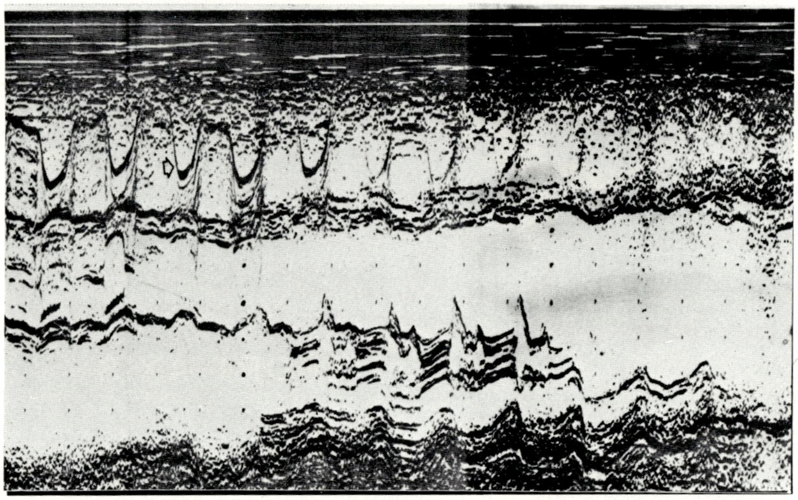

Figure 8-11

This is a M-mode echocardiogram taken in the coronary intensive care unit. The patient sustained a massive anterior myocardial infarction.

8-11.1. This echocardiogram demonstrates which of the following?

A. Left ventricular enlargement
B. Decreased ejection fraction
C. An arrow pointing to a catheter in the right ventricular outflow tract
D. Diminished or absent motion of the interventricular septum
E. Tricuspid valve prolapse (arrow)

David J. Mehlman

9

Vegetations, Thrombi, Myxomas, and Intracardiac Masses

VEGETATIONS

Vegetations are masses of fibrin and cellular debris adherent to valvular or other intracardiac structures. Though vegetations are most frequently infected and related to bacterial or fungal endocarditis, nonbacterial thrombotic endocarditis may occur in association with chronic illness, cancer, or collagen vascular disease. The detection of vegetations in the presence of unexplained bacteremia or stroke may explain the pathophysiology of the illness as well as guide therapeutic management. The surgical implications of finding a vegetation in the presence of bacterial endocarditis are unclear; although it appears that such a finding increases the likelihood that such a patient will require valvular surgery, the presence of a vegetation is not, in itself, an indication for such surgery.[1]

On M-mode echocardiograms, vegetations appear as shaggy, nonuniform structures in association with or in close proximity to a cardiac structure—usually a valve (Figures 9-1 and 9-2). Vegetations vary in size, although those due to fungal endocarditis frequently are quite large.[2] Vegetations as small as 2 or 3 mm may be detected by M-mode echocardiography.[3] As vegetations may adhere to the undersurface of valve leaflets, the vegetation may appear to prolapse into the valvular inflow tract during valve closure: for example, from the mitral valve into the left atrium during ventricular systole or from the aortic valve into the left ventricular outflow tract during ventricular diastole. Vegetations may be difficult to distinguish from prolapsing torn chordae tendineae and from thickened **myxomatous** mitral valves such as found in patients with mitral valve prolapse.

Two-dimensional echocardiography permits more accurate demonstration of the size of vegetations, as well as more accurate localization. A more complete examination of the tricuspid and pulmonary valves is possible with this technique.[4] Unlike M-mode echocardiography, this technique can determine on which leaflet of a valve a vegetation is present. Vegetations on the interventricular septum are also easier to recognize. Even with two-dimensional echocardiography, however, the failure to visualize vegetations does not exclude the possibility of vegetative endocarditis or of a cardiac source of emboli.[3,5]

The natural history of a vegetation is varied. During the course of infection, or thereafter, the vegetation may **embolize,** causing the echocardiographic pattern of the structure from which it originated to return to normal. On the other hand, the vegetation may undergo calcific changes, in which case focal calcification will be noted on the underlying cardiac structure.

THROMBI

Thrombi, or clots, may be present in any cardiac chamber, especially in association with relative stasis of blood, such as would occur with dilated cardiac chambers, stenotic valves, **atrial fibrillation,** or segmental myocardial wall dysfunction.[6] If the thrombus is attached to the heart via a stalk, its echocardiographic appearance could be similar to that of a vegetation, intracardiac tumor, or atrial myxoma. It is somewhat more difficult to identify mural thrombi. If a poorly moving cardiac wall exhibits localized thickening with different acoustic properties than the adjoining muscle, mural thrombus should be considered.[7,8] If serial echocardiograms show the cardiac structure both with and without additional echoes, the possibility is quite strong that thrombus is present. The visualization of a left atrial "shelf" frequently raises the possibility of thrombus in an M-mode echocardiogram with a large left atrium. Two-dimensional echocardiographic techniques usually permit the pulmonary veins to be identified and differentiated from atrial thrombus.[9] M-mode echocardiography is limited here due to an inability to image the left ventricular apex, the region where most ventricular thrombi are found. As the entire left ventricular myocardial surface can be examined by two-dimensional echocardiography, this method is preferred when mural thrombi are suspected.[8]

MYXOMAS AND INTRACARDIAC TUMORS

Myxomas account for approximately half of all primary cardiac tumors and are the most common intracavitary tumors.[10-12] Presenting symptoms depend upon the location of the tumor and may be consistent with other more common forms of heart disease, including valvular obstrucion, **constrictive pericarditis,** and **superior vena cava syndrome.** Some tumors may present with constitutional symptoms or with embolization.

Because three fourths of myxomas occur in the left atrium, M-mode echocardiography is particularly useful in their detection. Right atrial myxomas are also

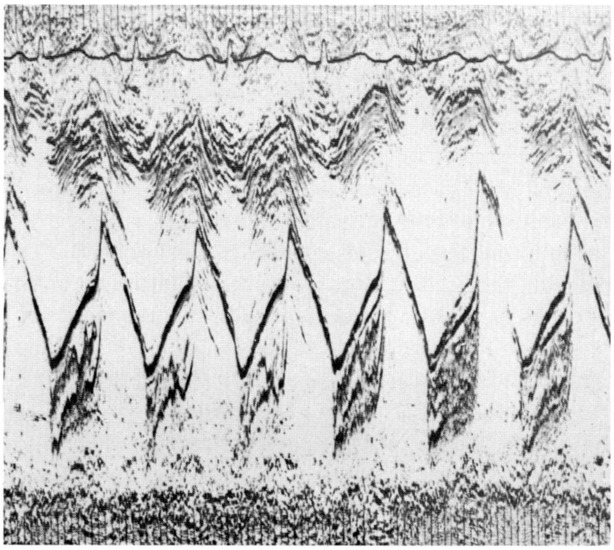

Figure 9-1

Mitral valve echocardiogram of a young male narcotics addict who presented with fever and a pansystolic murmur. Blood cultures grew *Neisseria gonorrheae.* Note the erratic vibration behind the anterior mitral leaflet during systole. Heavy, dense echoes are seen behind the anterior mitral leaflet during systole; during diastole, they disappear.

9-1.1. The erratic vibration noted during systole is most likely caused by:

A. Vegetations on the posterior mitral leaflet with a flail posterior leaflet
B. A flail anterior mitral leaflet
C. A thrombus in the left atrium
D. Atrial myxoma

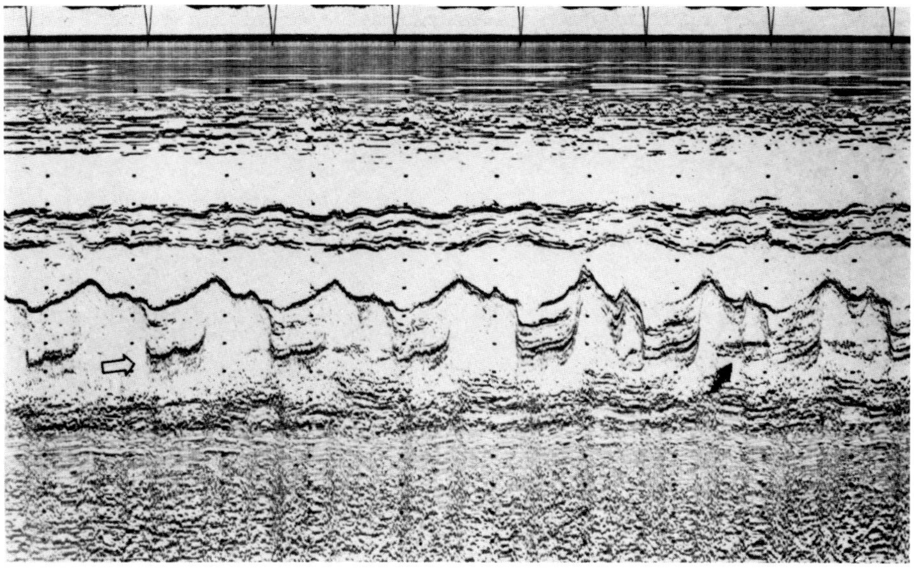

Figure 9-2

Echocardiogram of a 26-year-old female who presented with fever, leukocytosis, and a new systolic murmur.

9-2.1. The open arrow to the left of the tracing demonstrates:

A. Mitral prolapse into the left atrium
B. Systolic oscillation
C. Echoes that may be valve tissue or vegetation
D. All of the above

9-2.2. The closed arrow to the right of the tracing demonstrates:

A. Left ventricular posterior wall
B. Left atrium
C. Abnormal diastolic position of the posterior mitral leaflet
D. All of the above

9-2.3. Serial echocardiograms during antibiotic therapy may show:

A. No change in the size of the lesion
B. Slow resolution of the abnormality
C. Complete reversion to normal in 1 week
D. Both A and B

9-2.4. The most likely diagnosis in this patient is:

A. Mitral valve endocarditis
B. Mitral stenosis
C. Left atrial myxoma
D. None of the above

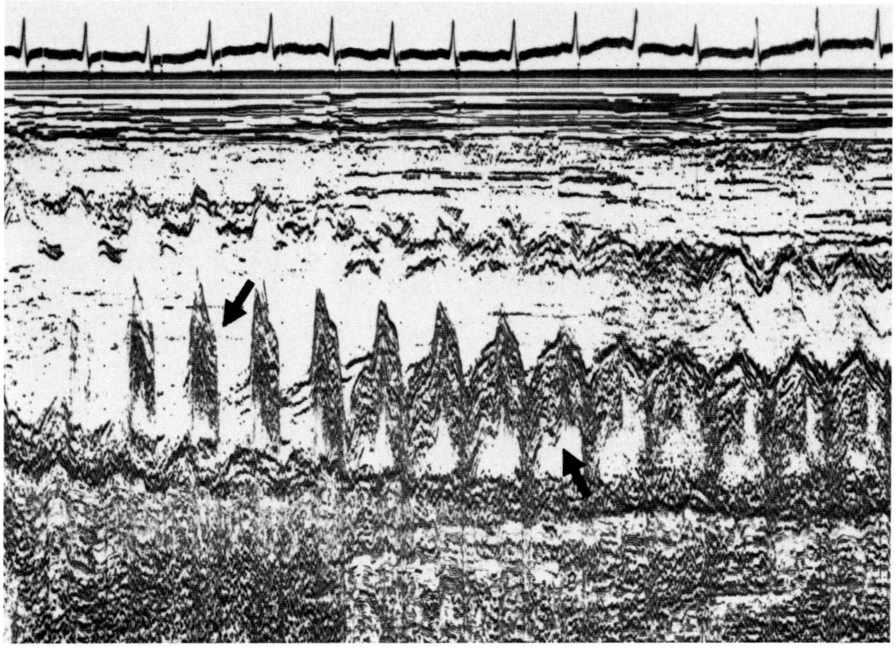

Figure 9-3

Echocardiogram taken from a patient who presented with fever, an embolic event, and a new diastolic murmur. The descending arrow shows a mass in the left ventricle during ventricular systole; the ascending arrow shows a mass in the left atrium during ventricular systole.

9-3.1. The correct diagnosis is:

A. Mitral stenosis
B. Left atrial myxoma
C. Mitral valve endocarditis
D. None of the above

9-3.2. Left atrial myxomas typically:

A. Move into the mitral orifice in diastole
B. Move into the mitral orifice in systole
C. Are immobile
D. None of the above

9-3.3. Left atrial clots typically:

A. Move into the mitral orifice in diastole
B. Move into the mitral orifice in systole
C. Are generally immobile
D. None of the above

9-3.4. If embolization occurs from atrial myxoma, the tumor:

A. No longer will be seen in the left atrium
B. May be unchanged by echo
C. Will be larger
D. None of the above

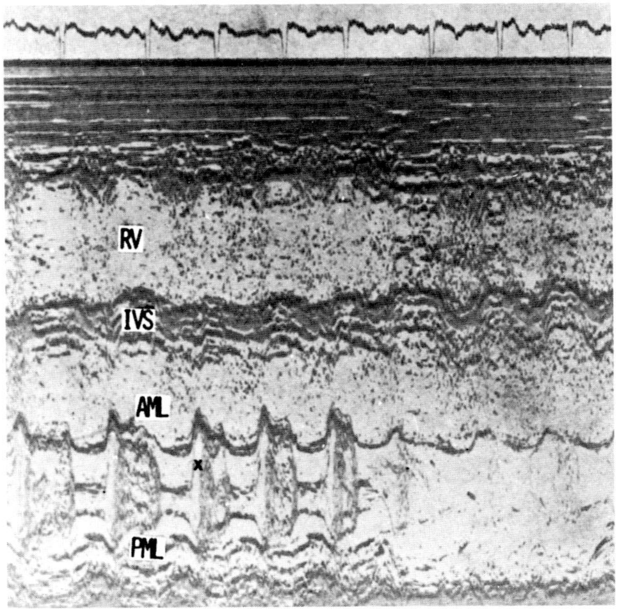

Figure 9-4

M-mode echocardiogram taken at the level of the mitral valve. Note the dense diastolic echoes seen behind the anterior mitral leaflet. Also note the clear space marked "x" between the anterior mitral leaflet and the diastolic mass.

9-4.1. The most likely diagnosis is:

A. Vegetations on the anterior mitral leaflet
B. Vegetations on the posterior mitral leaflet
C. Left atrial myxoma
D. Flail anterior leaflet

9-4.2. The area marked "x" is a clear space that represents:

A. Delay between mitral opening and tumor motion
B. A large mass fixed to the anterior mitral leaflet
C. A large mass fixed to the posterior mitral leaflet

encountered, but here two-dimensional echocardiography is more helpful.[13,14] Since the tumors are frequently multilobulated, a dense cloud of echoes is produced. In some instances, when the tumor surface is calcified, a discrete, well-defined echo may be seen. Most atrial myxomas are pedunculated masses, attached by a stalk to the interatrial septum near the **fossa ovalis.** During ventricular diastole, the left atrial myxoma prolapses from the left atrium into the left ventricle (Figure 9-3) so that a mass of echoes is seen posterior to the anterior mitral leaflet. This mass of echoes returns to the left atrium during ventricular systole. If one examines the M-mode echocardiogram carefully, one notes that, in early diastole, an echo-free space is present posterior to the anterior mitral valve leaflet. The tumor prolapses into the left ventricle after the mitral valve opens, so that the tumor echoes appear later in diastole. If the tumor mass is large, the diastolic closing velocity (E–F slope) of the mitral valve may be reduced (Figure 9-4). This may be due to decreased blood flow across the mitral valve or to mechanical factors.[12,13] Likewise, flutter of the mitral valve may be noted. It is the prolapsing feature of the atrial myxoma that permits visualization of the echoes behind the mitral valve leaflets during diastole. Following surgical removal of the myxoma, the mitral valve motion returns to normal.

With M-mode technique, tumors of the right and left ventricles have been noted as well. As two-dimensional echocardiography provides better orientation and more complete visualization of the various cardiac chambers, this technique is preferred when intracardiac tumors are suspected and M-mode echocardiography is unrevealing.[13,14]

REFERENCES

1. Millman AE, Federici EE, Miskovits C: Left atrial myxoma: Two-dimensional echocardiographic, angiographic, and pathological correlations. J Med Soc NJ 76:749–753, 1979

2. Mintz GS, Kotler MN, Segal BL, Parry WR: Comparison of two-dimensional and M-mode echocardiography in the evaluation of patients with infective endocarditis. Am J Cardol 43:738-744, 1979
3. Wann LS, Hallam CC, Dillon JC, Weyman AE, Feigenbaum H: Comparison of M-mode and cross-sectional echocardiography in infective endocarditis. Circulation 60:728-733, 1979
4. Berger M, Delfin LA, Jelveh M, Goldberg E: Two-dimensional echocardiographic findings in right-sided infective endocarditis. Circulation 61:855-861, 1980
5. Martin RP, Meltzer RS, Chia GL, Stinson EB, Rakowski H, Popp RL: Clinical utility of two-dimensional echocardiography in infective endocarditis. Am J Cardiol 46:379-385, 1980
6. Kramer NE, Rathod R, Chawla KK, Patel R, Towne WD: Echocardiographic diagnosis of left ventricular mural thrombi occurring in cardiomyopathy. Am Heart J 96:381-383, 1978
7. Ports TA, Cogan J, Schiller NB, Rapaport E: Echocardiography of left ventricular masses. Circulation 58:528-536, 1978
8. Meltzer RS, Guthaner D, Rakowski H, Popp RL, Martin RP: Diagnosis of left ventricular thrombi by two-dimensional echocardiography. Br Heart J 42:261-265, 1979
9. Mikell FL, Asinger RW, Rourke T, Hodges M, Sharma B, Francis GS: Two-dimensional echocardiographic demonstration of left atrial thrombi in patients with prosthetic mitral valves. Circulation 60:1183-1190, 1979
10. Ciraulo DA: Mitral valve fluttering: An echocardiographic feature of left atrial myxoma. Chest 76:95-96, 1979
11. Donahue JS, Weiss JL, Gardner TJ, Fortuin NJ, Brawley RK: Current management of atrial myxoma with emphasis on a new diagnostic technique. Ann Surg 189:763-768, 1979
12. Lappe DL, Buckley BH, Weiss JL: Two-dimensional echocardiographic diagnosis of left atrial myxoma. Chest 74:55-58, 1978
13. Moses HW, Nanda NC: Real-time two-dimensional echocardiography in the diagnosis of left atrial myxoma. Chest 78:788-791, 1980
14. Pernod J, Piwnica A, Duret JC: Right atrial myxoma: An echocardiographic study. Br Heart J 40:201-203, 1978

ADDITIONAL ILLUSTRATIONS AND EXERCISES

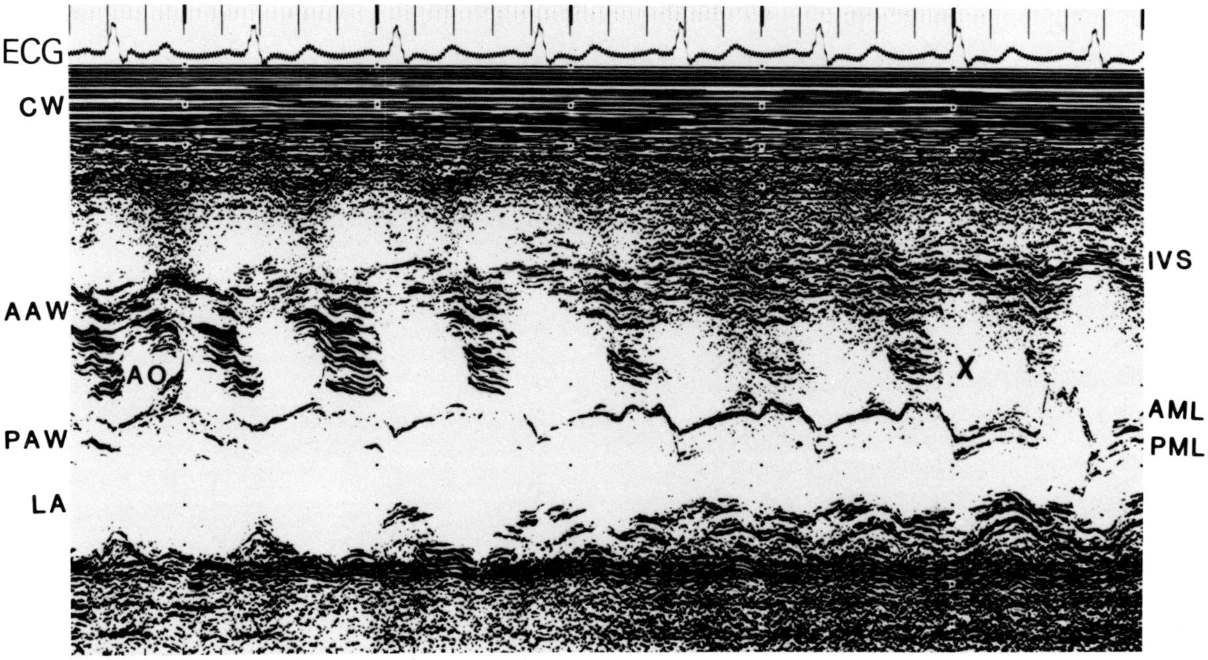

Figure 9-5

M-mode echocardiogram of a patient with healed *Staphylococcus aureus* aortic valve endocarditis. Scan is from the aortic valve to the left ventricular outflow tract. Note the mass of echoes in the left ventricular outflow tract (X), which represents a large, healed vegetation. The left ventricular echo demonstrates left ventricular volume overload.

9-5.1. The patient's clinical course is best described as:

- A. Afebrile with mumur of aortic stenosis
- B. Afebrile with murmur of aortic regurgitation
- C. Febrile with murmur of aortic stenosis
- D. Febrile with murmur of aortic regurgitation

9-5.2. Following treatment for vegetative endocarditis of the aortic valve:

- A. The vegetation may appear unchanged
- B. The vegetation may be reduced in size
- C. The vegetation may disappear
- D. The vegetation may become larger

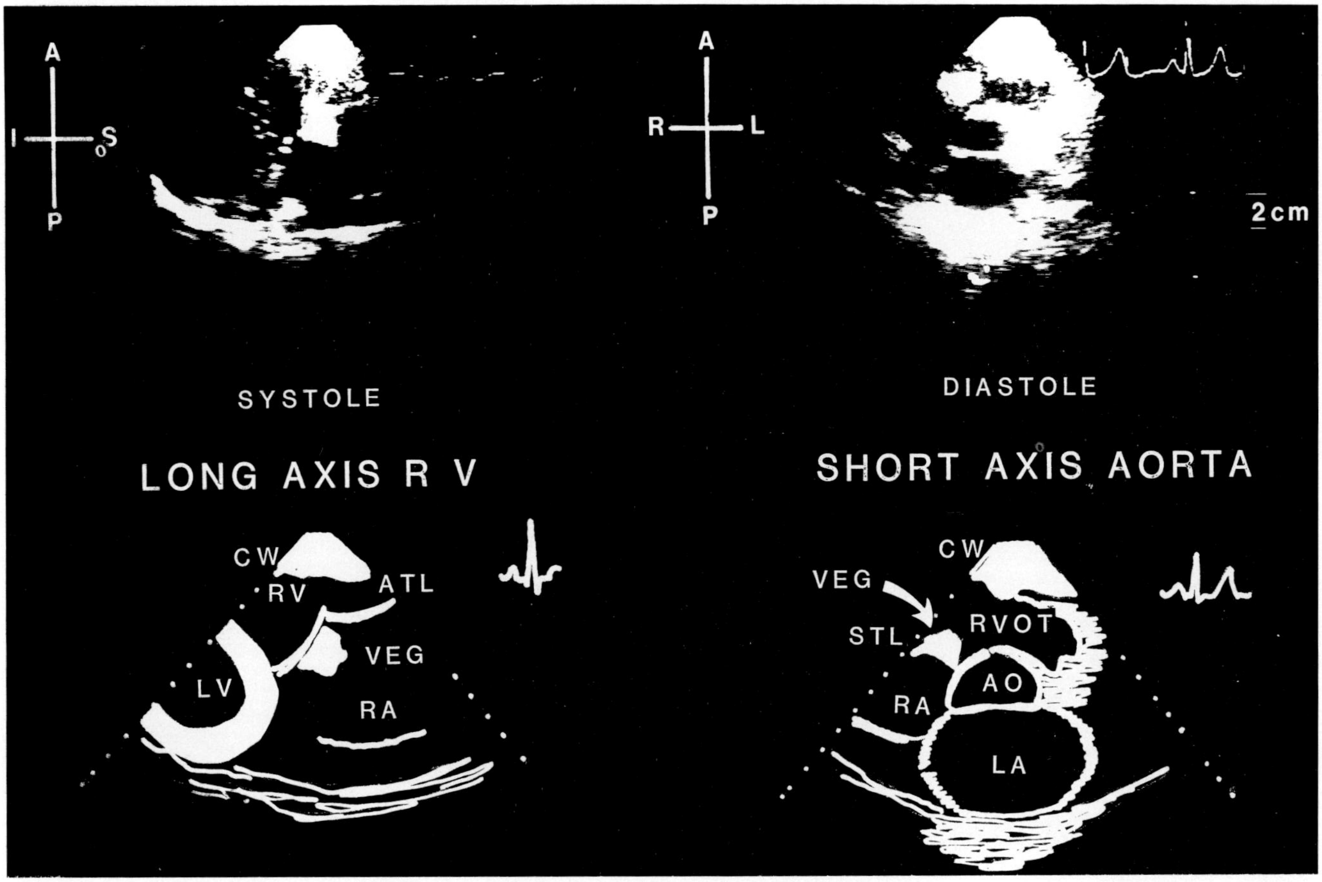

Figure 9-6

Phased-array 90° two-dimensional echocardiogram of a 56-year-old man with *Streptococcus viridans* endocarditis of the tricuspid valve. Views taken in long axis of the right ventricle during systole and in short axis at the aorta during diastole. Note vegetation (VEG) on the septal leaflet of the tricuspid valve.

9-6.1. As to right-side endocarditis, which of the following statements are true?

A. M-mode and two-dimensional echocardiography are both helpful, but M-mode is more useful localizing vegetations on the right heart.

B. M-mode and two-dimensional echocardiography are both helpful, but two-dimensional echocardiography is more useful for localizing vegetations on the right heart.

C. M-mode and two-dimensional echocardiography are equally helpful.

D. Two-dimensional echocardiography is superior in all aspects.

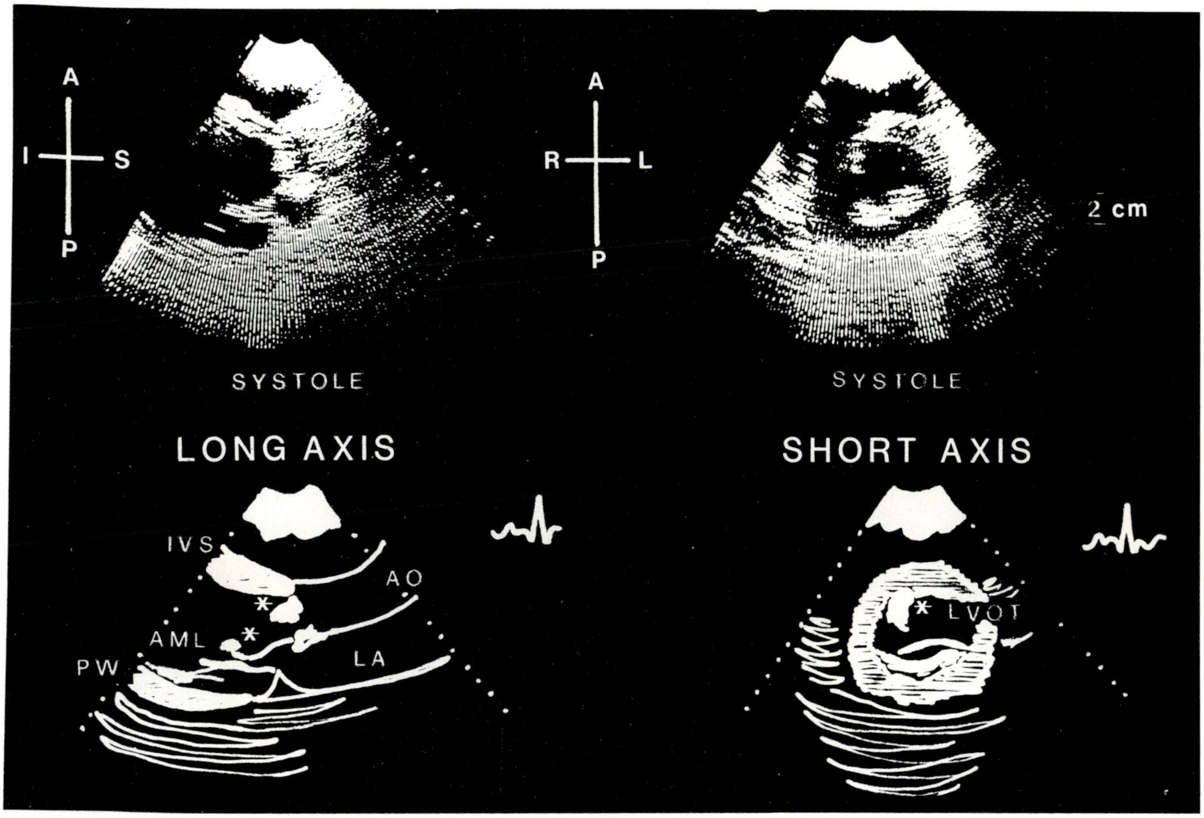

Figure 9-7

Mechanical 87° sector two-dimensional echocardiogram taken in long axis and short axis in systole of a 27-year-old female with *Streptococcus viridans* endocarditis with aortic valve vegetations and aortic regurgitation. Note a sessile vegetation (*) in the left ventricular outflow tract in long and short axis and a pedunculated "satellite" vegetation (*) on the anterior mitral leaflet.

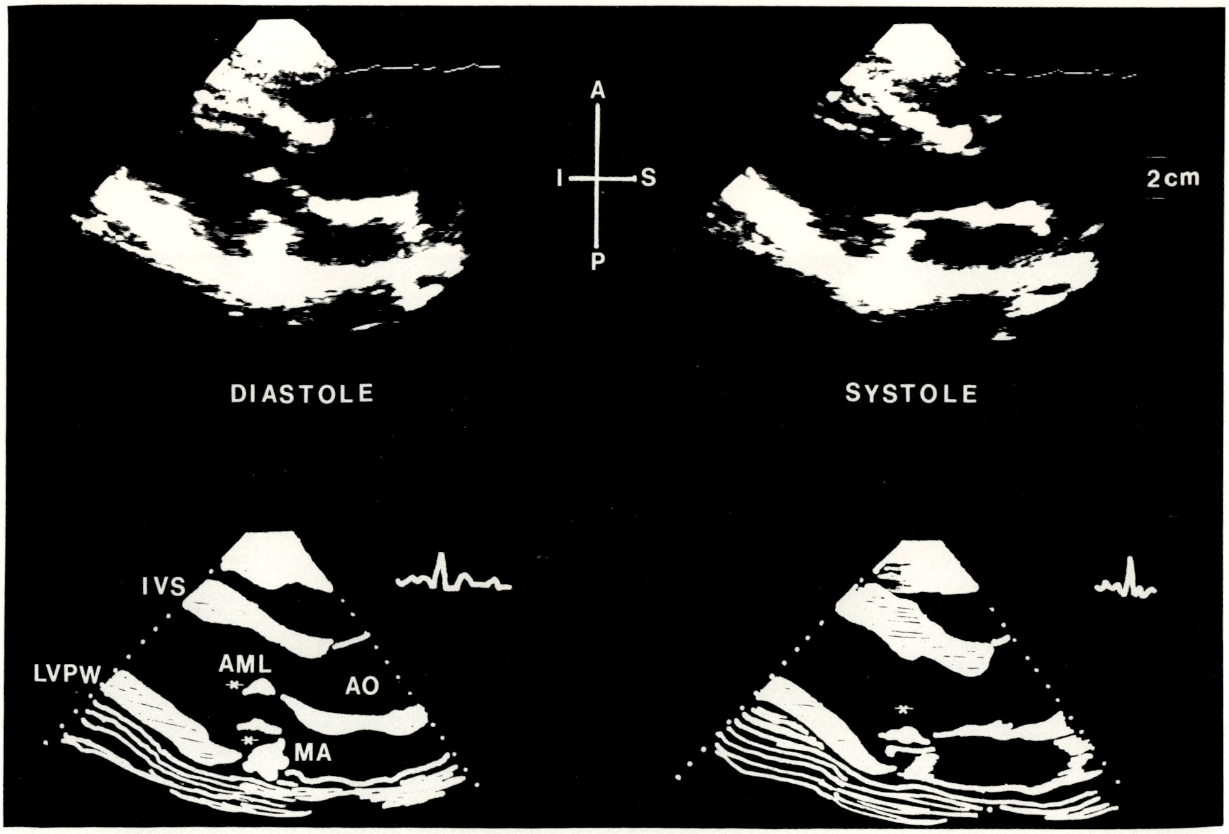

Figure 9-12

Phased-array 90° two-dimensional echocardiogram of a 26-year-old woman with systemic lupus erythematosus and *Streptococcus viridans* endocarditis of the mitral valve. The echocardiogram is taken in the long-axis view of the left ventricle during diastole and systole. Note the vegetations (*) on the anterior and posterior mitral leaflets. The mitral annulus (MA) is calcified. There is left ventricular enlargement and mitral regurgitation.

9-12.1. In systemic lupus erythematosus with infective endocarditis, which of the following statements is correct?

A. Echocardiography is quite helpful to distinguish infective from noninfective vegetations (Libman-Sacks lesions).

B. Echocardiography is often not helpful to distinguish infective vegetations from noninfective vegetations (Libman-Sacks lesions).

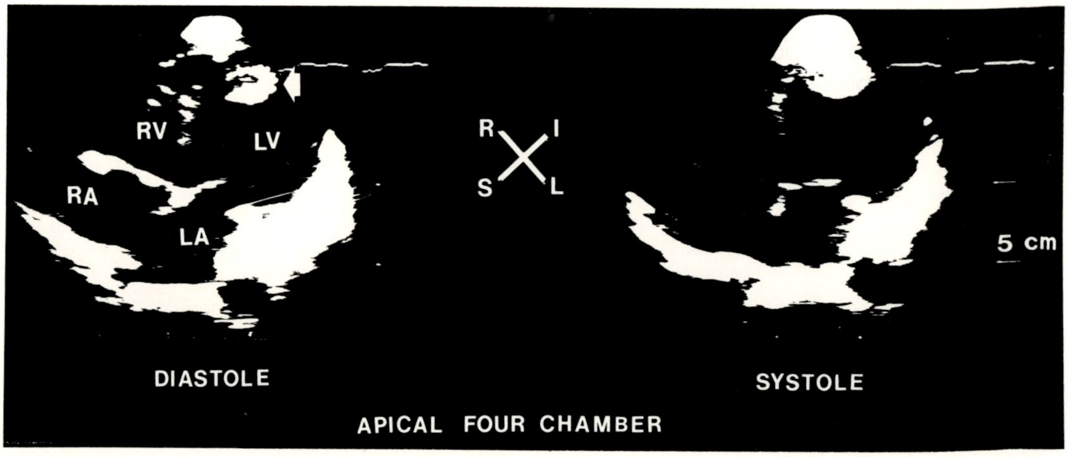

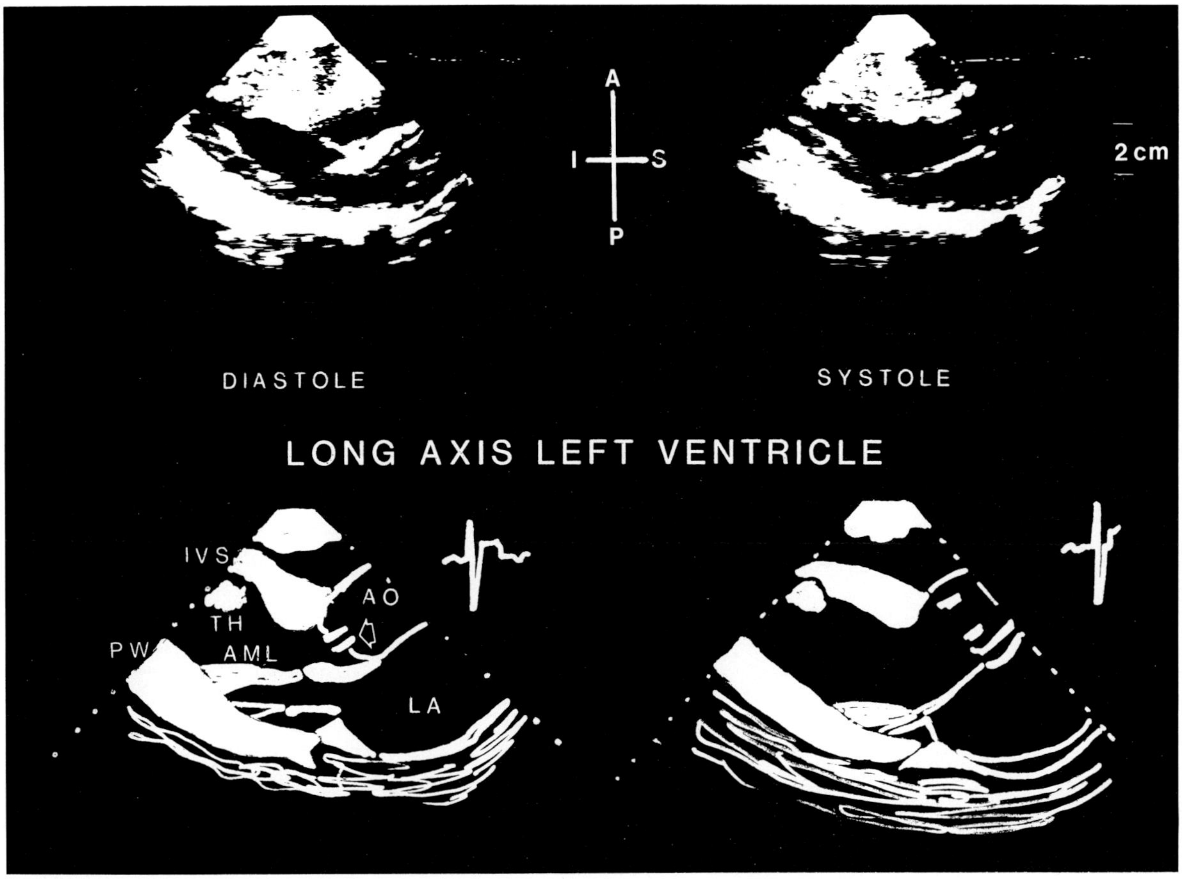

Figure 9-14

Phased-array 90° two-dimensional echocardiogram of a patient with anterior apical myocardial infarction and a left ventricular thrombus (TH), taken in long-axis view of the left ventricle in diastole and systole. Note mild thickening of the aortic valve and persistent separation of the aortic cusp in diastole. Patient also had aortic regurgitation.

9-14.1. With regard to thrombus detection by echocardiography, which of the following statements is true?

A. Two-dimensional echocardiography is most helpful because most thrombi are at the apex, an area poorly imaged by M-mode.

B. M-mode is quite helpful because most thrombi are at the base, an area well imaged by M-mode.

Figure 9-13

Phased-array 90° two-dimensional echocardiogram of a 56-year-old man with congestive cardiomyopathy and a large apical thrombus (arrow), taken in apical four-chamber view in diastole and systole. Note the position of the thrombus and the lack of change in diastolic and systolic of left ventricular size. The ejection fraction was calculated at 13 percent.

James V. Talano

10

Congenital Heart Diseases

LEFT VENTRICULAR PRESSURE OVERLOAD STATES

Congenital Bicuspid Aortic Valve

In the normal aortic valve, all three cusps meet in the midline of the aorta during diastole, allowing the dominant diastolic echoes to be equidistant from the anterior and posterior aortic walls. In the **congenital bicuspid aortic valve,** by contrast, only two cusps are present and these are of unequal size. When such a valve closes, the commissure between the two cusps is eccentrically located, being closer to either the anterior or the posterior aortic wall (Figure 5-3). Eccentricity of the diastolic aortic valve echo is therefore one echocardiographic criterion of congenital bicuspid aortic valve. When either of the aortic cusp echoes is seen to one side of the aorta (and migrates to the other) in diastole, or when multiple diastolic echoes occur from a redundant aortic cusp, a congenital bicuspid aortic valve should be suspected (Figure 10-1). This **eccentricity index** is reliable, provided an associated ventricular septal defect is not present.[1]

With two-dimensional echocardiography, the bicuspid aortic valve can be identified in the parasternal long-axis or short-axis view. In long axis, systolic doming of the bicuspid aortic valve is seen, with a cephlad bowing of the aortic valve cusps (Figure 10-1). In short axis, only two unequal-sized aortic leaflets are idenitified. Because of leaflet degeneration, these will most often thicken and calcify, causing **aortic valve stenosis.** The bicuspid aortic cusps are unequal in size and somewhat redundant, with the effect that portions of the leaflets do not approximate each other during diastole; **aortic regurgitation** is therefore inherent in these valves.

Discrete Subvalvular Aortic Stenosis

This disorder and its aortic valve manifestations on M-mode echocardiography have been discussed and illustrated in Chapter 5 (Figure 10-2). However, **accessory subvalvular aortic leaflets** have also been identified. Here, an accessory aortic valve leaflet attaches to the anterior mitral leaflet at its junction with the posterior aortic wall and to the interventricular septum in the left ventricular outflow tract. A subvalvular chamber with a subvalvular accessory valve is thus

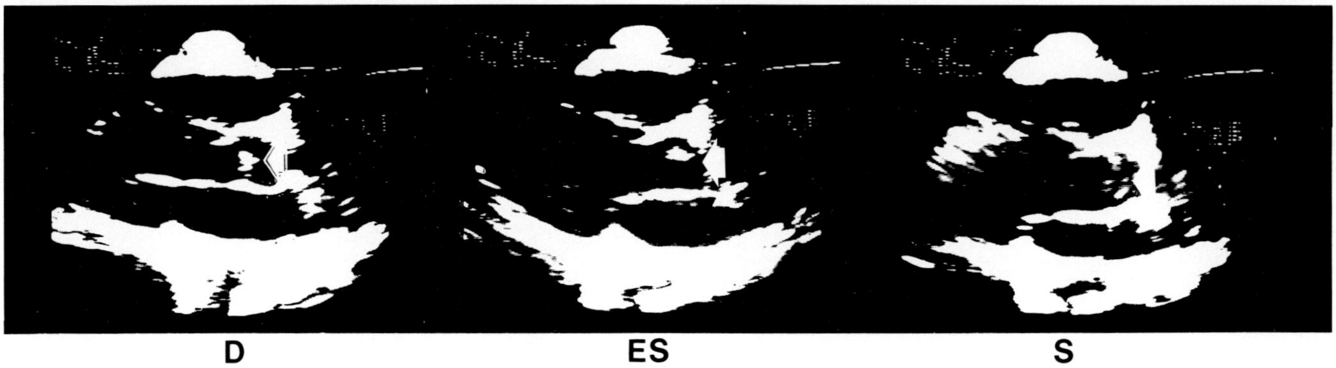

Figure 10-1

Two-dimensional 90° echocardiogram in long axis of the aortic valve in a patient with a congenital bicuspid aortic valve taken during diastole (D), early systole (ES), and systole (S). Note cephalad doming of the aortic valve during early systole (arrow) and incomplete opening of the bicuspid valve during systole.

formed (Figure 10-3). Distortion of the aortic annulus occurs, so that the trileaflet aortic valve is distorted during diastole. The predominant effect is aortic regurgitation. A trivial aortic valve gradient may be present.

RIGHT VENTRICULAR PRESSURE OVERLOAD STATES

Pulmonic Valve Stenosis

In pulmonic valve stenosis, the hemodynamic change in the right heart is an increase in right ventricular systolic pressure at the same time that pulmonary artery systolic pressure is normal or reduced. Right ventricular end-diastolic pressure also is elevated; this increased end-diastolic pressure exceeds pulmonary artery diastolic pressure, so that pronounced presystolic opening of the

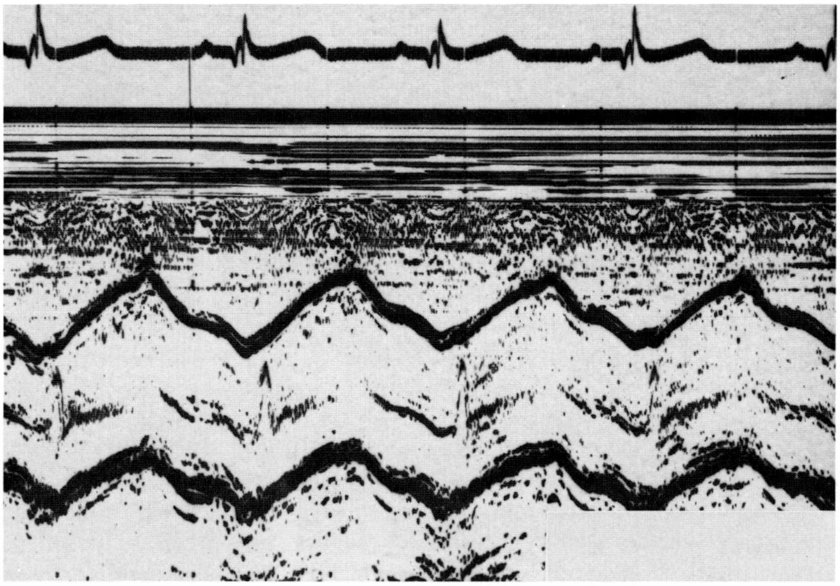

Figure 10-2

Echocardiogram of the aorta taken at the level of the aortic valve of a 12-year-old child who presented with a systolic ejection murmur.

10-2.1. The most likely diagnosis is:

- A. Aortic valvular stenosis
- B. Idiopathic hypertrophic subaortic stenosis
- C. Supravalvular aortic stenosis
- D. Discrete membranous subvalvular aortic stenosis

pulmonic valve occurs. The M-mode echocardiographic finding is an exaggerated pulmonic valve a-wave, one which exceeds 6 mm (Figure 10-4).[2] Pulmonic valve echocardiograms may be normal in some children with pulmonic valve stenosis, however, and exaggerated a-waves have also been seen in adults with normal pulmonic valves who have sinus bradycardia and large right ventricular stroke volumes.

In two-dimensional echocardiography, systolic doming of the pulmonic leaflets can be seen when pulmonic valve stenosis is present. Most often, the posterior pulmonic leaflet is seen. On occasion, the domed anterior and posterior pulmonic valve leaflets can be visualized within the main pulmonary artery in the short-axis view at the aorta (Figure 10-5).

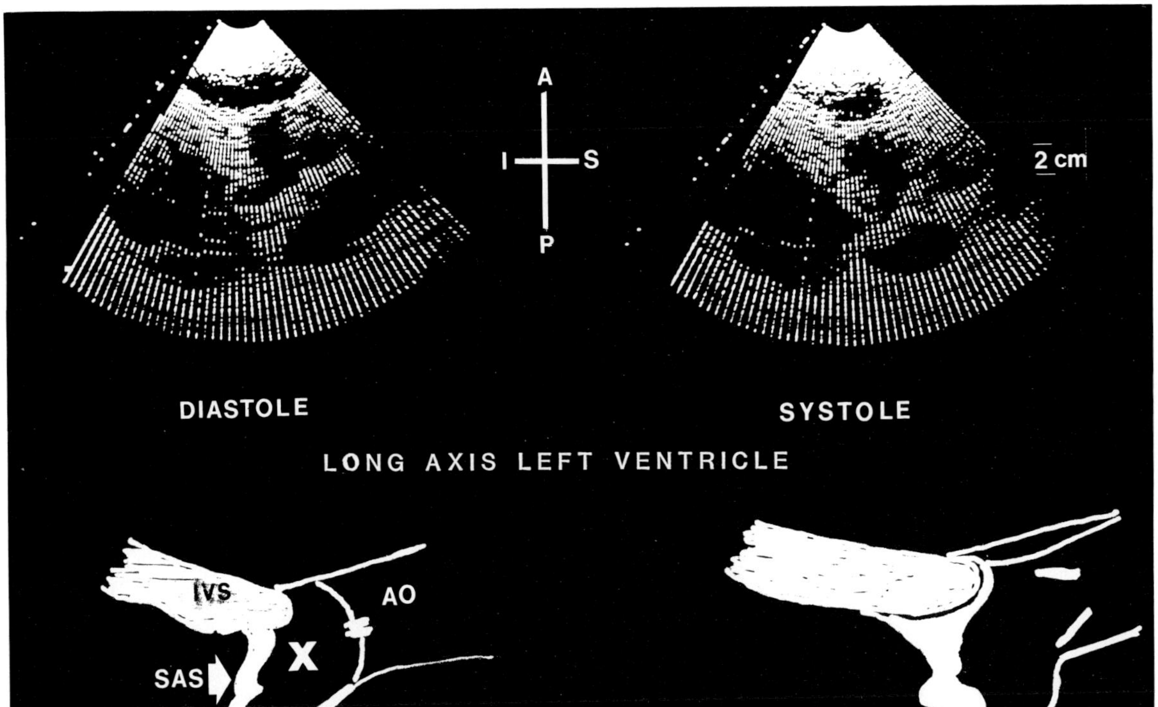

Figure 10-3

Mechanical 90° scan taken in long axis of a man with subvalvular aortic stenosis from an accessory subaortic leaflet. Note the subvalvular membrane (SAS) attached to the septum, and anterior mitral valve. A subvalvular chamber (X) is present during diastole.

10-3.1. With regard to subvalvular aortic stenosis due to accessory aortic leaflets, the predominant valvular lesion is:

A. Aortic valve stenosis
B. Aortic subvalvular stenosis
C. Aortic regurgitation due to a congenital bicuspid aortic valve
D. Aortic regurgitation due to distortion of the aortic valve ring

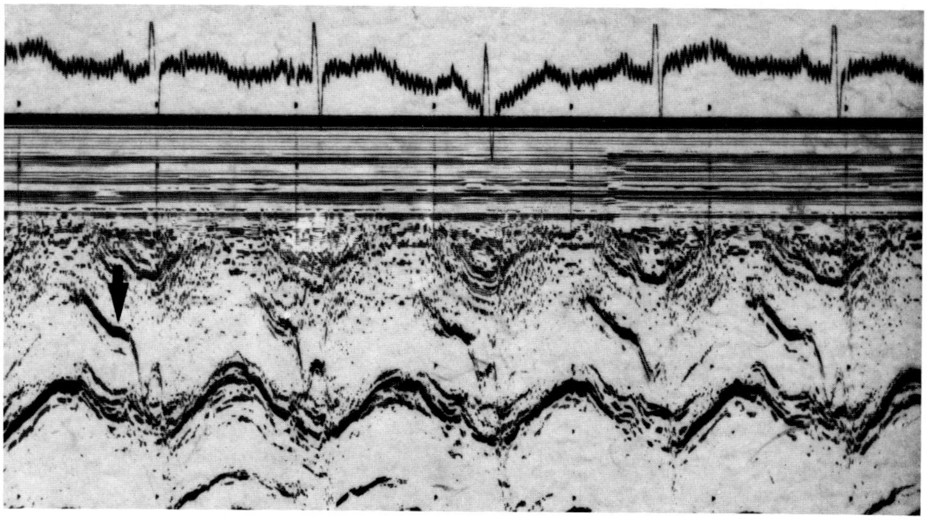

Figure 10-4

M-mode echocardiogram (courtesy of Dr. K. Aziz) of the posterior pulmonic valve cusp (arrow) in a 14-year-old female who presented with a systolic murmur at the second left intercostal space. A systolic thrill also is palpable at the first and second left intercostal spaces. The chest x-ray shows a normal aortic root, with dilitation of the main pulmonary artery. The pulmonary vascular markings are normal to slightly decreased.

10-4.1. The most likely diagnosis in this patient is:

A. Atrial septal defect
B. Pulmonary hypertension
C. Infundibular pulmonic stenosis
D. Congenital pulmonic valve stenosis
E. Pulmonary regurgitation

RIGHT VENTRICULAR VOLUME OVERLOAD STATES

Atrial Septal Defect

An **atrial septal defect** with a significant left-to-right shunt can be suspected whenever the M-mode echocardiogram shows a pattern of right ventricular volume overload (abnormal interventricular septal motion and increased right ventricular dimension). In the normal heart, the interventricular septum moves posteriorly and thickens with the onset of systole—just as the posterior left ventricular wall thickens and moves anteriorly. In the presence of right ventricular volume overload, however, the interventricular septum moves paradoxically—anteriorly at the onset of systole and then posteriorly at the end of it (Figure 10-6). In addition, the right ventricle is enlarged. Using two-dimensional echocardiography, Weyman and co-workers have found that the paradoxical motion of the interventricular septum in these patients appears to be related to the indenting of the left ventricle during diastole by the enlarged right ventricle.[2] The interventricular septum thickens during systole, a finding that distinguishes this paradoxical motion from that observed in the presence of an interventricular septal aneurysm—the result of ischemic heart disease and scar formation in the septum.

In atrial septal defect, the right ventricular diastolic dimension is increased because of the excessive blood flow into the ventricle from the left-to-right interatrial shunt. When this left-to-right shunt is very large, the separation between the anterior and posterior tricuspid leaflets during diastole may significantly exceed that between the anterior and posterior mitral leaflets in the same patient; this increased separation is due to increased trans-tricuspid valve flow. The finding of right ventricular volume overload pattern is nonspecific, however, and may be observed in the presence of other congenital or acquired lesions: tricuspid regurgitation, pulmonary valve regurgitation, partial anomalous pulmonary venous drainage, total anomalous pulmonary venous drainage (in the absence of pulmonary hypertension due to pulmonary venous obstruction), constrictive pericarditis, and anomalous origin of the left coronary artery.[3,4] Contrast studies using saline

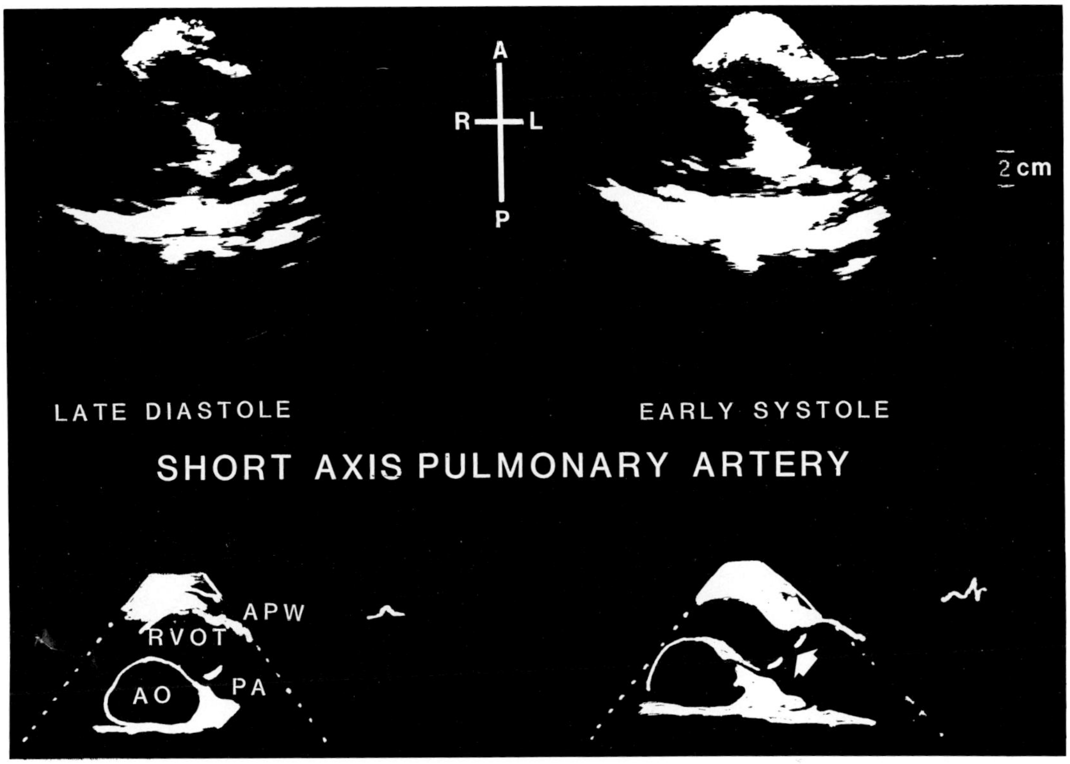

Figure 10-5

Phased-array 90° two-dimensional echocardiogram in short axis of an 18-year-old woman with a systolic murmur and thrill at the second left intercostal space. The right ventricular outflow tract and pulmonary artery lie as a sausage-shaped structure above the aorta. Note the doming of the pulmonic valve (arrow) into the pulmonary artery during systole. Dilatation of the main pulmonary artery is present.

10-5.1. The most likely diagnosis in this patient is:

A. Infundibular pulmonary stenosis
B. Congenital pulmonic valve stenosis
C. Pulmonary hypertension
D. Atrial septal defect

injections into a peripheral vein can be used to detect intra-atrial left-to-right and right-to-left shunts (Figure 10-7).

Ostium Primum Atrial Septal Defect

The pattern just described is most commonly seen with **ostium secundum atrial septal defect.** An increased right ventricular diastolic dimension occurs in **ostium primum atrial septal defect** as well; the paradoxical interventricular septal motion may be masked, however, due to associated abnormalities of the mitral valve and the presence of significant mitral regurgitation. The M-mode echocardiogram in ostium primum atrial septal defect may also show the anterior mitral leaflet abnormally positioned in the left ventricular outflow tract, close to the interventricular septum; this is due to an abnormal insertion of the anterior leaflet on the interventricular septum (Figure 10-8). This is different from the pattern of insertion of the mitral valve in the **complete atrioventricular canal,** wherein the mitral anterior leaflet appears to cross the interventricular septum during diastole.[5] In the latter defect, the interventricular septum may appear "fragmented" or absent near the aorta, due to the **ventricular septal defect** in the **endocardial cushion.** Other findings in ostium primum atrial septal defect include multiple echoes of the mitral valve during systole, anterior motion of the mitral valve in late systole, and a lack of continuity between the mitral and tricuspid valves (each valve is seen separately).

Ebstein's Anomaly

Ebstein's anomaly is a congenital lesion, the major pathologic features of which are myxomatous deformity of the tricuspid valve and abnormal inferior

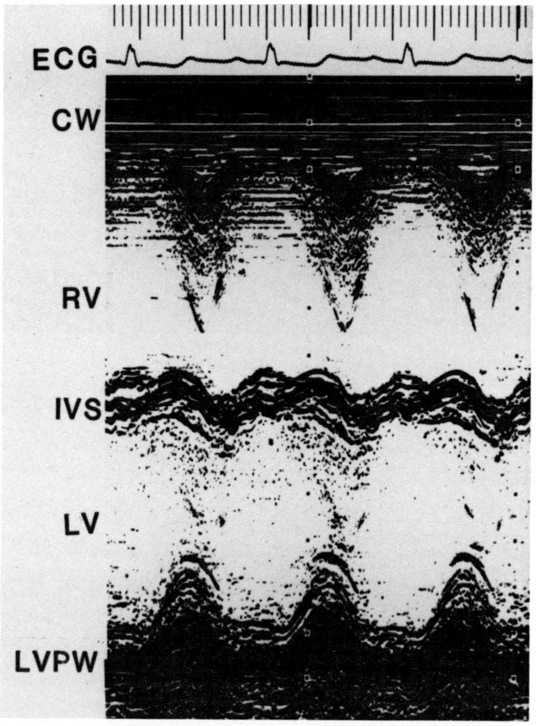

Figure 10-6
M-mode echocardiogram of a 29-year-old woman with a large secundum atrial septal defect. Note the enlarged right ventricle, the relatively smaller left ventricle, and the paradoxical motion of the septum. Also note the increased amplitude of the right ventricular anterior wall.

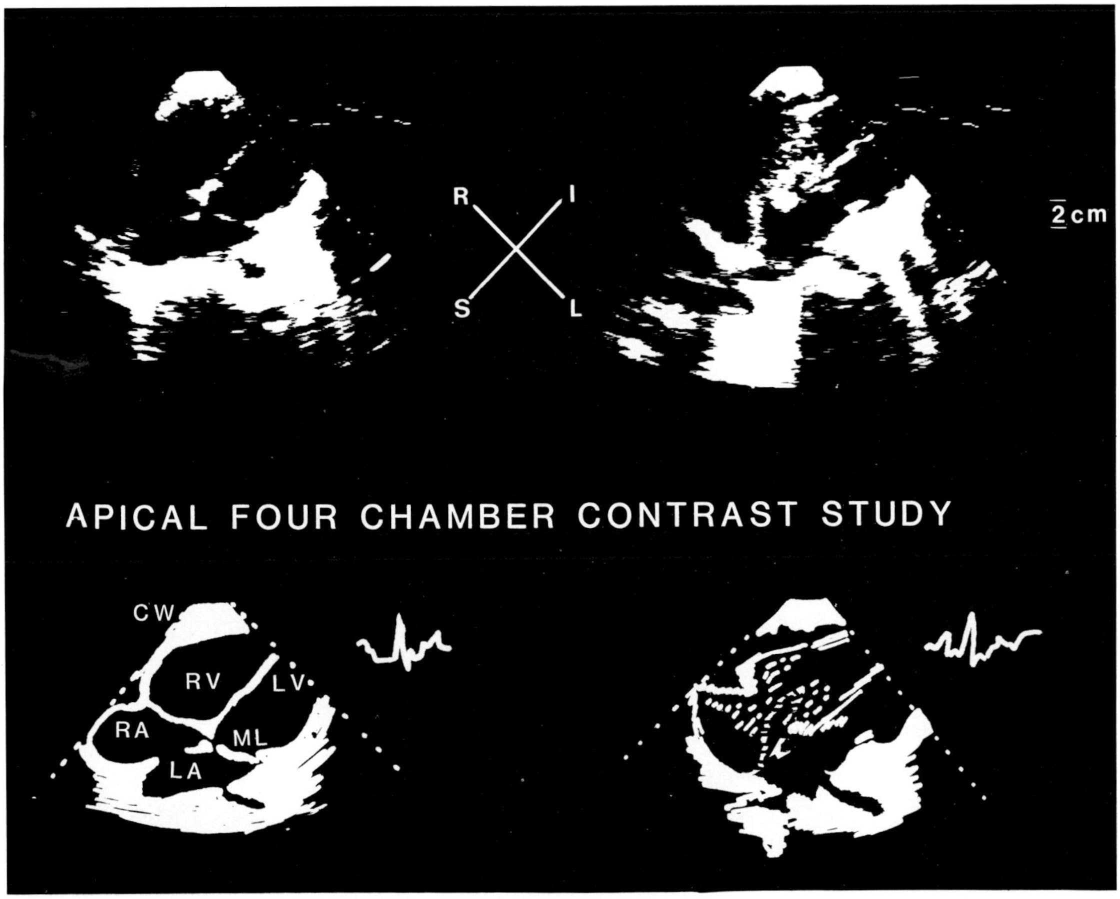

Figure 10-7

Apical four-chamber study using a 90° two-dimensional echocardiogram of the patient in Figure 10-6. In the left panel, note the break in continuity of the interatrial septum separating the left and the right atria. There is also right ventricular enlargement. In the right panel, an injection of normal saline is seen as small microbubbles in the right atrium. The left-to-right shunt at the interatrial septum (arrow) displaces the microbubbles in the right atrium.

10-7.1. Following peripheral injection for detection of left-to-right shunts in an atrial septal defect, which of the following occurs?

A. Micro-bubbles in the right atrium are displaced by noncontrast blood from the left atrium at the atrial septal defect.

B. Micro-bubbles in the left atrium are displaced by noncontrast blood in the right atrium at the atrial septal defect.

displacement of the valve into the right ventricle. The tricuspid valve is displaced leftward of the usual position in the chest cavity and is more easily recorded. The amplitude of the valve's movement may be increased, and its closure follows mitral valve closure by a greater than normal interval (greater than 55 msec). Two-dimensional echocardiography permits the abnormal inferior attachment of the tricuspid valve to be visualized; it is best seen in the apical four-chamber view (Figure 10-9).

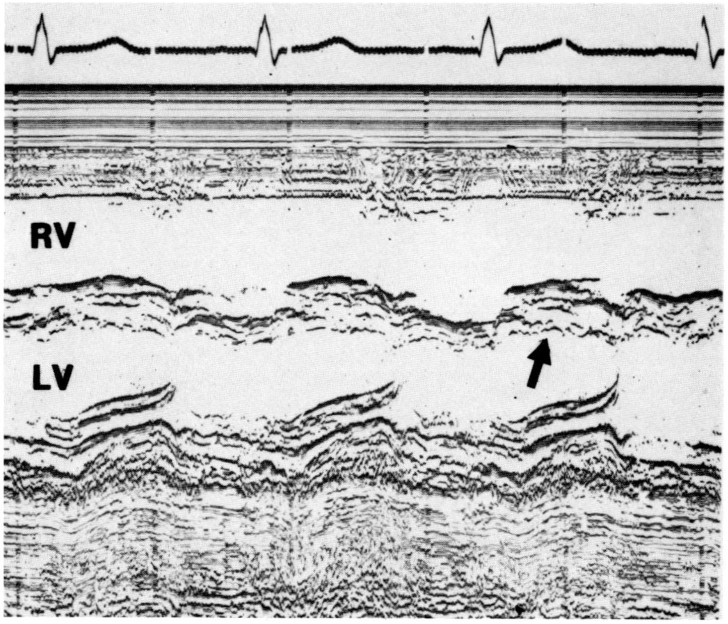

Figure 10-8

Echocardiogram taken at the level of the left and right ventricles. There is right ventricular enlargement. Note the systolic septal motion (arrow).

10-8.1. Interventricular septal motion is:

A. Normal
B. Abnormal
C. Unimportant
D. None of the above

10-8.2. The correct diagnosis is:

A. Right ventricular volume overload
B. Atrial septal defect
C. Cardiomyopathy
D. A and B

10-8.3. The distinction between atrial septal defect and the paradoxical septal motion that normally follows cardiac surgery could be made by:

A. Historical information and accurate clinical examination
B. Thallium scan
C. Nuclear magnetic resonance
D. CT scan

LEFT VENTRICULAR VOLUME OVERLOAD STATES

Ventricular Septal Defect

In isolated ventricular septal defect, unless the defect is very large, the discontinuity between the interventricular septum and anterior aortic wall is usually not apparent on the M-mode echocardiogram. The indirect effects of the ventricular septal defect can be seen on M-mode, however, the primary one being the increase in left ventricular and left atrial dimensions that results from increased left

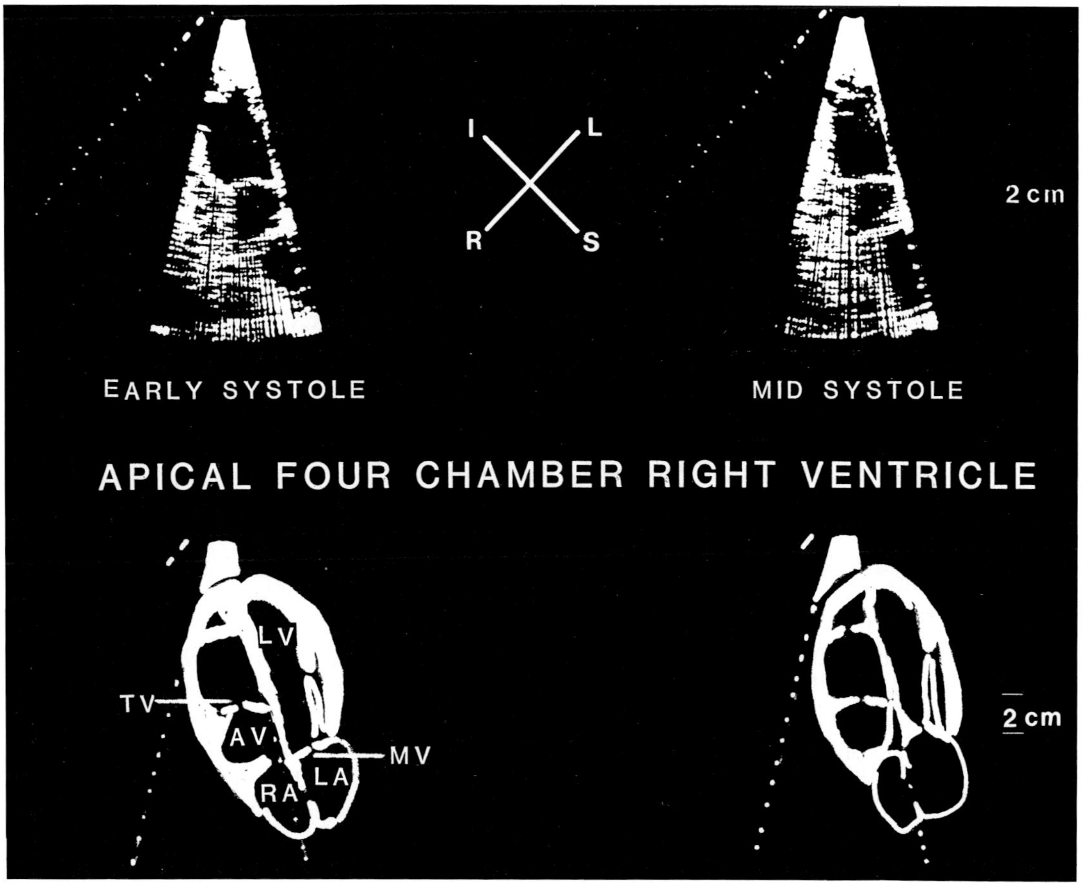

Figure 10-9

Mechanical 30° sector echocardiogram of a 48-year-old man with atrial flutter, Wolff-Parkinson-White syndrome, and Ebstein's anomaly of the tricuspid valve. The four-chamber view is taken to image the right ventricle and right atrium. Note the inferior displacement of the tricuspid valve and the resulting atrialized portion of the right ventricle (AV). The tricuspid valve (TV) is usually large and myxomatous in Ebstein's anomaly.

ventricular volume overload in these chambers (Figure 10-10). An increase in the ratio of the left atrial diameter to the aortic root diameter occurs if the left-to-right shunt is large. Two-dimensional echocardiography may be helpful in identifying large ventricular septal defects. In high (supracrista) ventricular septal defect, discontinuity of the anterior aortic wall is occasionally noted on the M-mode echocardiogram (Figure 10-11).

Patent Ductus Arteriosus

A large **patent ductus arteriosus** causes a significant left-to-right shunt from the aorta to a pulmonary artery and may be demonstrated on M-mode by an increased left atrial dimension and the pattern of left ventricular volume overload.

In normal adults, the left atrial-aortic root dimension ratio (LA/Ao) has been reported to be 0.87-1.11;[6] in full-term infants the ratio is 0.74 ± 0.13; and in premature infants it is 0.86 ± 0.10. By contrast, in infants with a large patent ductus arteriosus and significant left-to-right shunt, the LA/Ao ratio increases to

Figure 10-12

Echocardiogram of a 2-week-old cyanotic infant. Note the overriding of the aorta over the septum and the continuity of the anterior mitral leaflet with the aorta.

10-12.1. What is the most likely diagnosis?

A. Single ventricle
B. Tetralogy of Fallot
C. Endocardial cushion defect
D. Ebstein's anomaly

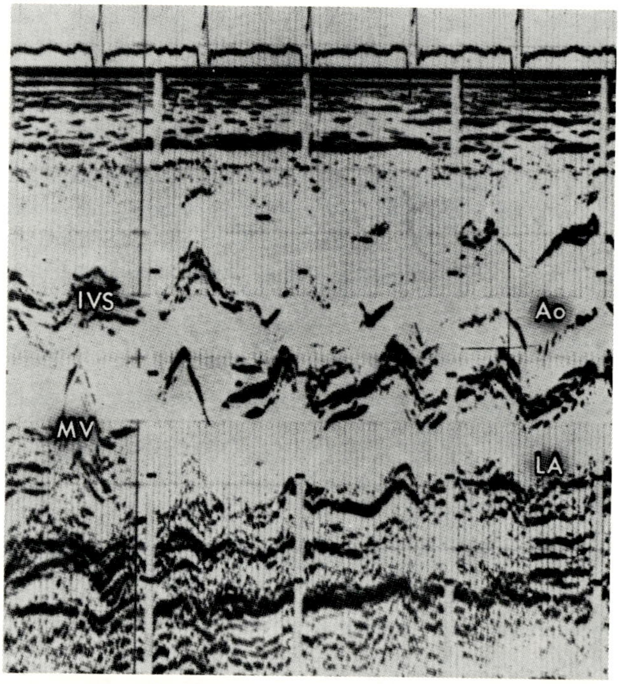

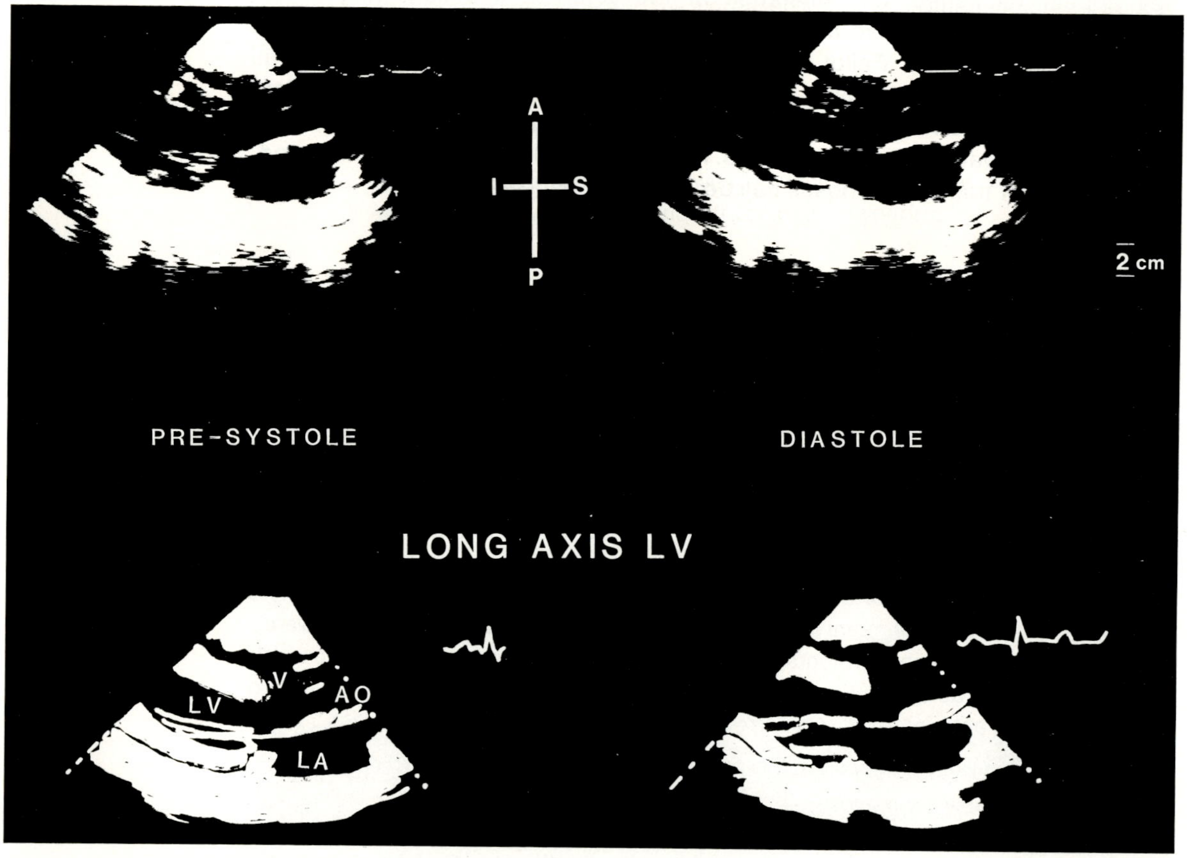

Figure 10-13
(See legend facing page)

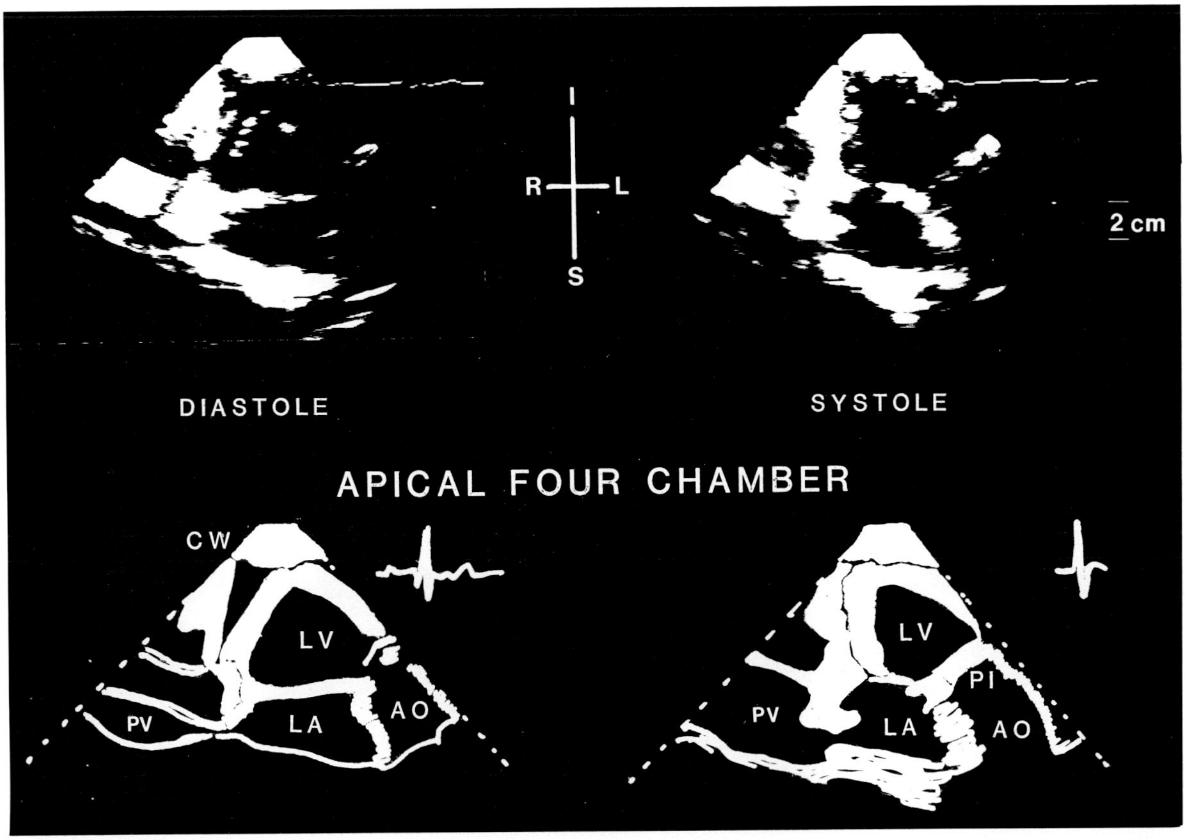

Figure 10-14

Phased-array 90° two-dimensional echocardiogram of a 29-year-old man with a single ventricle in apical four-chamber view. There is transposition of the aorta, which arises from the right ventricular outflow tract or pulmonary infundibulum (PI). The tricuspid valve is missing. A pulmonary vein communicates with the left atrium.

echocardiogram the two artioventricular valves are seen to empty into the single, large ventricular chamber, on the same side as the interventricular septum (Figure 10-14). A hypoplastic right ventricle with a small interventricular septum and right ventricular outflow tract is sometimes seen. A patient with a single ventricle occasionally may have only one atrioventricular valve, making the diagnosis of single ventricle difficult.

Figure 10-13

Phased-array 90° two-dimensional echocardiogram of a patient with tetralogy of Fallot. In systole, note the large ventricular septal defect (V) just below the aortic valve with the large overriding aorta. The right ventricular outflow tract (anterior to the aorta) is almost obliterated.

10-13.1. In tetralogy of Fallot, which of the following abnormalities are generally present?

A. Ventricular septal defect
B. Large overriding aorta
C. Pulmonary valve stenosis
D. Atrial septal defect

Transposition of the Great Vessels

The normal pulmonary artery originates anterior to and then descends posteriorly and to the left of the aorta. This can be seen in an M-mode scan as the ultrasonic beam is moved from the aortic valve leftward to the pulmonic valve. In the scan the posterior pulmonic cusp is recorded to the left of the anterior wall of the aorta, with the pulmonic valve positioned somewhat superior to the aortic valve. Rarely are both cusps of the pulmonic valve recorded simultaneously; usually only the posterior pulmonic cusp is recorded.

In **transposition of the great vessels,** by contrast, the aorta and pulmonary artery lie parallel to each other. Both **semilunar** valves (aortic and pulmonic) are at the same level (superior to the heart), so that the M-mode beam transects both valves simultaneously. Thus, the two great vessels are recorded in parallel, the aorta being transposed anterior to the pulmonary artery. In a scan from one great vessel to another, the anterior outflow tract and great vessels (aorta) fail to dip

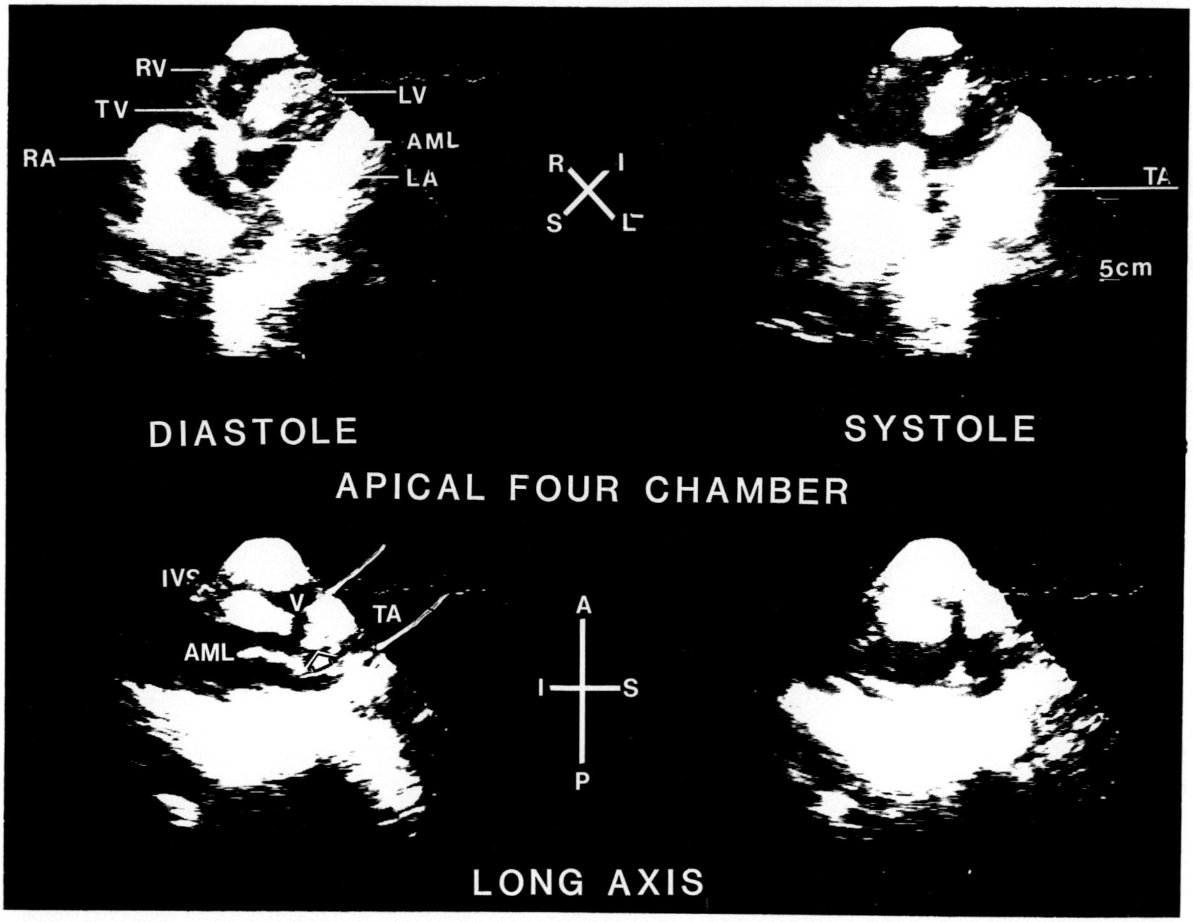

Figure 10-15

Two-dimensional phased-array echocardiogram in the apical four-chamber and long-axis view in diastole and systole in a patient with truncus arteriosus. No pulmonary valve could be identified. The left pulmonary artery was seen to take off from the ascending truncus vessel. Note the ventricular septal defect (V) in the four-chamber and long-axis views. Note the large truncus valve (TV) (arrow) and the overriding truncus artery (TA). The anterior mitral leaflet is in continuity with the posterior truncus artery wall.

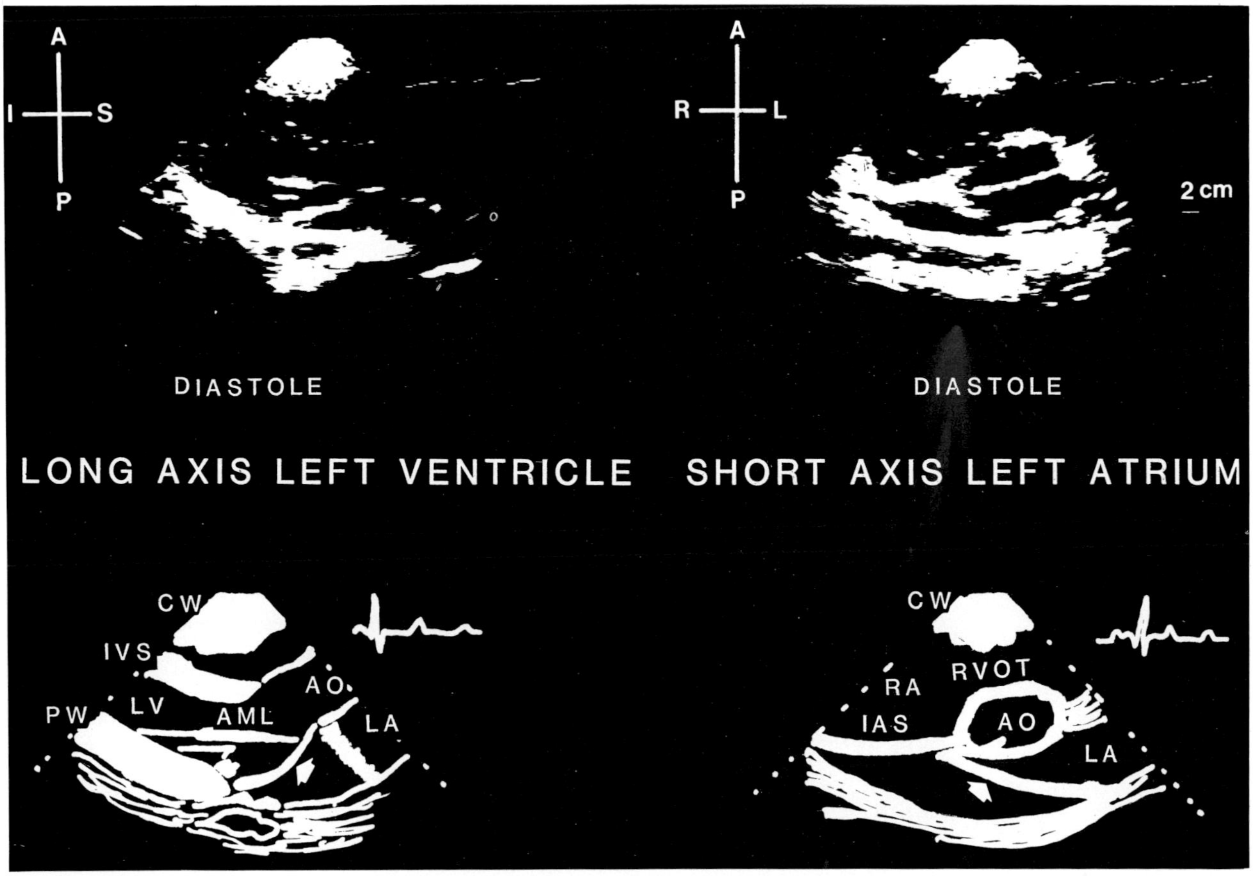

Figure 10–16

Phased-array 90° two-dimensional echocardiogram of a 19-year-old woman with partial cor triatriatum, taken in long axis of the left ventricle in diastole and in short axis of the aorta and left atrium in diastole. In long axis, note the membrane within the left atrium, which extends from the posterior aortic wall to the atrioventricular groove (arrow). In short axis, the membrane attaches anteriorly to the interatrial septum to the lateral posterior left atrial wall (arrow). Note the separation of the left atrium into an anterior superior chamber and posterior inferior chamber. No atrial septal defect was detected.

posteriorly. The echoes from the aortic and pulmonic semilunar valves are superimposed.

In a two-dimensional echocardiogram, the normal pulmonary artery is seen to dip posteriorly and to the left of the aorta (Figure 10-5). When the great vessels are transposed, however, the two vessels do not intertwine; the aorta is situated anteriorly and to the right, the pulmonary artery is situated posteriorly and to the left,[8,9] and the two arteries parallel each other and do not cross. In two-dimensional echocardiography, the parallel position of the two great vessels and the common level at which both semilunar valves are found are diagnostic of transposition. The spatial orientation of two-dimensional echocardiography helps to diagnose this disorder more readily.[10]

Truncus Arteriosus

Truncus arteriosus, like tetralogy of Fallot, is characterized by a large aorta overriding a ventricular septal defect. The truncus artery is larger, however, and overrides the septum to a greater extent. In tetralogy of Fallot infundibular or pulmonic valve stenosis generally is evident, whereas, in truncus, the pulmonary valve is altogether absent. Either the main pulmonary artery is a branch of the truncus artery (type 1), or both pulmonary arteries originate separately from the truncus artery. The truncus valve is a single, large semilunar valve. Aortic regurgitation is always present. On two-dimensional echocardiography the large truncus artery is seen to override the large ventricular septal defect, a large, single semilunar valve is present, and only one great vessel is detected (Figure 10-15).

Cor Triatriatum

In this condition, the left atrium is divided by an intraatrial membrane into two chambers: a cephalad posterior chamber and an inferior anterior chamber. Frequently, a left-to-right interatrial shunt also is present. The M-mode echocardiogram shows a linear density within the left atrium. The posterior left atrial chamber can be confused with either a large coronary sinus or a common pulmonary vein, as seen in total anomalous pulmonary venous return. Two-dimensional studies show the intraatrial membrane within the left atrium. A contrast study can be used to demonstrate the left-to-right interatrial shunt. Occasionally this membrane can be partially complete, as shown in Figure 10-16.

REFERENCES

1. Nanda NC, Gramiak R, Manning J, Mahoney EB, Lipchik EO, DeWeese JA: Echocardiographic recognition of the congenital bicuspid aortic valve. Circulation 49:870-875, 1974
2. Weyman AE, Dillon JC, Feigenbaum H, Cheng C: Echocardiographic differentiation of infundibular from valvular pulmonic stenosis. Am J Cardiol 36:21-29, 1975
3. Bierman FZ, Williams RG: Subxiphoid two-dimensional imaging of the interatrial septum in infants and neonates with congenital heart disease. Circulation 60:80-90, 1979
4. Fraker TD Jr, Harris PJ, Behar VS, Kisslo JA: Detection and exclusion of interatrial shunts by two-dimensional echocardiography and peripheral venous injection. Circulation 59:379-384, 1979
5. Bass JL, Bessinger FB Jr, Lawrence C: Echocardiographic differentiation of partial and complete atrioventricular canal. Circulation 57:1144-1150, 1978
6. Silverman NH, Lewis AB, Heymann MA, Rudolph AM: Echocardiographic assessment of ductus arteriosis in premature infants. Circulation 50:821-828, 1974
7. Allen DH, Sahn DJ, Goldberg SJ: New serial contrast technique for assessment of left to right shunting patent ductus arteriosus in the neonate. Am J Cardiol 41:288-294, 1978
8. Henry WL, Maren BJ, Griffith JM, Redwood DR, Epstein SE: Differentiated diagnosis of anomalies of the great vessels by real-time two-dimensional echocardiography. Circulation 51:283-287, 1975
9. Gramiak R, Nanda NC: Ultrasonic assessment of transposition of the great vessels. Prog Cardiovasc Dis 21:43-52, 1978
10. Dillon J, Feigenbaum H, Koneche LL, Keutel J, Horwitz RA, Davis RH, Chang S: Echocardiographic manifestation of two-dimensional transposition of the great vessels. Am J Cardiology 32:74-81, 1973

ADDITIONAL ILLUSTRATIONS AND EXERCISES

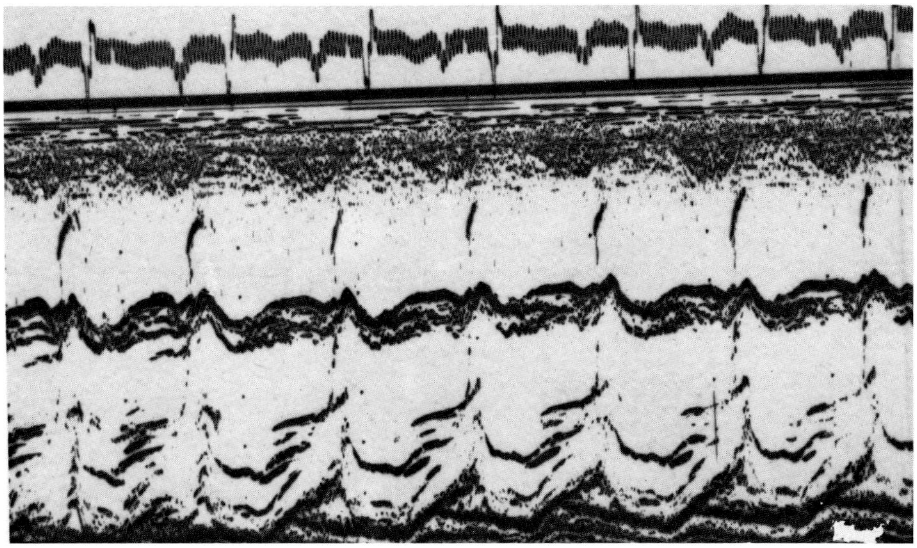

Figure 10-17

M-mode echocardiogram taken at the level of the right and left ventricles of a 4½-year-old infant with a loud systolic murmur and cardiomegaly. Note the right ventricular enlargement, abnomal interventricular septal motion, and multiple systolic echoes of the mitral valve. A portion of the anterior mitral leaflet appears to traverse the septum.

10-17.1. The most likely diagnosis of this congenital anomaly is:

A. Secundum atrial septal defect
B. Primum atrial septal defect
C. Coarctation of the aorta
D. Ventricular septal defect

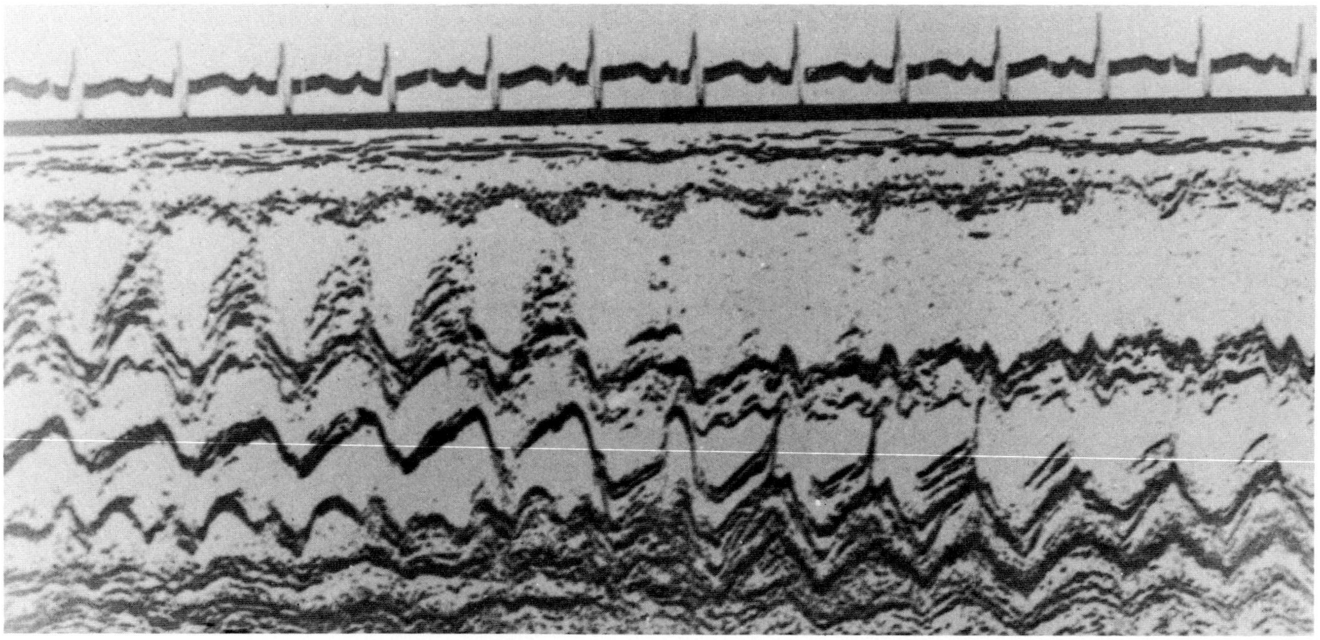

Figure 10-18

M-mode echocardiogram of a child who presents with left-to-right intracardiac shunt. The echocardiogram is taken at the level of the aortic valve with a slow-speed scan down into the cavity of the left ventricle. Note the undulating structure in the middle of the left atrium behind the aortic root.

10-18.1. The most likely diagnosis in this patient is:

A. Atrial septal defect, secundum type
B. Cor triatriatum
C. Pulmonary venous drainage into the coronary sinus
D. Congenital mitral stenosis

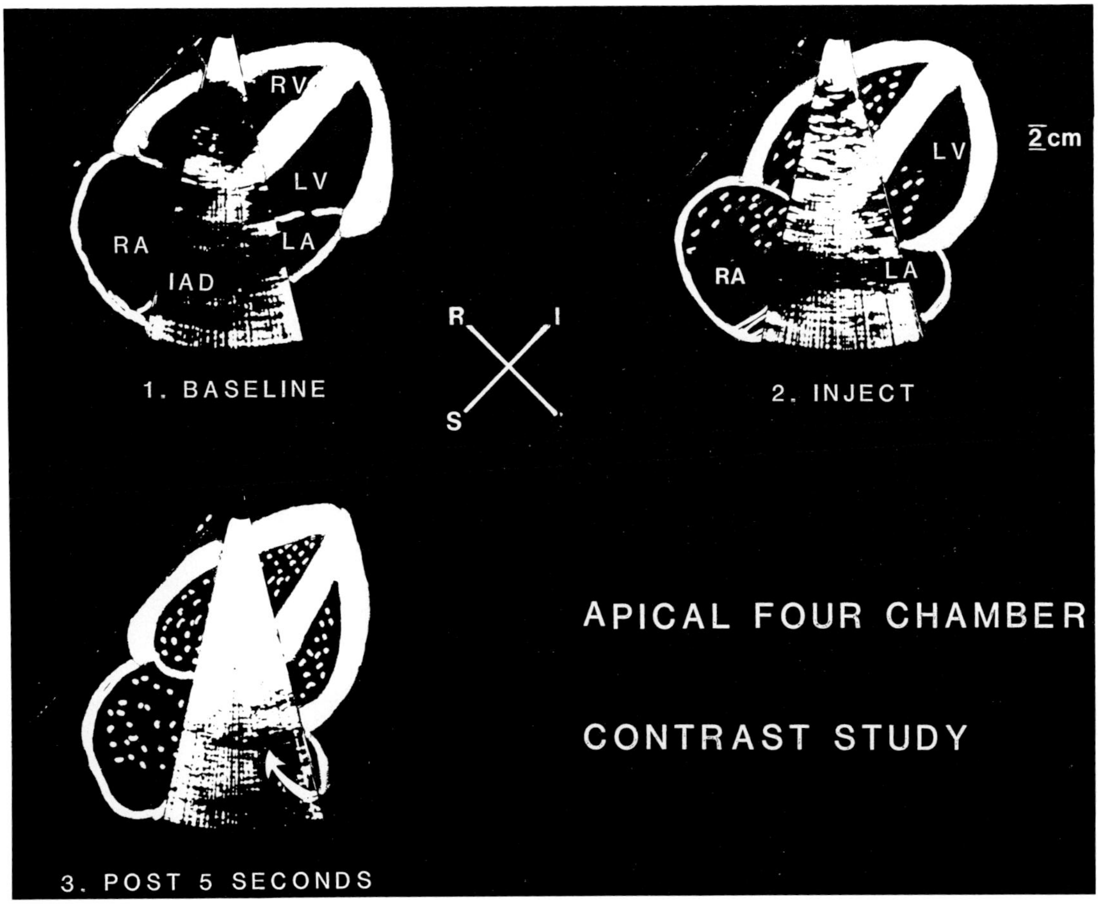

Figure 10-19

Mechanical 30° scan of a 45-year-old man with a large atrial septal defect and severe pulmonary hypertension (Eisenminger's syndrome). An apical four-chamber study was performed. (1) A baseline study demonstrates a large interatrial defect (IAD). (2) After a injection of normal saline, micro-bubbles are seen to fill the right atrium and right ventricle and to enter the left atrium and left ventricle (right-to-left-shunt). (3) After the micro-bubbles fill the right heart (5 seconds), a negative shadow is seen (arrow) in the left atrium, which crosses the interatrial defect and displaces micro-bubbles in the right atrium (small left-to-right shunt).

10-19.1. With respect to peripheral injection of saline in atrial septal defects and pulmonary hypertension:

A. Micro-bubbles are seen in the right atrium and then traverse the interatrial defect and are seen principally in the left atrium and ventricle (right-to-left shunt).

B. Micro-bubbles are seen in the right atrium and do not traverse the interatrial defect but are seen principally displaced by noncontrast blood entering from the left atrium (left-to-right shunt).

David J. Mehlman

11
Prosthetic Heart Valves

Noninvasive graphic techniques such as echocardiography and phonocardiography frequently assist the clinician in the recognition of prosthetic valve dysfunction. Although routine history and physical examination are useful in assessing prosthesis function, in many cases both can be misleading. For example, small changes in the timing of specific cardiac events may be crucial in the recognition of prosthesis obstruction, but these changes may not be apparent by auscultation. Likewise, in certain situations such as rhythm disturbances[1] or low cardiac output states, auscultatory events may be difficult to correlate with valvular function. Echocardiography and phonocardiography have been useful in assessing a number of complications of valve replacement, including paravalvular leak,[2] transvalvular regurgitation due to thrombus,[3] bioprosthetic leaflet disruption,[4] prosthesis stenosis due to thrombus,[5] inappropriately small prosthesis orifice,[6] obstruction to poppet movement,[7] stiffening of bioprosthetic leaflets,[8] thromboembolism, endocarditis,[9] and mechanical dysfunction such as ball variance[10] or disc escape.[11] Seventy percent of 118 patients operated upon for prosthetic valve dysfunction had abnormal echocardiograms or phonocardiograms preoperatively.[12]

During the past two decades of cardiac valve replacement, several different types of prosthetic valves have been developed in an effort to optimize hemodynamic characteristics and to minimize complications. All commercially available cardiac prostheses have a circular base ring, or sewing ring, by which the prosthesis is anchored to the valve annulus. This ring also supports the remaining portions of the valve. Mechanical prostheses are frequently subdivided into types on the basis of their "poppet"—the mobile part of the valve which permits blood to pass through the valve orifice. A number of prostheses, such as Braunwald-Cutter (Cutter Biomedical, San Diego), Smeloff-Cutter (Cutter Biomedical) and many Starr-Edwards (Edwards Laboratories, Santa Ana, CA) valves, employ a ball as a poppet. The ball moves from its seated position on the base ring to the apex of a relatively tall cage. As a small ventricle is not able to accommodate a ball-in-cage prosthesis in the atrioventricular position, "low-profile" prostheses were developed, in which the poppet is a disc. Several different types of disc valves have been in use. In the disc-in-cage prosthesis, the disc remains parallel to the plane of the base ring as it moves to the apex of the flattened cage. The Beall (Surgitool, Pittsburgh) and Kay-Shiley (Shiley Laboratories, Irvine, CA) valves are of this type. To preserve more centralized blood flow through the orifice, tilting-disc valves have been utilized. These valve types, such as the Bjork-Shiley (Shiley Laboratories) or Lillehei-Kaster (Medical Inc, Inver Grove Heights, MN) prosthetic valves, have a single tilting disc, which maneuvers on hinge points within or near the plane of the base ring. To maximize central flow, a double-tilting-disc valve, the St. Jude valve (St. Jude Medical, St. Paul, MN), has been designed. In this valve two hemicircular discs pivot along a diameter of the base ring. In bioprosthetic valves, delicate porcine aortic valve leaflets or pericardial tissues are suspended on a stent and fashioned into a trileaflet valve.

Phonocardiographic and echocardiographic findings differ for each valve type. To properly evaluate a patient with a prosthetic valve, the examiner must know the type of prosthesis being imaged. If this information is not available, a chest x-ray can show characteristic radiographic silhouettes.[13] As valve prostheses are best examined when the M-mode ultrasound beam is parallel to the major axis of poppet motion, the optimal transducer position will depend partly on the type of prosthesis to be examined. Excellent images are frequently obtained from the apical or suprasternal positions. As cardiac prostheses are often composed of highly reflective materials, extraneous echoes ("ringing") are frequently noted around the surrounding structures, particularly those behind the reflective object. These echoes may mimic pathologic findings such as thrombus or vegetation. Examining the same structures from different chest wall positions and comparing the echogram with previous ones may help distinguish artifact from pathology.

Auscultation and phonocardiography reveal that ball-in-cage prostheses produce relatively loud, frequently metallic-like sounds on opening and closing. The early models of the normally functioning Starr-Edwards aortic ball prostheses have an opening sound amplitude at least half (and often equal to or greater than) that of the closing sound.[14] Multiple additional clicks may be produced by the normally functioning aortic or mitral ball-in-cage prosthesis in the open position as it "bounces" on the apex or sides of the cage. The low-profile disc-in-cage valves produce relatively loud opening and closing sounds as well. On the other hand, the tilting-disc valves may produce a low-amplitude opening sound, though the closing sound remains loud and of high frequency. The bioprosthetic valves may produce very low-amplitude opening sounds. The closing sounds are similar in quality to native valve sounds.

With prostheses in the mitral position, the interval between aortic valve closure and mitral valve opening (A2–MVO), measured by phonocardiographic or echophonocardiographic techniques, is a potentially useful noninvasive index of prosthetic valve function. As with native mitral stenosis, the A2–MVO interval of the prosthetic mitral valve reflects the aortic pressure at the time of aortic valve closing, the rate at which the left ventricular pressure falls during late systole, and, particularly, the left atrial pressure at the time of mitral valve opening. Fortunately, significant changes in left ventricular or aortic valve function over a short period of time are relatively unusual, and their presence may well be indicated on an echocardiogram. With increasing left atrial pressure (as would occur with either prosthetic valve orifice obstruction or paravalvular or transvalvular regurgitation), the A2–MVO interval generally decreases.[15] On the other hand, if the poppet or leaflets in the mitral prosthesis cannot move freely, the valve is likely to open late or erratically, reflected by a prolonged or variable A2–MVO interval.[16] A2–MVO intervals of less than 0.07 or more than 0.12 sec suggest possible valve dysfunction. These findings have considerably more meaning if changes in serial recordings can be demonstrated.

Echocardiographically, the status of a prosthesis can be determined directly by examining the prosthesis itself or indirectly by examining the other cardiac structures. Postoperatively, the interventricular septal motion is usually paradoxical; although septal motion may normalize in some patients with passage of time, *normal* septal motion in the period shortly after aortic or mitral valve replacement is suggestive of paravalvular or transvalvular regurgitation.[17] Prosthetic aortic regurgitation can produce fluttering of the anterior mitral valve leaflet or interventricular septum, or, if massive, can cause premature closure of the mitral valve. Narrowing of the orifice of a mitral prosthesis would be expected to decrease the emptying rate of the left atrium and thus affect posterior aortic wall motion.[18] Obstruction across the mitral valve would produce similar changes in the diastolic motion of the posterior left ventricular wall.[19] Narrowing of the left ventricular outflow tract (the distance between the anterior portion of a mitral valve prosthesis and the interventricular septum) might explain a low cardiac output in the early postsurgical period.[20] After valve replacement, depending on the clinical situation, one expects enlarged cardiac chambers to stabilize or return towards normal in size. If, for example, left atrial size continues to increase after valve replacement for mitral stenosis, or if a left ventricular overload pattern persists or worsens after valve replacement for mitral regurgitation, valve dysfunction or left ventricular dysfunction might be suspected. Complications such as atrial thrombi can be detected by M-mode or two-dimensional echocardiography.[21] With two-dimensional echocardiographic techniques, disturbances in left ventricular wall motion are more easily evaluated. Since left ventricular dysfunction may mimic the signs and symptoms of prosthetic valve dysfunction,[22] a two-dimensional echocardiogram is a very useful diagnostic test in this patient group. In all of these situations, as well as those to follow, the importance of serial studies cannot be overemphasized. Each patient undergoing valve replacement should have a noninvasive postoperative evaluation to establish a baseline valve profile for future studies.

BALL-IN-CAGE PROSTHESES

Figure 11-1 shows an echocardiogram of a Starr-Edwards aortic valve, which is similar echocardiographically to the Smeloff-Cutter (Cutter Biomedical), Magovern (Surgitool, Pittsburgh), and other ball-in-cage prostheses. This valve is imaged from the cardiac apex; in other patients adequate studies could be obtained from the supraclavicular or suprasternal positions. The electrocardiogram is recorded with the prosthesis tracing in order to identify the onset of ventricular systole. At the end of the QRS complex, the ball moves away from the sewing ring; since the transducer is at the cardiac apex, this is recorded as movement away from the transducer. The opening velocity can be determined by measuring the slope of the echo that represents ball motion. On reaching maximal excursion, the ball hits the apex of the cage, thus producing the aortic opening sound. The ball is seen to move several millimeters towards the sewing ring before reopening fully, at which time an additional sound is produced. The distance between the sewing ring and the ball echo in systole represents the excursion of the ball. The ball remains in the open position until the end of systole, at which time it moves towards the sewing ring; it merges with the ring throughout diastole. The closing velocity is the slope of the line representing movement of the ball towards the sewing ring. When the ball merges with the sewing ring, a closing sound is produced. The opening sound of the valve is as great in amplitude as the closing sound.

Similar echoes are produced by the ball valves in the tricuspid or mitral positions, although valve opening is, of course, a diastolic event. As sound travels slowly through silastic, balls frequently produce posterior echo "ghosts," giving the false impression that a large ball is located behind the valve's posterior structures.[23]

Early silastic balls infrequently absorbed blood lipids, causing the poppet to swell, split, or fracture, producing "ball variance" and impeding poppet movement.[24] For ball valves in the aortic position this was recognized with noninvasive techniques as an absent or diminished aortic opening sound.[14] Although false positives and false negatives occurred with phonocardiography,[25] many patients whose opening sound was less than half the amplitude of the closing sound were demonstrated to have poppet malfunction.[14] In the mitral position, ball variance produced a delay in mitral valve opening, causing a variable or prolonged A2–MVO interval. Echocardiographically, this phenomenon was represented as delayed, erratic, or partial valve opening.[10] Any structure that interferes with poppet motion, such as thrombus on the sewing ring or cage, septal or papillary muscle within the cage, or vegetation, could produce similar findings.

DISC-IN-CAGE PROSTHESES

As in the ball-in-cage valve, the disc, cage, and sewing ring of the disc-in-cage prosthesis each produce prominent echoes. As shown in Figure 11-2, the sewing ring moves slowly anteriorly at the end of diastole, and the disc echo merges with the sewing ring. At the time of mitral valve opening, the disc begins to move rapidly forward and the sewing ring and cage move slowly posteriorly; the disc echo merges during diastole with the strut or cage echo. If free movement of the disc is impaired, its rapid forward movement at the beginning of diastole is

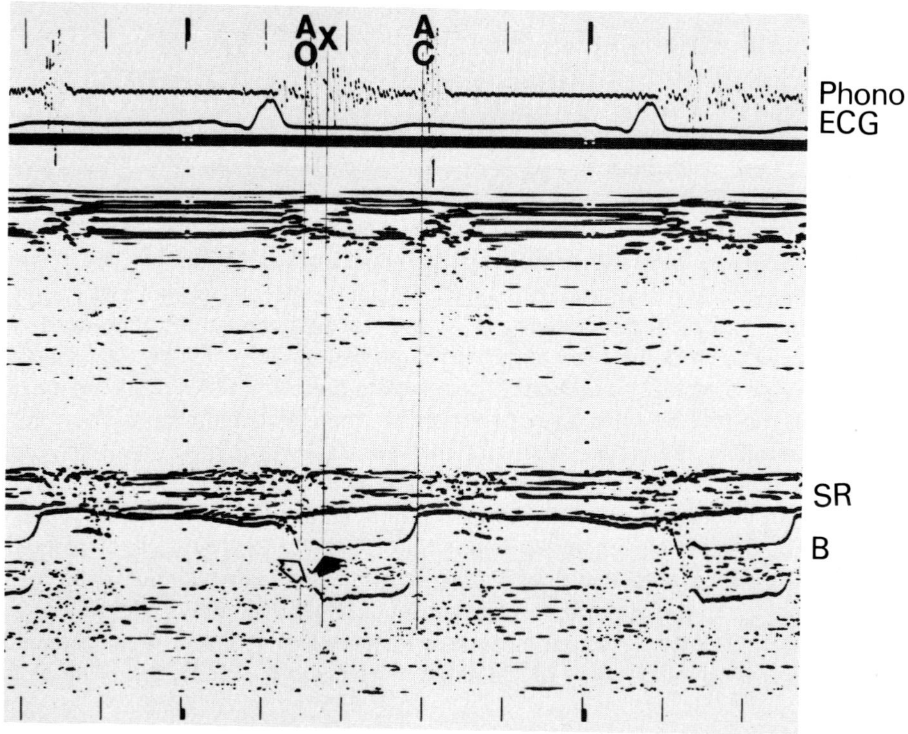

Figure 11-1
Starr-Edwards ball-in-cage prosthesis in the aortic position, imaged from the cardiac apex. The open arrow indicates initial ball movement to the open position at the onset of systole. The ball moves slightly towards the closed position, and then fully opens again, as indicated by the solid arrow. The vertical lines show that the cardiac sound representing aortic valve opening (AO), aortic valve reopening (X), and aortic valve closure (AC) correspond to ball movement. (SR, sewing ring; B, ball.)

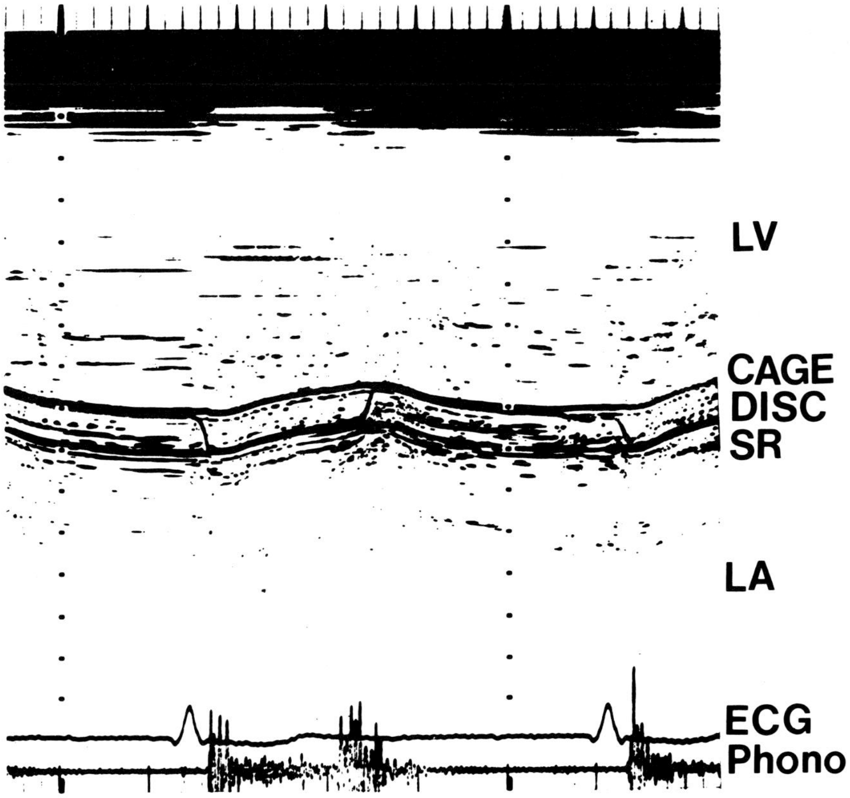

Figure 11-2

Beall disc-in-cage prosthesis in the mitral position imaged from the cardiac apex.

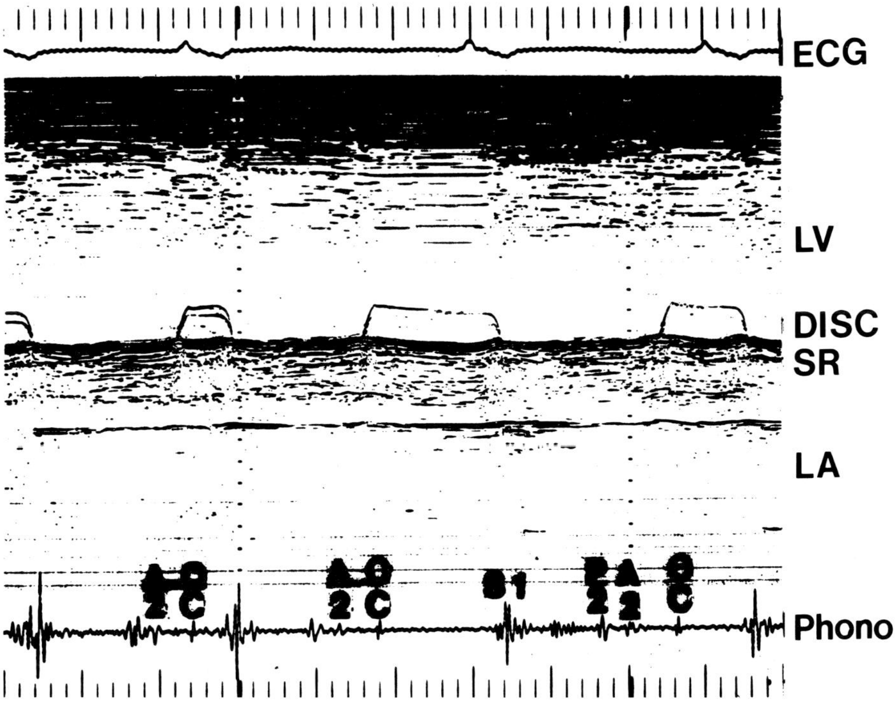

Figure 11-3

Bjork-Shiley tilting-disc prosthesis in the mitral position imaged from the cardiac apex. The excursion of the disc is approximately 9 mm. The patient has left bundle branch block with reversed splitting of the second heart sound. As a result, A2 (aortic valve closure) follows P2 (pulmonary valve closure). The origin of the sound was confirmed by echophonocardiography (not shown). (S1, first heart sound; OC, mitral opening sound.)

delayed. An exaggerated anterior early diastolic movement ("hump") of the disc, cage, and ring has been described in several patients with paravalvular or transvalvular regurgitation.[26]

TILTING-DISC PROSTHESES

The echogram of the tilting disc valve reveals the sewing ring and disc, as shown in Figure 11-3. Disc motion is limited by small structures (not seen on the echogram) within the plane of the sewing ring. Because of asymmetry of the valve, a variety of different echoes can be obtained, some of which are not interpretable. Infrequent cases of valve thrombosis have been reported in inadequately anticoagulated patients. Echograms of these valves reveal reduced or absent disc movement, with dense echoes from the thrombus filling the area where disc motion would be expected.[27,28]

DOUBLE-TILTING-DISC PROSTHESES

The St. Jude prosthetic valve has a characteristic echographic pattern in which two "parallel" lines are seen within the sewing ring when the valve is open. The parallel lines represent the two hemicircular disc leaflets. When the valve leaflets are closed, the lines are no longer seen (Figure 11-4).

BIOPROSTHETIC VALVES

Bioprosthetic valves have large sewing rings and stents from which the leaflets are suspended. The sewing ring and stent are very reflective, so that in

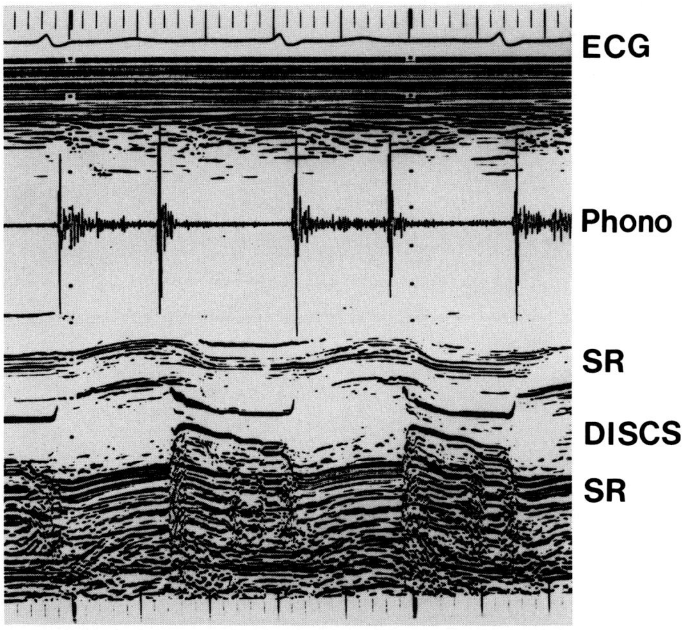

Figure 11-4
St. Jude double-tilting disc valve in the mitral position, showing the "parallel" motion of the two leaflets while the valve is open. The phonocardiogram shows a loud closing sound due to the prosthesis, but the opening sound is of low amplitude.

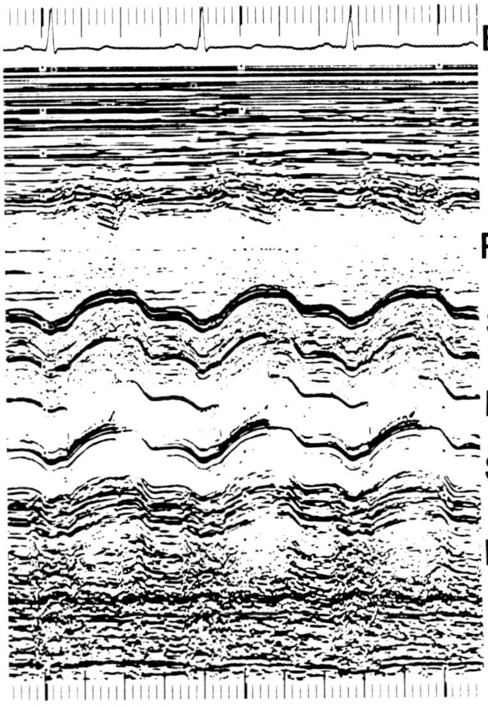

Figure 11-5

Ionescu-Shiley pericardial valve (Shiley Laboratories) in the aortic annulus imaged from the left parasternal position. The boxlike opening is demonstrated during systole.

examining the struts and sewing ring it is sometimes necessary to increase reject and damping; the reverse may be needed to visualized the valve leaflets.[29] As shown in Figure 11-5, anterior and posterior stents are recorded with the valve leaflets. In both the aortic and mitral positions, leaflet motion produces echoes similar to the trileaflet echo of the normal native aortic valve opening. Frequently, the entire trapezoid cannot be recorded (Figure 11-6). Immobility of the leaflets due to calcification or thrombosis of these valves has been demonstrated (Figure

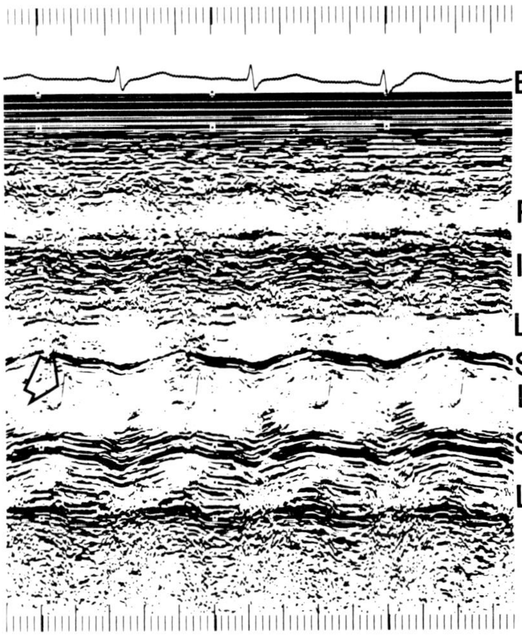

Figure 11-6

Hancock porcine heterograft valve (Hancock Lab, Anaheim, CA) in the mitral annulus, imaged from the left parasternal chest wall. The box-like opening is demonstrated during diastole. However, only the initial portion of the valve leaflet motion (open arrow) is clearly seen.

Figure 11-7

Hancock porcine heterograft valve in the aortic position, imaged from the left parasternal position, in a patient with prosthetic aortic valve regurgitation and stenosis. Dense echoes in the anterior portion of the aortic root seen during late diastole and early systole represent calcification on the aortic valve prosthesis. There is persistent separation of the aortic valve leaflets during diastole, with fine flutter related to severe aortic regurgitation. The boxlike opening of the leaflets during systole is reduced and displaced posteriorly, probably related to aortic stenosis. (AAR, anterior aortic root; ?Ca^{++}, calcification of prosthetic leaflets; PAR, posterior aortic root.)

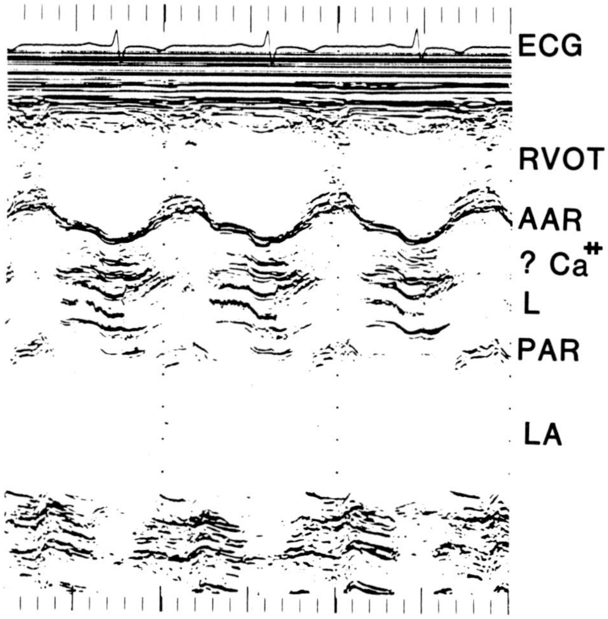

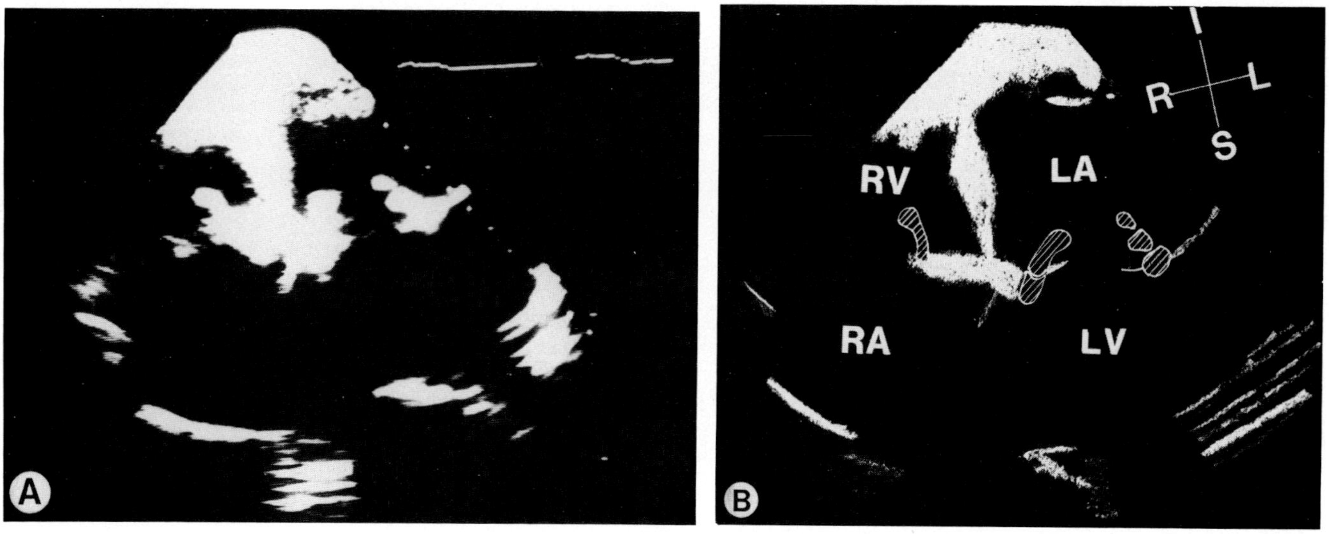

Figure 11-8

Two-dimensional echocardiogram (A) and line drawing (B) of mitral and tricuspid Hancock heterograft valves in the four-chamber apical view during diastole. Two mitral prosthesis stents (cross-hatched areas) are seen, with a small portion of the valve leaflets. Only one of the tricuspid prosthesis stents (cross-hatched area) is imaged.

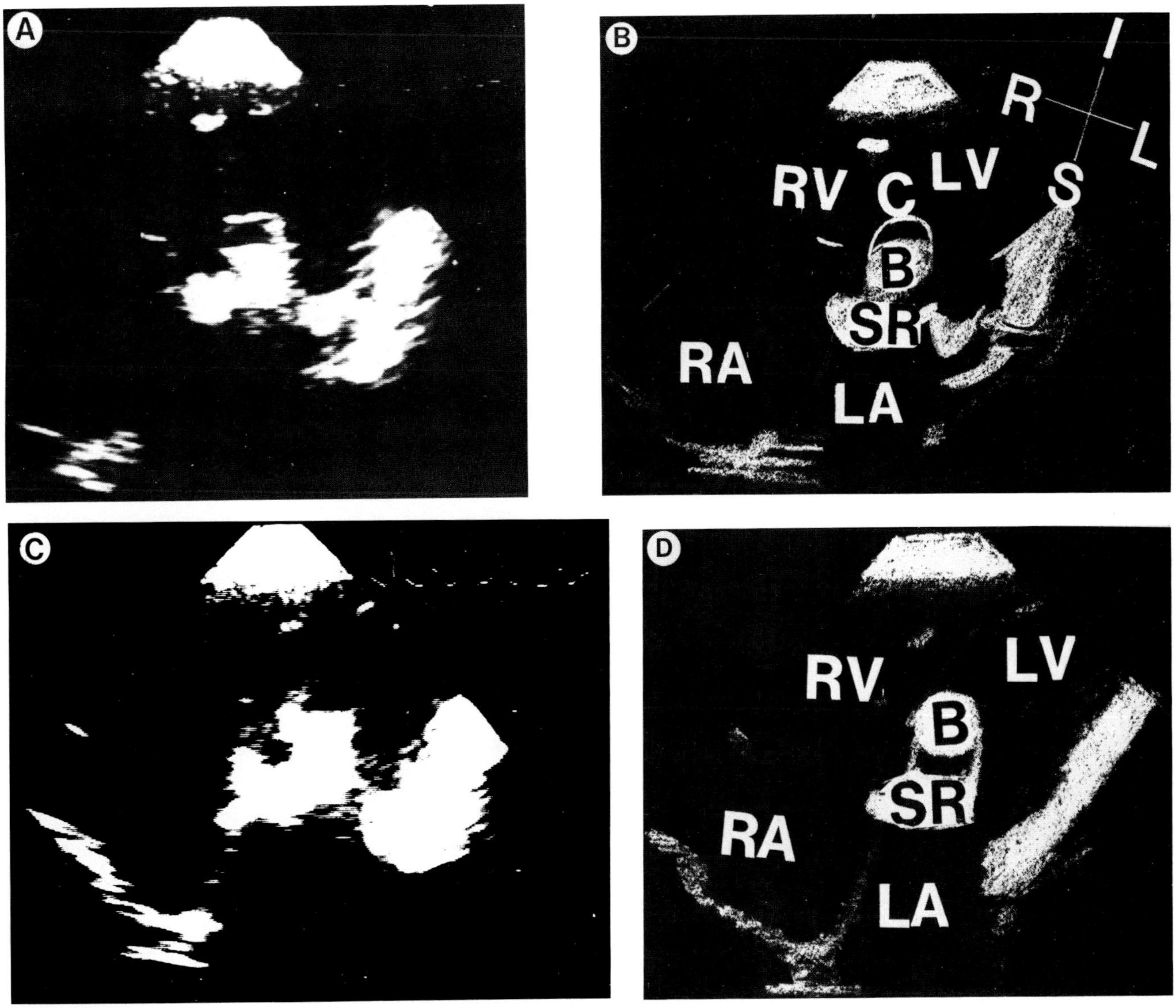

Figure 11-9

Two-dimensional echocardiograms and line drawings of a Starr-Edwards ball-in-cage mitral valve during systole (A, B) and diastole (C, D). (C, cage; B, ball.)

11-7), and abnormal leaflet flutter or prolapse has been noted in patients with disrupted leaflets.[8]

TWO-DIMENSIONAL ECHOCARDIOGRAPHY

Two-dimensional techniques can provide additional information concerning valve function. Representative two-dimensional echocardiograms from patients with bioprosthetic and mechanical prosthetic valves are shown in Figures 11-8 and 11-9. The rocking motion of a partially dehiscent valve is more easily detected with this technique,[22] although it can also be detected with M-mode echocardiography.[30] Certain complications of valve replacement such as left atrial clots[21] or left ventricular dysfunction[22] also may be more easily detected with this method. As spatial relationships are more clearly defined with two-dimensional echocardiography, suspected abnormalities may be more accurately localized and quantitated. In addition, extraneous echoes (such as reverberations) may often be distinguished from pathologic echoes (such as clots). In patients with more than one prosthetic valve, two-dimensional echocardiographic techniques permit definitive identification of the annular position of the prosthesis being examined. With many two-dimensional echocardiographs, one may place an M-mode cursor through the imaged two-dimensional plane, so that an M-mode tracing from a specifically identified valve annulus can be obtained.

REFERENCES

1. Brown DF: Decreased intensity of closure sound in a normally functioning Starr-Edwards mitral valve prosthesis. Am J Cardiol 31:93-97, 1973
2. Miller HC, Gibson DB, Stephens JD: Role of echocardiography and phonocardiography in diagnosis of mitral paraprosthetic regurgitation with Starr-Edwards prostheses. Brit Heart J 35:1217-1225, 1973
3. Bloch WN, Felner JM, Wickliffe C, Symbas PN: Echocardiographic diagnosis of thrombus on a heterograft in the mitral position. Chest 70:399-401, 1976
4. Bloch WN, Felner JM, Schlant RC, Symbas PN, Jones EL: The echocardiogram of the porcine aortic bioprosthesis in the aortic position. Chest 72:640-646, 1977
5. Fernandez J, Samuel A, Yang SS, Sumathisena S, Gooch A, Maranhao V, et al: Late thrombosis of the aortic Bjork-Shiley prosthesis. Chest 70:12-16, 1976
6. Wise JR Jr, Webb-Peploe M, Oakley CM: Detection of prosthetic mitral valve obstruction by phonocardiography. Am J Cardiol 28:107-110, 1971
7. Pfeifer J, Goldschlager N, Sweatman T, Gerbode F, Selzer A: Malfunction of mitral ball prosthesis due to thrombus. Am J Cardiol 29:95-99, 1972
8. Alam M, Madrazo AC, Magilligan DJ, Goldstein S: M-mode and two-dimensional echocardiographic features of porcine valve dysfunction. Am J Cardiol 43:502-509, 1979
9. Schelbert HR, Muller OF: Detection of fungal vegetations by means of ultrasound. Vascular Surg 6:20-25, 1972
10. Schluger J, Mannix EP, Wolf RE: Auscultatory and phonocardiographic sign of ball variance in a mitral prosthetic valve. Am Heart J 91:809-816, 1971
11. Schaeffer JW, Marks SD, Wolf PS, Shander D, Craddock LD, Blount SG Jr: Systemic embolization of the disk occluder of the Wada-Cutter prosthetic valve. Chest 71:44-46, 1977
12. Cunha CLP, Giuliani ER, Callahan JA, Pluth JR: Echophonocardiographic findings in patients with prosthetic valve malfunction. Mayo Clin Proc 55:231-242, 1980
13. Mehlman DJ, Resnekov L: A guide to the radiographic identification of prosthetic heart valves. Circulation 57:613-623, 1978
14. Hylen JC, Kloster FE, Starr A, Griswold HE: Aortic ball variance: Diagnosis and treatment. Ann Int Med 72:1-8, 1970
15. Willerson JT, Kastor JA, Dinsmore RE, Mundth E, Buckley MJ, Austen WG, et al: Non-invasive assessment of prosthetic mitral paravalvular and intravalvular regurgitation. Brit Heart J 34:561-568, 1972
16. Kawai N, Segal BL, Linhart JW: Delayed opening of Beall mitral prosthetic valve detected by echocardiography. Chest 67:239-241, 1975
17. Burggraf GW, Craige E: Echocardiographic studies of left ventricular wall motion and dimensions after valvular heart surgery. Am J Cardiol 35:473-480, 1975
18. Strunk BL, London EJ, Fitzgerald J, Popp RL, Barry WH: The assessment of mitral

stenosis and prosthetic valve obstruction, using the posterior aortic wall echocardiogram. Circulation 55:885-891, 1977

19. Wise JR Jr: Echocardiographic evaluation of mitral stenosis using diastolic posterior left ventricular wall motion. Circulation 61:1037-1042, 1980
20. Nanda NC, Gramiak R, Shah PM, DeWeese JA, Mahoney EB: Echocardiographic assessment of left ventricular outflow width in the selection of mitral valve prosthesis. Circulation 48:1208-1214, 1973
21. Mikell FL, Asinger RW, Rourke T, Hodges M, Sharma B, Francis GS: Two-dimensional echocardiographic demonstration of left atrial thrombi in patients with prosthetic mitral valves. Circulation 60:183-190, 1979
22. Schapira JN, Martin RP, Fowles RE, Rakowski H, Stinson EB, French JW: Two-dimensional echocardiographic assessment of patients with bioprosthetic valves. Am J Cardiol 43:510-519, 1979
23. Johnson ML, Paton BC, Holmes JH: Ultrasonic evaluation of prosthetic valve motion. Circulation 41, 42(suppl 2):-3-7, 1970
24. McHenry MM, Smeloff EA, Fong WY, Miller GE Jr, Ryan PM: Critical obstruction of prosthetic heart valves due to lipid absorption by Silastic. J Thor Cardiovasc Surg 59:413-425, 1970
25. Delman AJ, Attai LA, Naida S, Robinson G: Limitations of phonocardiographic assessment of ball variance. Ann Thor Surg 10:278-284, 1970
26. Yuste P, Aza V, Minguez I, Asin E, Martinez-Bordiu C: Echocardiographic evaluation of mitral valve prosthesis malfunction, in Kazner E, deVlieger M, Muller HR, McCready VR (eds): Ultrasonics in Medicine. Amsterdam, Excerpta Medica, 1975, 239-244
27. Ben-Zvi J, Hildner FJ, Chandraratna PA, Samet P: Thrombosis on Bjork-Shiley aortic valve prosthesis. Am J Cardiol 34:538-544, 1974
28. Copans H, Lakier JB, Kinsley RH, Colsen PR, Fritz VU, Barlow JB: Thrombosed Bjork-Shiley mitral prosthesis. Circulation 61:169-174, 1980
29. Chandraratna PAN, San Pedro SB: Echocardiographic features of the normal and malfunctioning porcine xenograft valve. Am Heart J 95:548-554, 1978
30. Berndt TB, Goodman DJ, Popp RL: Echocardiographic and phonocardiographic confirmation of suspected caged mitral valve malfunction. Chest 70:221-230, 1976

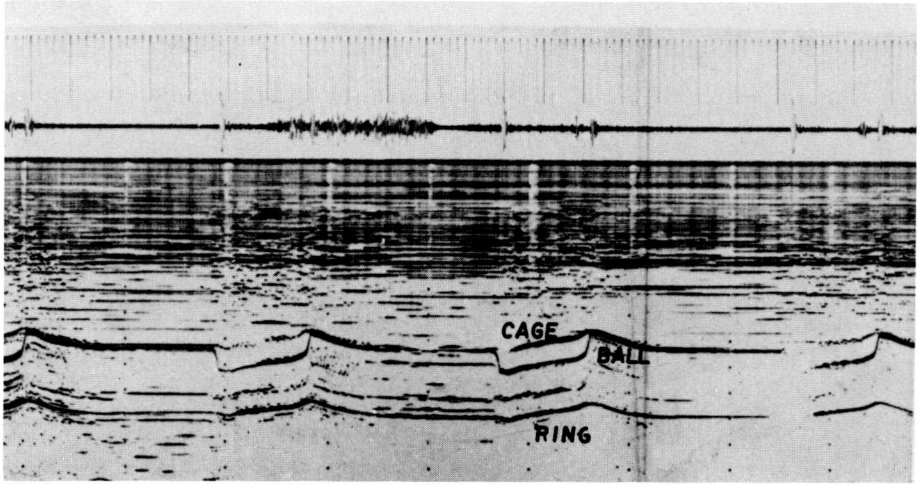

Figure 11-10

Starr-Edwards ball-in-cage mitral valve. Note the phonocardiogram taken at the apex of the left ventricle.

11-10.1. With respect to the caged-ball mitral valve, which of the following statements are correct?

A. The closing velocity of the ball should always be greater than the opening velocity.

B. The excursion of the ball during diastole should be constant from beat to beat.

C. In a normally functioning mitral caged-ball valve, the aortic closure to opening click interval should be variable.

D. For correct visualization of the caged-ball valve, the transducer should be placed at the apex and oriented parallel to the opening direction of the valve.

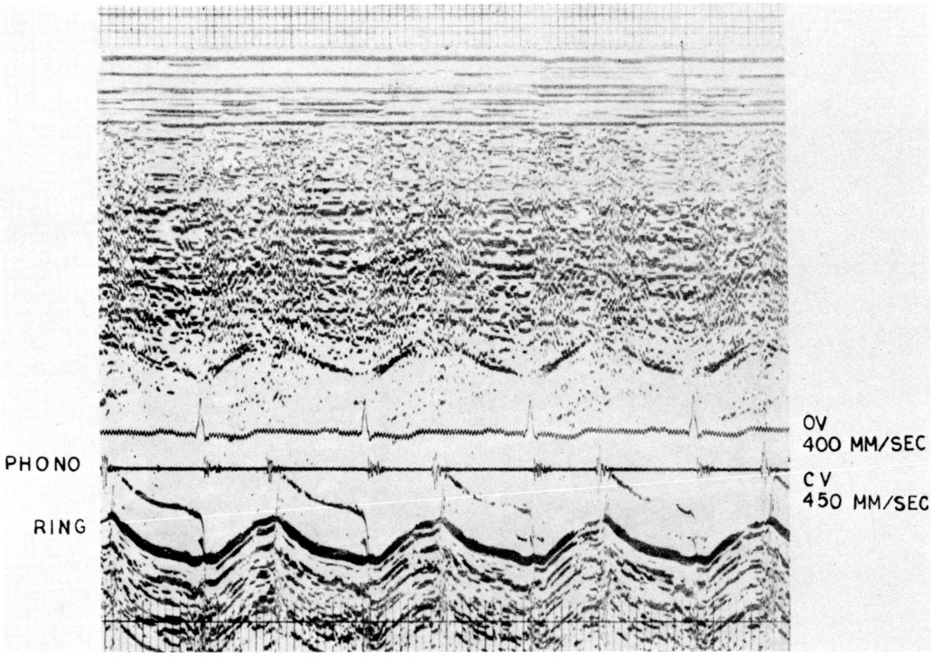

Figure 11-11

Normal Bjork-Shiley tilting-disc mitral valve. The phonocardiogram is recorded at the apex. The ring of the valve is marked, the disc excursion is seen during diastole. (OV, opening velocity; CV, closing velocity.)

11-11.1. With respect to the tilting-disc valve, which of the following statements are correct?

A. The closing click of the valve is generally heard.
B. The opening click of the valve is generally not heard.
C. A sewing ring and cage echo are commonly seen.
D. The disc excursion could be variable.

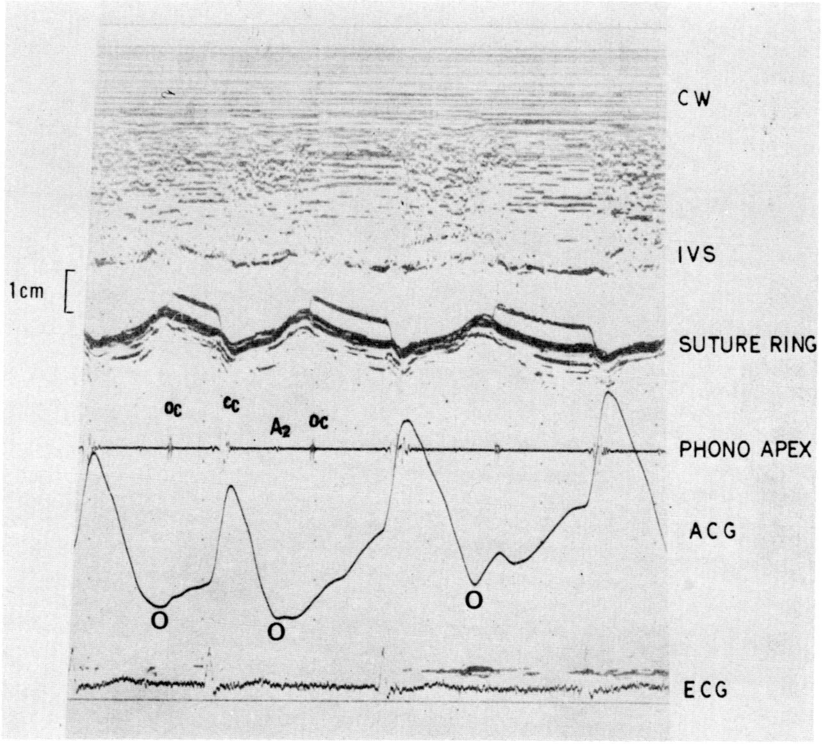

Figure 11-12

This is a prosthetic Beall disc-in-cage mitral valve taken from an asymptomatic patient. The echocardiogram is shown with a phonocardiogram taken at the left ventricular apex, an apex cardiogram (ACG) to demonstrate the opening click (OC) of the mitral valve, and the electrocardiogram. (A2, aortic second sound; CC, closing click of the valve.)

11-12.1. With respect to this valve, which of the following statements are correct?

A. There is a delay in opening of the disc.

B. The A2 to opening click interval is variable and abnormal.

C. The opening click of the valve occurs after the 0 point of the apex cardiogram, which is abnormal.

D. There is early sticking of the disc.

E. All of the above.

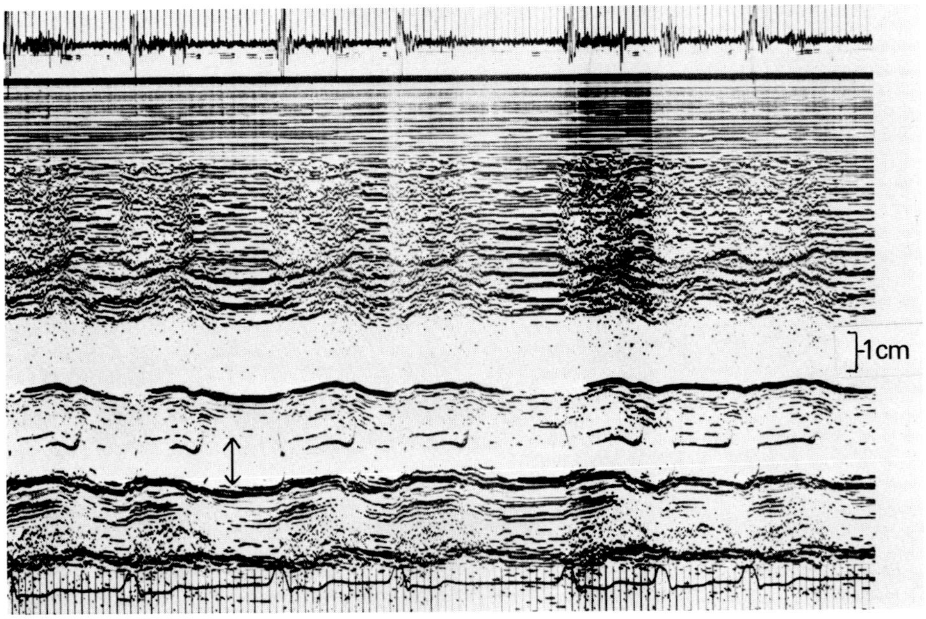

Figure 11-13

Echocardiogram of a 57-year-old man who underwent porcine heterograft mitral valve replacement for idiopathic hypertrophic subaortic stenosis. The echocardiogram shows the porcine mitral valve with a phonocardiogram from the apex.

11-13.1. With respect to the heterograft mitral valves, which of the following statements are correct?

A. The duration of the heterograft mitral valve opening is variable due to malfunctioning of the porcine valve.

B. The opening duration of the mitral valve is variable due to the atrial arrhythmia.

C. The heterograft mitral valve has a diminished excursion (arrows).

D. The heterograft mitral valve appears stenotic.

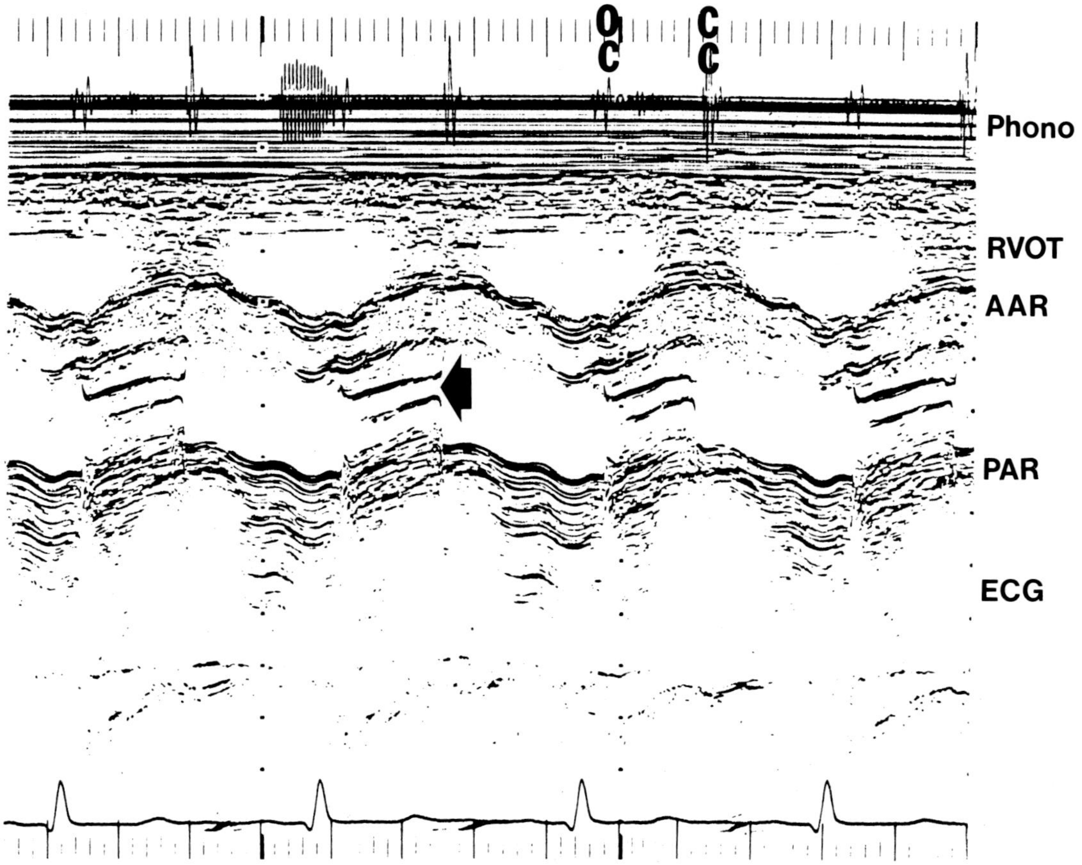

Figure 11-14

Echocardiogram of a 33-year-old male who underwent aortic valve replacement with a St. Jude double-tilting disc aortic valve. The two leaflets are seen to converge during valve opening. While the valve is open, the two leaflets appear as parallel lines in the middle of the aortic root, indicated by the large arrow. (AAR, anterior aortic root, PAR, posterior arotic root.)

11-14.1. With respect to the prosthetic valve, which of the following statements are correct?

A. The opening sound of the aortic valve is commonly heard.

B. The closing sound of the aortic valve is commonly heard.

C. The opening velocity and closing velocity appears delayed.

D. The opening velocity and closing velocity appears normal.

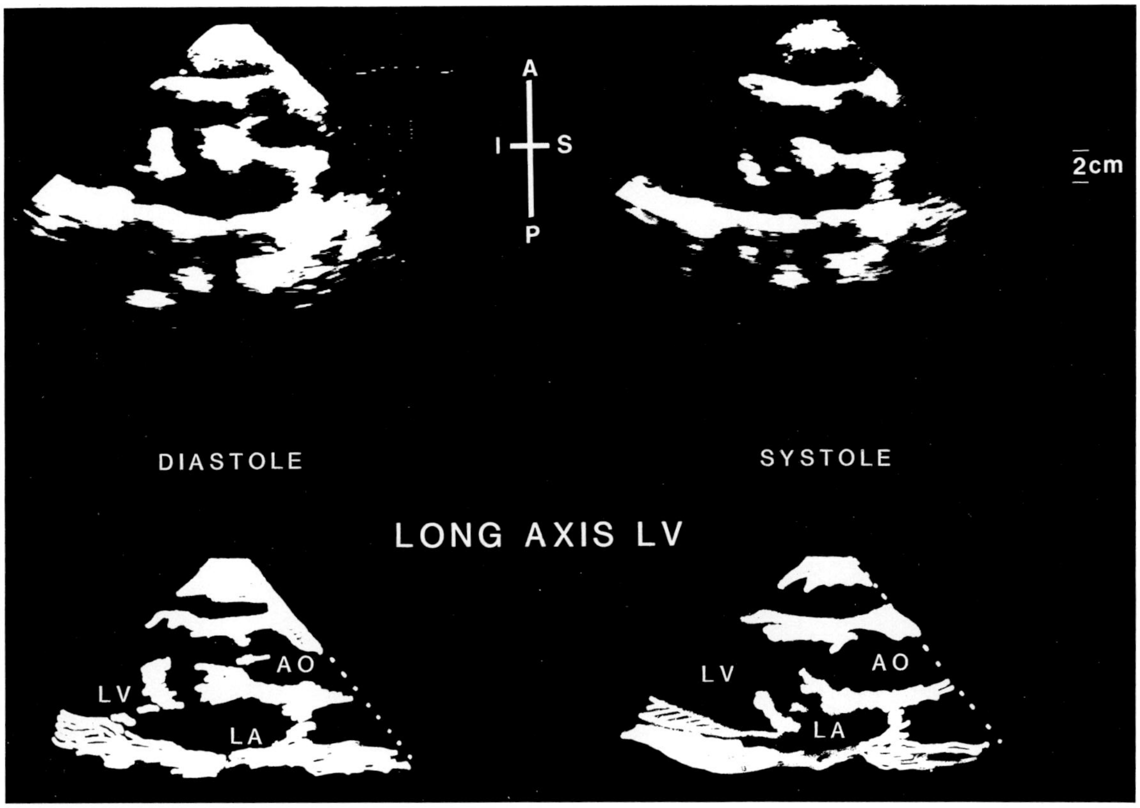

Figure 11-15

Phased-array 90° echocardiogram of a 29-year-old man who underwent mitral valve replacement for bacterial endocarditis and ruptured chordae tendineae. The mitral valve was replaced with a porcine heterograft valve. Echocardiogram was taken in long axis of the left ventricle. Note the prominent valve stents anteriorly and posteriorly. During systole, note the procine leaflets in the closed position.

11-15.1. With respect to the heterograft mitral valve, which of the following statements are correct?

A. The leaflets can become obstructed by thrombus.
B. The leaflets can calcify.
C. The leaflets can become flail.
D. The leaflets can develop prolapse.
E. All of the above.

James V. Talano

12

Left Ventricular Function by Two-Dimensional Echocardiography

M-mode echocardiography is useful in estimation of left ventricular function. However, the formulas used assume the ellipsoid configuration to the ventricle. As the ventricle enlarges in valvular or segmental myocardial disease, the changes in configuration are less predictable and the method of estimation by M-mode becomes less valid. Several methods of determining left ventricular function by two-dimensional echocardiography have been developed. This chapter will describe the single-plane ellipsoid method, the biplane ellipsoid method, and Simpson's rule method (modified).

SINGLE-PLANE ELLIPSOID METHOD

In this method, the apical long-axis view of the left ventricle is obtained by selecting the apical four-chamber view and then rotating the transducer 90° counterclockwise from the apical four-chamber view. The right ventricular structures will be out of the scan plane which cuts through the anterior and inferior myocardial walls. Stop frames are taken at end diastole (onset QRS complex) and end systole (systolic chamber size). The endocardial surface is then traced for each frame either directly from the screen or from a polaroid or silver-processed printout, and the grid method of calculation (a transparent grid consisting of 3 × 3 cm squares) is made from the calibration marks recorded from the two-dimensional image. The construction grid is then planimetered* and a correction factor calculated according to the following formula:

$$K = \frac{\text{number of cm}^2 \text{ of grid}}{\text{planimetered area of the grid}}$$

where K = correction factor.

*Use calibration marks on screen or paper to measure length (L).

The area of the left ventricular cavity is then planimetered each for a diastolic and systolic frame. The planimetered area (A_P) is then corrected for the true area (A_{LV}) by the formula.

$$A_{LV} = A_P \times K$$

The long axis of the left ventricle (L) is obtained by measuring the length from the apex to the left ventricle to the midpoint of the mitral valve.* The area (A_{LV}) and length (L) are then used for calculation of left ventricular volume (V) in diastole and systole by the following formula:

$$V = \frac{8\,(A_{LV})^2}{3\pi L}$$

$$EDV = \frac{8\,(A_{Ld})^2}{3\pi L_d}$$

$$ESV = \frac{8\,(A_{L_s})^2}{3\pi L_s}$$

$$EF = \frac{EDV - ESV}{EDV}$$

where A_{L_d} is the area of left ventricle in diastole, A_{L_s} is area of left ventricle in systole, L_d is length of the left ventricle in diastole, L_s is length of the left ventricle in systole, EDV is end-diastolic volume, ESV is end-systolic volume, and EF is ejection fraction.

BIPLANE ELLIPSOID METHOD

Two left ventricular projections are selected. This method assumes that the left ventricle is an ellipsoid. As with the single-plane method, the apical four-chamber view is utilized for one projection, and the short-axis view taken at the mitral valve is selected for the second projection. The recorded projections are taken at end diastole (onset of QRS complex) and end systole (smallest systolic size or at the end of the T wave). The area of the left ventricle is outlined and planimetered in each view in both diastolic and systolic frames. The planimetered areas are corrected using the previously obtained correction factor (K):

$$A_{LV_{sx}} = A_P \text{ (short axis)} \times K$$

$$A_{LV_{AP}} = A_P \text{ (four chamber)} \times K$$

where

$A_{LV_{SX}}$ = short-axis area of the left ventricle
$A_{LV_{AP}}$ = apical-view area of the left ventricle

The areas are then substituted using the biplane formula of Sandler and Dodge. The minor axis in apical view (D_{AP}) is calculated from the following formula:

$$D_{AP} = \frac{4(A_{LV_{AP}})}{\pi L_{LV}}$$

*Use calibration marks on screen or paper to measure length (L).

The long axis of the left ventricle (L_{LV}) is measured from the apex to the midpoint of the mitral valve in the apical four-chamber view. The minor axis short-axis view (D_{SX}) is calculated from the following formula:

$$D_{sx} = \frac{4(A_{LV_{SX}})}{\pi d_s}$$

where d_s is measured from the endocardial surface of the posterior lateral left ventricle to the endocardial surface of the interventricular septum. Therefore, the left ventricular volumes are calculated by the following formula:

$$EDV = \frac{\pi}{6} L_{LV}(D_{AP})\,(D_{SX})$$

$$\text{Ejection fraction} = \frac{EDV - ESV}{EDV}$$

LEFT VENTRICULAR VOLUME USING MODIFIED SIMPSON'S RULE

Simpson's rule is a method used to calculate an area under a curve by dividing it into multiple sections and solving for each individual section. The sum of the section approximates the entire area under the curve. To determine left ventricular volumes using Simpson's method, three two-dimensional views are utilized: (1) the apical four-chamber view, (2) the parasternal short-axis view of the left ventricle at the base of the papillary muscle, and (3) the parasternal short-axis view at the mitral valve. The views are taken and recorded. The endocardial surface is traced in both a systolic and diastolic frame for the left ventricular cavity from the short-axis left ventricular view (A_{PM}) and the short-axis mitral valve view (A_{MV}) by planimetering the left ventricular traces. The true area is obtained by using the calculated correction factor (K). The apical four-chamber view is used to measure the longest length of the left ventricle by measuring from the apex to the midpoint of the mitral valve. The three sections are used to calculate the left ventricular volume according to the Simpson's rule with the assumption that the left ventricle from base to apex is a composite of a cylinder, a truncated cone, and a cone. The formulas using the three sections are:

(1) cylinder is $V = (\pi r^2)h$

(2) truncated cone is $V = \dfrac{(\pi r^2 a + \pi r^2 b)h}{2}$

(3) cone is $V = 1/3(\pi r^2)h$

where h is height of the ventricle and r is the radius of the left ventricle. Assuming that each section is equal in length, then $h = L/3$. Therefore the left ventricular volumes can be solved by the formula:

$$V = \frac{(\pi r^2)\,L/3 + (\pi r^2 a + \pi r^2 b)\,L/3 + 1/3(\pi r^2)\,L/3}{2}$$

$$\text{Ejection fraction} = \frac{EDV - ESV}{EDV}$$

Appendix A

Indications for M-Mode and Two-Dimensional Echocardiography*

Table A-1
Indications in Which M-Mode Echocardiography Usually Provides a Definitive Diagnosis

Rheumatic mitral valve disease*
Mitral valve prolapse (Barlow's syndrome)
Pericardial effusion
Pericardial thickening
Left atrial myxoma
Congestive cardiomyopathy
Hypertrophic nonobstructive and obstructive cardiomyopathy
Aortic regurgitation
Flail mitral leaflet
Mitral annular calcification*
Flail aortic leaflet
Atrial thrombus
Calcific aortic valve disease*
Right ventricular volume overload
Left ventricular hypertrophy
Segmental myocardial disease

*Not applicable in pediatric populations.

*All tables in Appendix A have been reprinted with permission from Guidelines for the Practice of Echocardiography, Echocardiography Study Group, Diagnostic Committee of the Chicago Heart Association, 1981.

Table A-2
Indications in which M-Mode Echocardiography is Helpful in the Diagnosis

Aortic stenosis
Constrictive pericarditis
Prosthetic mitral and aortic valve dysfunction
Aortic root dissection
Secundum atrial septal defect
Primum atrial septal defect
Single ventricle
Ebstein's anomaly
Pulmonic valve stenosis*
Indundibular pulmonic stenosis*
Supravalvular aortic stenosis
Discrete subvalvular (fixed) aortic stenosis
Tetralogy of Fallot
Common atrioventricular canal
Patent ductus arteriosus (relative size)
Bicuspid aortic valve
Endocarditis (vegetation)
Segmental myocardial disease* (except apical and anteriorlateral left ventricle)
Cardiomyopathy
Tricuspid valve prolapse
Mural thrombus in left ventricle or atrium
Mediastinal mass anterior or posterior to the heart
Intracardiac tumors
Sinus of Valsalva aneurysm

*Not applicable in pediatric population

Table A-3
Indications in which Two-Dimensional Echocardiography Usually Provides a Definitive Diagnosis

Intracardiac mural thrombus
Intracardiac tumors
All valvular vegetations
Ventricular aneurysms
Left ventricular wall motion abnormalities
Right ventricular and right atrial size
All cyanotic congenital cardiac defects
Ebstein's anomaly of the tricuspid valve
All varieties of atrioventricular canal defects
Atrial septal defects
Ventricular septal defects
Mitral stenosis (especially determination of valve area)
Mediastinal masses
Hypertrophic cardiomyopathy (including idiopathic hypertrophic subartic stenosis)
Tricuspid valve stenosis
Tricuspid valve prolapse
Loculated or localized pericardial effusions
Flail mitral leaflet
Flail aortic leaflet
Flail tricuspid leaflet
Flail pulmonic leaflet
Corrected transposition of the great vessels
Bioprosthetic valve vegetations or thrombus
Left ventricular pseudoaneurysms

Table A-4
Indications in which Two-Dimensional Echocardiography Appears Promising but Is Still Under Investigation

Estimating left ventricular function
Stenotic and aneurysmal lesions of the ascending aorta and aortic arch
Mitral valve prolapse
Aortic valve stenosis
Pulmonic valve stenosis
Detection of proximal coronary artery stenosis
Detection of anomolous coronary artery origin
Prosthetic valve vegetation or thrombus
Patent ductus arteriosus

Appendix B
Echocardiographic Form

Ordering physician ______________________ ______________________
Attending Resident

Reason for test ______________________________

Height ________ cm Weight ________ kg ________ m^2 Age ________ M ________ F ________

Identification No. ______ ______________________ ________ Room No. _____ Lab _____ Bed _____
H/C Social Security No. Visit No.

Approach A _____ SX _____ SS _____ E _____ Values ( ) Corrected for BSA*

	Patient Value	Normal Values		Patient Value	Normal Values
RV size-dias. sup.	( ) cm	0.7-2.3 cm	Aortic		
LV size-syst. sup.	( ) cm	2.3-3.4 cm	Root dia.	( ) cm	2.0-3.7 cm
LV size-dias. sup.	( ) cm	3.5-5.1 cm	Valve opening	( ) cm	1.5-2.6 cm
Fractional shortening	( )	30-45%	Mitral valve		
LV post. wall thick.	( ) cm	0.65-1.1 cm	Excur.	( ) cm	1.6-2.8 cm
LV post. wall excur.	( ) cm	0.9-1.6 cm	E-F slope	( ) mm/sec	70-180 mm/sec
IV septal wall thick.	( ) cm	0.5-1.0 cm	Tricuspid valve		
			E-F slope	( ) mm/sec	60-125 mm/sec
IV septal wall excur.	( ) cm	0.6-1.1 cm	Pulmonic valve		
LA diam.	( ) cm	1.9-4.0 cm	A-wave depth	( ) cm	0.2-0.7 cm

Impressions and Comments:

Appendix C
Equations List

Fractional Shortening (% *FS*)

$$\%FS = \frac{EDD - ESD}{EDD} \times 100$$

where EDD = left ventricular end-diastolic dimension
ESD = left ventricular end-systolic dimension

Left Ventricular End-Diastolic Volume (*EDV*)

$$EDV = \left(\frac{\pi}{3}\right)(EDD)^3$$

or

$$= (EDD)^3$$

or

$$= \left(\frac{7.0}{2.4 + EDD}\right)(EDD)^3$$

Left Ventricular End-Systolic Volume (*ESV*)

$$ESV = \left(\frac{\pi}{3}\right)(ESD)^3$$

or

$$= (ESD)^3$$

or

$$= \left(\frac{7.0}{2.4 + ESD}\right)(ESD)^3$$

Mean Velocity of Circumferential Shortening ($\bar{V}_{cf}$)

$$\bar{V}_{cf} = \left(\frac{EDD - ESD}{EDD}\right) \times \mathrm{ET}$$

where ET = left ventricular ejection time (measured from the onset of opening to closure of the aortic valve or from systolic time intervals.

Left Ventricular Ejection Fraction (*EF*)

$$EF = \frac{SV}{EDV} = \frac{EDV - ESV}{EDV}$$

where SV = stroke volume

Single-Plane Ellipsoid Method

$$K = \frac{\text{number of cm}^2 \text{ of grid}}{\text{planimetered area of the grid}}$$

where K = correction factor

$$A_{LV} = A_P \times K$$

where A_{LV} = true area and A_P = planimetered area

The long axis of the left ventricle (L) is obtained by measuring the length from the apex to the left ventricle to the midpoint of the mitral valve. (Use calibration marks on screen or paper to measure length.) The area (A_{LV}) and length are then used for calculation of left ventricular volume in diastole and systole by the following formula:

$$V = \frac{8\,(A_{LV})^2}{3\pi L}$$

$$EDV = \frac{8\,(A_{LD})^2}{3\pi L_d}$$

$$ESV = \frac{8\,(A_{LS})^2}{3\pi L_s}$$

$$EF = \frac{EDV - ESV}{EDV}$$

where A_{Ld} is the area of the left ventricle in diastole, A_{Ls} is the area of the ıeft ventricle in systole, L_d is the length of the left ventricle in diastole, L_s is the length of the left ventricle in systole, EDV is the end-diastolic volume, ESV is the end-systolic volume, and EF is the ejection fraction.

Biplane Ellipsoid Method

$$D_{AP} = \frac{4\,(A_{LV_{AP}})}{L_{LV}}$$

where D_{AP} = minor axis in apical view, $A_{LV_{AP}}$ = apical view area of the left ventricle, and L_{LV} = long axis of the left ventricle

The long axis of the left ventricle (L_{LV}) is measured from the apex to the midpoint of the mitral valve in the apical four-chamber view. The minor axis short-axis view (D_{SX}) is calculated from the following formula:

$$D_{SX} = \frac{4\ (A_{LV_{AX}})}{d_S}$$

where d_s is measured from the endocardial surface of the posterior lateral left ventricle to the endocardial surface of the interventricular septum. Therefore, the left ventricular volumes are calculated by the following formula:

$$EDV = \frac{\pi}{6} L_{LV}\ (D_{AP})\ (D_{SX})$$

$$\text{Ejection fraction} = \frac{EDV - ESV}{EDV}$$

Left Ventricular Volume Using Simpson's Rule

The left ventricular volume (V) can be solved by the formula:

$$V = \frac{(\pi r^2)L/3 + (\pi r^2 a + \pi r^2 b)L/3 + 1/3(\pi r^2)L/3}{2}$$

$$\text{Ejection fraction} = \frac{EDV - ESV}{EDV}$$

Appendix D
Echocardiographic Tips for the Technologists

- A directed echocardiographic examination is more productive and yields more information for the referring physician. Know what your physician wants, what he or she is looking for, and how you plan to obtain the information.
- Recording of brachial arterial blood pressure will help the interpretation, especially in left ventricular hypertrophy, cardiomegaly, and aortic stenosis. In the presence of left ventricular hypertrophy, it is best to know whether the patient is normotensive (implying hypertrophic cardiomyopathy) or hypertensive (implying hypertensive heart disease). Left ventricular hypertrophy with a calcified aortic valve and normal blood pressure may indicate significant aortic stenosis.
- Use plenty of coupling gel and always maintain good contact of the transducer with the chest wall. Angulating the transducer off the chest wall may produce an artifact.
- For optimal grey scale, use maximal damping and minimal reject to first outline the endocardium. Then adjust these settings to best identify cardiac structures in your patient.
- Use time-gain compensation to set the ramp at the interventricular septum. Once the cardiac structures have been identified, you can set the ramp at a more rapid slope, or lower the near-field time-gain compensation. Reduce time-gain compensation 2 to 3 centimeters posterior to the posterior wall to prevent blooming in this area.
- After obtaining an echocardiographic window, locate the long-axis view of the left ventricle. This may take considerable repositioning of the transducer on the chest wall, due to the variable anatomic position of the heart and great vessels in the chest wall. You may have to rotate the transducer 90° to the left from a vertical parasternal position for a vertical heart in a thin patient to a horizontal chest wall position for a horizontal-lying heart in a large patient.
- Calibration lines should be set at the initiation of the study and kept there throughout. However, if the image has calibration lines throughout the entire image, record them for a few frames for each cardiac position obtained. It is important to maintain them throughout the study for determination of ventricular volume or valve areas.
- Remember to record a minimum of 7 to 10 seconds for each cardiac position. Too rapid a change in position does not allow for proper visualization of the structure; too long a recording allows for wastage of videotape time and is unnecessary.

- For suspected vegetations or thrombi on cardiac valves, place the damping and reject settings at minimal levels. If the suspected lesions are not seen, readjust the settings to *just* identify the weakly reflective endocardium.
- For determination of left ventricular volume or mitral valve area, a stop-frame or trigger-mode is helpful. For left ventricular volumes, trigger the *end-diastolic* frame at the onset of the QRS, and the *end-systolic* frame at the end of the T wave or smallest chamber size, whichever comes first. For mitral valve orifice, the trigger is best set for early diastole (just after the end of the T wave).
- Remember that proper gain settings and transducer positions vary from patient to patient. First obtain an image of the heart in long axis. Set gain settings, reject, and damping to best suit your patient. Then obtain the best position in long-axis view. You may have to readjust the settings with each change in position. Once the view and settings are acceptable, record that view and go on to the next. Be flexible in positioning and angulating the transducer. Sometimes a slight repositioning of the transducer or a slight change in angulation will give you the proper view.
- Patients with chronic lung disease and elderly patients are at times difficult to image in parasternal views. Here *apical* four- and five-chamber views and *subcostal* four-chamber and short-axis views can be frequently obtained for evaluation of cardiac size and wall motion. Chamber size, dimensions, and wall motion can be estimated from these views. The postoperative open heart patient is difficult to image immediately following surgery, due to the median sternotomy incision. If possible, delay study for at least 2 to 3 weeks.

Appendix E
Suggested Additional References

CHAPTER 1: Echocardiographic Techniques and Measurements

Bennett DH, Rowlands DJ: Test of reliability of echocardiographic estimation of left ventricular dimensions and volumes. Br Heart J 38:1133-1139, 1976

Bhatt DR, Jones JB, Villoria GJ, Nakazawa M, Yabek SM, Marks RA, et al: Accuracy of echocardiography in assessing left ventricular dimensions and volume. Circulation 57:699-707, 1978

Bommer W, Weinert L, Neumann A, Neef J, Mason DT, DeMaria A: Determination of right atrial and right ventricular size by two-dimensional echocardiography. Circulation 60:91-100, 1979

Carr KW, Engler RL, Forsythe JR, Johnson AD, Gosink B: Measurement of left ventricular ejection fraction by mechanical cross-sectional echocardiography. Circulation 59:1196-1206, 1979

Halliday H, Hirschfeld S, Riggs T, Leibman J, Faranogg A: Echographic ventricular systolic time intervals in normal term and preterm neonates. Pediatrics 62:317-321, 1978

Johnson ML, Kisslo JA: Basic diagnosis of echocardiography. DM 23:1-58, 1976

Kisslo JA, VonRamm OT, Thurstone FL: Techniques for real-time two-dimensional echocardiography. Cardiovasc Clin 9:21-38, 1978

Kossoff G: Principles of two-dimensional echocardiography and real-time imaging. Med J Aust 1:7-8, 1977

Kotler MN, Segal BL, Mintz G, Parry WR: Pitfalls and limitations of M-mode echocardiography. Am Heart J 94:227-249, 1977

Martin RP: Two-dimensional echocardiography: Methodology and application in clinical cardiology. Adv Cardiol 27:17-39, 1980

Mason SJ, Fortuin NJ: The use of echocardiography for quantitative evaluation of left ventricular function. Prog Cardiovasc Dis 21:119-132, 1978

Matsumoto M, Matsuo H, Kitabatake A, Inque M, Hamanaka Y, Tamura S, et al: Three dimensional echocardiograms and two-dimensional echocardiographic images at desired planes by a computerized system. Ultrasound Med Biol 3:163-178, 1980

Popp RL, Rubenson DS, Tucker CR, French JW: Echocardiography: M-mode and two-dimensional methods. Ann Intern Med 93:844-56, 1980

Prakash R, Linsday P: Determination of right ventricular wall thickness by echocardiogram, JAMA 239:638-640, 1978

Quiniones MA, Pickering E, Alexander JK: Percentage of shortening of the echocardiographic left ventricular dimension: Its use in determining ejection fraction and stroke volume. Chest 74:59-65, 1978

Sahn DJ, Bom N, Lancee CT, Van Egmond FC, Roelandt J: A dual M-mode system for simultaneous time motion analyses of cardiac structures and evaluation of cardiac function: Initial clinical applications, in Bom N, (Ed): Echocardiology. The Hague, Martinus Nijhoff Medical Division, 1977

Seward JB, Tajik AJ: Two-dimensional echocardiography. Med Clin North Am 64:177-203, 1980
Tomoda H, Okabe S, Kawada S, Shostsu A, Sasamoto H: An experience in clinical applicaiton of real-time two-dimensional echocardiography. Jpn Heart J 17:437-444, 1976
Vogel JA, Ligtvoet C, Bom N, VanZieten G, Hugenholtz PG: Processing equipment for two-dimensional echocardiographic data. Ultrasound Med Biol 2:171-179, 1976
Waggoner AD, Adyanthaya AV, Quinones MS, Alexander JK: Left atrial enlargement: Echocardiographic assessment of electrocardiographic criteria. Circulation 54:553-557, 1976
Weyman AE: The cross-sectional echocardiogram in clinical cardiology: Applications and relationship to the M-mode technique. Acta Med Scand, Suppl 627, pp 25-40, 1979
Wilcken DE, Paoloni HG, Dadd M, Carpenter D, Kossoff G: The clinical applications of two-dimensional echocardiography. Med J Aust Suppl 1, p 8, 1977

CHAPTER 3: Mitral Valve Disease

Ahmad S, Kleiger RE, Connors J, Krone R: The echocardiographic diagnosis of a rupture of a papillary muscle. Chest 73:232-234, 1978
Baker DW: The present role of Doppler techniques in cardic diagnosis. Prog Cardiovasc Dis 21:79-91, 1978
Chandraratna PA, Aronow WS: Incidence of ruptured chordae tendineae in the mitral valvular prolapse syndrome: An echocardiographic study. Chest 75:334-339, 1979
Cohen IS, Wharton TP Jr, Neill WA; Pathophysiologic observations on premature opening of the aortic valve utilizing a technique for multiplane echocardiographic analysis. Am Heart J 97:766-772, 1979
Hall RJ, Clarke SE, Brown D: Evaluation of posterior aortic wall echogram in diagnosis of mitral valve disease. Br Heart J 41:522-528, 1979
Heger JJ, Wann LS, Weyman AE, Dillon JC, Feigenbaum H: Long-term changes in mitral valve area after successful mitral commisurotomy. Circulation 59:443-448, 1979
Hirschfeld DS, Rogriguez HJ, Schiller NB: Duplication of aortic wall seen by echocardiography. Br Heart J 38:843-850, 1976
Karnegis JN, Heinz J: Case report: Factors involved in the production of the presystolic murmur in a patient with mitral stenosis and atrial trigeminy: Correlation of echocardiographic, phonocardiographic, and hemodynamic data. Am J Med Sci 276:341-347, 1978
Koga Y, Toshima H, Kimura N, Ohishi K, Koga M: Preoperative evaluation of the structural lesion of the mitral valve by M-mode scan echocardiography. Nippon Junkankigaku Shi 41;975-982, 1977
Kronzon I, Mitchell J, Shapiro J, Winer HE, Newman P: Two-dimensional echocardiography in mitral annulus calcification. Am J Radiol 134:355-358 1980
Kushner FG, Lam W, Morganroth J: Apex sector echocardiography in evaluation of the right atrium in patients with mitral stenosis and atrial septal defect. Am J Cardiol 42:733-737, 1978
Milo S, Ho SY, Macartney RJ, Wilkinson JL, Becker AE, Wenink AC, Gittenberger de Groot AC, Anderson RH: Straddling and overriding atrioventricular valves: Morphology and classification. Am J Cardiol 44:1122-1134, 1979
Mintz GS, Kotler MN, Segal BL, Parry WR: Two-dimensional echocardiographic evaluation of patients with mitral insufficiency. Am J Cardiol 44:670-678, 1979
Rosenthal R, Kleid JJ, Cohen MV: Abnormal mitral valve motion associated with ventricular septal defect following acute myocardial infarction. Am Heart J 98.638-641, 1979
Sasayama S, Takahashi M, Osakada G, Hirose K, Hamashima H, Nishimura E, Kawai C: Dynamic geometry of the left atrium and left ventricle in acute mitral regurgitation. Circulation 60:177-186, 1979.
Tajik AJ, Seward JB, Habler DH, Mair DD, Lie JT: Two-dimensional real-time ultrasonic

imaging of the heart and great vessels; Technique, image orientation, structure identification, and validation, Mayo Clin Proc 53:271-303, 1978

CHAPTER 4: Mitral Valve Prolapse

Barnett HJ, Boughner DR, Taylor DW, Cooper PE, Kostuk WJ, Nichol PM: Further evidence relating mitral valve prolapse to cerebral ischemic events. N Engl J Med 302:139-148, 1980
Cohen MV: Real time sector scan study of the mitral valve prolapse syndrome. Br Heart J 40:964, 1978
Desser KB, Promisloff SD, Yellen LG, Venchimol A: Stress electrocardiography in Uhl's anomaly with mitral valve prolapse. Chest 70:529-531, 1976
Dillon JC, Haine CL, Chang S, Feigenbaum H: Use of echocardiography in patients with prolapsed mitral valve. Circulation 43:503-507, 1971
Forbes RB, Morton GH: Ventricular fibrillation in a patient with unsuspected mitral valve prolapse and a prolonged Q-T interval. Can Anaesth Soc J 26:424-427, 1979
Gilbert VW, Schatz RA, Vonramm DT, Behar VS, Kisslo JA: Mitral valve prolapse: Two-dimensional echocardiographic and angiographic correlation. Circulation 54:716-723, 1976
Greenwald JG: Autonomic dysfunction in women with mitral valve prolapse. Circulation 60:910-913, 1979
Liedtke A Jr, Babb JD, DeJoseph RL: Mitral valve echoes in patients with mitral valve prolapse syndrome. Am Heart J 97:286-290, 1979
Ogawa S, Hubbard FE, Mardelli TJ, Driefus LS: Cross-sectional echocardiography spectrum of papillary muscle dysfunction. Am Heart J 97:312-321, 1979
Popp R, Brown OR, Silverman JE, Harrison DC: Echocardiographic abnormalities in the mitral valve prolapse syndrome. Circulation 49:428-433, 1974
Saffro R, Talano JV: Transient ischemic attack associated with mitral systolic clicks. Arch Intern Med 139:693-694, 1979
Sahn DJ, Wood J, Allen HD, Peoples W, Goldberg SJ: Echocardiographic spectrum of mitral valve motion in children with and without mitral valve prolapse: The nature of false positive diagnosis. Am J Cardiol 39:422-431, 1977
Watson RT: TIA stroke and mitral valve prolapse. Neurology 29:886-889, 1979

CHAPTER 5: Diseases of the Aorta and Great Vessels

Abdulla AM, Frank MJ, Canedo MI, Stefadouros MA: Limitations of echocardiography in the assessment of left ventricular size and function in aortic regurgitation. Circulation 61:148-155 1980
Baker DW: The present role of Doppler techniques in cardiac diagnosis. Prog Cardiovasc Dis 21:79-91, 1978
Bass JL, Einzig S, Hong CY, Moller JH: Echocardiographic estimation of peak left ventricular pressure in aortic stenosis (letter). Am J Cardiol 44:82-87, 1979
Bass JL, Einzig S, Hong CY, Moller JH: Echocardiographic screening to assess the severity of congenital aortic valve stenosis in children. Am J Cardiol 44:82-87, 1979
Blackwood RA, Bloom KR, Williams CM: Aortic stenosis in children: Experience with echocardiographic prediction of severity. Circulation 52:263-268, 1978
Borer JS, Rosing DR, Kent KM, Bacharach SL, Green MV, McIntosh CJ, Morrow AG, et al: Left ventricular function at rest and during exercise after aortic valve replacement in patients with aortic regurgitation. Am J Cardiol 44:1297-1305, 1979
Cunha CL, Guiliani ER, Fuster V, Seward JB, Brandenburg RO, McGoon DC: Preoperative M-mode echocardiography as a predictor of surgical results in chronic aortic insufficiency. J Thorac Cardiovasc Surg 79:256-265, 1980
Das G, Lee CC, Weissler SM: Echocardiographic manifestations of ruptured aortic valvular

leaflets in the absence of valvular vegetations. Chest 72:161-168, 1977
El Shahawy M, Graybell R, Pepine CJ, Conti CR; Diagnosis of aortic valvular prolapse echocardiography. Chest 69:411-413, 1976
Flanigan RJ, Cazzola EB, Goris GB, Jenny DB: Echocardiographic evaluation of the aortic valve. Circulation 58:1214-1215, 1978
Fowles RE, Martin RP, Abrams, JM, Schapira JN, French JW, Popp RL: Two-dimensional echocardiographic features of bicuspid aortic valve. Chest 75:434-440, 1979
Gewitz MH, Werner JC, Keinman CS, Hellenbrand WE, Talner NS: Role of echocardiography in aortic stenosis: Pre- and postoperative studies. Am J Cardiol 43:54-59, 1979
Joswig BC, Pick RA, Vieweg WV, Hagan AD: Flutter of the mitral valve associated with a diastolic murmur in the absence of disease. Am Heart J 97:635-638, 1979
Kligfield P, Okin P: Effect of ventricular function on left ventricular ejection time in aortic stenosis. Br Heart J 42:438-441, 1979
Matsumoto M, Kirschner M, Strom J, Frishman W, Sonnenblick E: Two-dimensional echocardiographic diagnosis of a prolapsing aortic root aneurysm after aortic valve replacement. JCU 8:504-510, 1980
Matsumoto M, Matsuo H, Ohara T, Yoshioka Y, et al: A two-dimensional echocardiographic approach to dissecting aneurysms of the aorta to prevent false-positive diagnoses. Radiology 127:491-499, 1978
McDonald IG, Jelinek VM: Serial M-mode echocardiography in severe chronic aortic regurgitation. Circulation 62:1291-1296, 1980
Mintz GS, Kotler MN, Segal BL, Parry WR: Two-dimensional echocardiographic recognition of the descending thoracic aorta. Am J Cardiol 44:232-238, 1979
Reeves WC, Ettinger U, Thomson K, Nanda N, Gramiak R, DE Weese J, Stewart S: Limitations in the echocardiographic assessment of aortic root dimensions in the presence of aortic valve disease. Radiology 132:411-413, 1979
Shemin RJ, Kent KM, Roberts WC: Syndrome of valvular pulmonary stenosis and valvular aortic stenosis with atrial septal defect. Br Heart J 42:442-446, 1979
Sher RF, Kimbiris D, Segal BL, Iskandrian AS, Bemis CE: Aneurysm of the sinus of valsalva: Its natural history. Postgrad Med 65:191-193, 1979
Shiu MF, Coltart DJ, Braimbridge MV: Echocardiographic findings in prolapsed aortic cusp with vegetation. Br Heart J 41:118-120, 1979
Way RC, Bloom KR, Izukawa T: Aoritc valve prolapse associated with ventricular septal defect: Echocardiographic features. Can Med Assoc J 121:62-64, 1979

CHAPTER 6: Pericardial Effusion and Pericardial Disease

Alimurung BN, Felner JM Schlant RC: Echocardiography in the diagnosis of idiopathic hypertrophic subaortic stenosis coexisting with pericardial effusion. Chest 76:187-192, 1979
Bowie PR, Teixeiera OH, Carpenter B: Malignant thymoma in a nine-year-old boy presenting with pleuropericardial effusion. J Thorac Cardiovasc Surg 77:777-781, 1979
Chandraratna PA, Aronow WS: Limitations of surgical methods of pericaridal drainage: Echocardiographic observations. JAMA 242:1062-1063, 1979
D'Cruz IA, Bhatt GR, Cohen HC, Glick G: Echocardiographic detection of cardiac involvement in patients with chronic renal failures. Arch Intern Med 138:720-724, 1978
Defalque RJ, Campbell C: Cardiac tamponade from central venous catherers. Anesthesiology 50:249-252, 1979
Hancock EW: Cardiac tamponade. Med Clin North Am 63:223-237, 1979
Hochberg MS, Merrill WH, Gruber M, McIntosh CL, Henry WL, Morrow AG: Delayed cardiac tamponade associated with prophylactic anticoagulation in patients undergoing coronary bypass grafting: Early diagnosis with two-dimensional echocardiography. J Thorac Cardiovasc Surg 75:777-781, 1978
Jacobs WR, Talano JV: Cardiomegaly and paradoxical pulse. Arch Int Med 138:1125-1126, 1978

of tricuspid valve endocarditis: An M-mode and two-dimensional study. Am J Cardiol 38:502-507, 1976

Lew W, Karliner JS: Assessment of pulmonary valve echogram in normal subjects and in patients with pulmonary arterial hypertension. Br Heart J 42:147-161, 1979

Nagai Y, Komatsu Y, Nakamura K, Sato Y, Takao A: Echocardiographic findings of congenital absence of the pulmonary valve with tetralogy of Fallot. Chest 65:481-486, 1979

Takahaski O, Eshaghpour E, Kotler MN: Tricuspid and pulmonic valve echoes in tricuspid and pulmonary atresia. Chest 76:437-440, 1979

Vecht RJ, Carmichael DJ, Gopal R, Philip G: Uhl's anomaly. Br Heart J 41:676-682, 1979.

CHAPTER 9: Vegetations, Thrombi, Myxomas, and Intracardiac Masses

Acquatella H, Schiller NB, Sharpe DN, Chatterjee K: Lack of correlation between echocardiographic pulmonary valve morphonology and simultaneous arterial pressure. Am J Cardiol 43:946-950, 1979

Assey ME, Usher BW: Development of aortic valvular vegetations during appropriate antibiotic therapy: Demonstration through serial echocardiograms. Chest 76:223-225, 1979

Bamrah VS, Williams GW, Hughes CV, Rose HD, Tristani FE: *Haemophilus parainfluenzae* mitral valve vegetation without hemodynamic abnormality. Demonstration by angiography and serial echocardiography. am J Med 66:543-546, 1979

Bulkley BH, Hutchins GM: Atrial myxomas: A fifty year review. Am Heart J 97:639-643, 1979

Bulkley H, Weiss JL: Atrial myxomas: Triumph of machine over man (editorial). Chest 75:537-539, 1979

Clements SD Jr, Perkins JV: The M-mode echocardiogram and endocarditis. J Med Assoc GA 68:321-323, 1979

Come PC, Kurland GS, Vine HS: Two-dimensional echocardiography in differentiating right atrial and tricuspid valve mass lesions. Am J Cardiol 44:1207-1212, 1979

Crawford FA Jr, Wechsler AS, Kisslo JA: Tricuspid endocarditis in a drug addict: Detection of tricuspid vegetations by two-dimensional echocardiography. Chest 74:473-475, 1978

DeMaria AN, Bommer W, Neumann A, Grehl T, Weinart L, Denardo S, et al: Left ventricular thrombi identified by cross-sectional echocardiography. Ann Intern Med 90:14-18, 1979

Dzindzio BS, Meyer L, Osterholm R, Hopeman A, Woltjen J, Forkner AD: Isolated gonococcal pulmonary valve endocarditis: Diagnosis by echocardiography. Circulation 59:1319-1324, 1979

Geyer SJ, Franzini DA: Myxomatous degeneration of the mitral valve complicated by nonbacterial thrombotic endocarditis with systemic embolization. Am J Clin Pathol 72:489-492, 1979

Gilbert BW, Haney RS, Crawford F, McClellan J, Gallis HA, Johnson ML, Kisslo JA: Two-dimensional echocardiographic assessment of vegetative endocarditis. Circulation 55:346-353, 1977

Gregoratos G, Karliner JS: Infective endocarditis: Diagnosis and management. Med Clin North Am 63:173-199, 1979

Jaffe CC, Kelley MJ, Taunt KA: Two-dimensional echocardiographic identification of a right ventricle tumor. Radiology 129:471-472, 1978

Kisslo J, Von Ramm DT, Haney R, Jones R, Juk SS, Behar VS: Echocardiographic evaluation of tricuspid valve endocarditis: An M-mode and two dimensional study. Am J Cardiol 38:502-507, 1976

Lappe DL, Bulkley BH, Weiss JL: Two-dimensional echocardiographic diagnosis of left atrial myxoma. Chest 74:55-58, 1978

Lee YC, Magram MY: Nonprolapsing left atrial tumor. The M-mode echocardiographic

diagnosis. Chest 78:332–333, 1980
LeJemtel TH, Factor SM, Koenigsberg M, O'Reilly M, Frater R, Sonnenblick EH: Mural vegetations at the site of endocardial trauma in infective endocarditis complicating hypertrophic subaortic stenosis. Am J Cardiol 44:569-574, 1979
Lundstrom NR, Bjorkhem G: Mitral and tricuspid valve vegetations in infancy diagnosed by echocardiography. Acta Paediatr Scand 68:345–350, 1979
Martin RP: Clinical utility of two-dimensional echocardiography in the detection of intracardiac mass lesions. Adv Cardio 58–70, 1980
Melendez JL, Sears GA, Coles JC: Right ventricular tumor demonstrated by echocardiography. Can Med Assoc J 118:62–63, 1978
Meltzer RS, Guthaner D, Rakowski H, Popp RL, Martin RP: Diagnosis of left ventricular thrombi by two-dimensional echocardiography. Br Heart J 42:261–265, 1979
Mintz GS, Kotler MN, Parry WR: Wide splitting of the first heart sound secondary to tricuspid valve endocarditis: A phonocardiographic-echocardiographic study. Am J Med 66:523-527, 1979
Mintz GS, Kotler MN, Segal BL, Parry WR: Comparison of two dimensional and M-mode echocardiography in the evaluation of patients with infective endocarditis. Am J Cardiol 43:738–744, 1979
Mintz GS, Kotler MN, Segal BL, Parry WR: Survival of patients with aortic valve endocarditis: The prognostic implications of the echocardiogram. Arch Intern Med 139:862-866, 1979
O'Neill MB Jr, Grehl TM, Hurley EJ: Cardial myxomas: A clinical diagnostic challenge. Am J Surg 138:68–76, 1979
Petty BG: M-mode vs. cross-sectional echo for bacterial endocarditis, letter. Circulation 61:1057, 1980
Powers JC, Falkoff M, Heinle RA, Nanda NC, Ong LS, Weiner RS, et al: Familial cardiac myxoma: Emphasis on unusual clinical manifestations. J Thorac Cardiovasc Surg 77:782–788, 1979
Rajpal RS, Leibsohn JA, Liekweg WG, Gross CM, et al: Infected left atrial myxoma with bacteremia simulating infective endocarditis. Arch Intern Med 139:1176–1178, 1979
Reeves WC, Nanda NC, Barold SS: Echocardiographic evaluation of intracardiac pacing catheters; M-mode and two-dimensional studies. Circulation 58:1049–1056, 1978
Sandrasagra FA, Oliver WA, English TA: Myxoma of the mitral valve. Br Heart J 42:221–223, 1979
Schoolmeester WL, Kelley JW, Sawyer CG: Multivalvular vegetations in a patient with enterococcal endocarditis diagnosed by echocardiography. South Med J 71:644-648, 1978
Sharratt GP, Grover ML, Monro JL: Calcified left atrial myxoma with floppy mitral valve. Br Heart J 42:608–610, 1979
Shemin RJ, Kent KM, Roberts WC: Syndrome of valvular pulmonary stenosis and valvular aortic stenosis with atrial septal defect. Br Heart J 42:442–446, 1979
Sonotani N: Conventional and two-dimensional real-time echocardiographic diagnses of left heart tumors: Three cases of left atrial myxoma. Bull Osaka Med Sch 25:128–138, 1979
Sonotani N, Takatsu T, Sawada K: Conventional and two-dimensional real-time echocardiographic diagnosis of osteosarcoma. A case report. Jpn Heart J 21:281–288, 1980
Stafford A, Wann LS, Dillon JC, Weyman AE, Feigenbaum H: Serial echocardiographic appearance of healing bacterial vegetations. Am J Cardiol 44:754–760, 1979
Ward C, Naik DR, Johnstone MC: Tricuspid endocarditis complicating pacemaker implantation demonstrated by echocardiography. Br J Radiol 52:501–502, 1979
Stewart JA, Warnica JW, Kirk ME, Winsberg F: Left atrial myxoma: False negative echocardiographic findings in a tumor demonstrated by coronary arteriography. Am Heart J 98:228–32, 1979
Yarnal JR, Smiley WH III: Right atrial mass simulated echocardiographically by a Swan-Ganz catheter letter. Chest 74:478–479, 1978
Sunagawa K, Orita Y, Tanaka S., et al: Left atrial ball thrombus diagnosed by two-dimensional echocardiography. Am Heart J 100:89–94, 1980

Yoshikawa J, Sabah I, Yanagihara K, Owaki T, Kato H, Tanemoto K: Cross-sectional echocardiographic diagnosis of large left atrial tumor and extracardiac tumor compressing the left atrium: Limitation of M-mode echocardiography in distinguishing the two lesions. Am J Cardiol 42:853-857, 1978

CHAPTER 10: Congenital Heart Diseases

Ahmad M, Hallidie-Smith KA: Assessment of left-to-right shunt and left ventricular function in isolated ventricular septal defect: Echocardiographic study. Br Heart J 41:147-158, 1979

Aziz KU, Paul MH, Bharati S, Lev M, Shannon K: Echocardiographic features of total anomalous pulmonary venous drainage into the coronary sinus. Am J Cardiol 42:108-113, 1978

Bass JL, Ben-Shachar G, Edwards JE: Comparison of M-mode echocardiography and pathologic findings in the hypoplastic left heart syndrome. Am J Cardiol 45:79-86, 1980

Beppu S, Nimura Y, Nagata S, Tamai M, Matsuo H: Diagnosis of endocardial cushion defect with cross-sectional and M-mode scanning echocardiography: Differentiation from secundum atrial septal defect. Br Heart J 1976; 38:911-20

Beppu S, Nimura Y, Tamai M, Nagata S, Matsuo H, Kawashima Y, et al: Differentiation from other hypoplastic right heart syndromes and common atrioventricular canal. Br Heart J 40:1174-1183, 1978

Bierman FZ, Williams RG: Prospective of D-transposition of the great arteries in neonates by subxiphoid, two-dimensional echocardiography. Circulation 60:1496-1502, 1979

Bommer W, Weinert L, Neumann A, Neef J, Mason DT, DeMaria A: Determination of right atrial and right ventricular size by two-dimensional echocardiography. Circulation 60:91-100, 1979

Botvinick EH, Schiller NB: The complementary roles of M-mode echocardiography and scintigraphy in the evaluation of adults with suspected left-to-right shunts: Additional observations on the role of two-dimensional echocardiography. Circulation 62:1070-1079, 1980

Daniel W, Rathsack P, Walpurger G, Kahle A, Gisbertz R, Schmitz J, et al: Value of M-mode echocardiography for non-invasive diagnosis of Ebstein's anomaly. Br Heart J 43:38-44, 1980

Disessa TG, Hagan AD, Pope C, Samtoy L, Friedman WF: Two-dimensional echocardiographic characteristics of double-outlet right ventricle. Am J Cardiol 44:1146-1154, 1979

Draulans-Noe HA, Voogd PJ, Ligtvoet DM, Ridder J, Wenink AC: Two-dimensional echocardiography in atrioventricular canal malformation: A diagnostic approach. Acta Med Scand, suppl 627, pp 196-202, 1979

Fraker TD Jr, Harris PJ, Behar VS, Kisslo JA: Detection and exclusion of interatrial shunts by two-dimensional echocardiography and peripheral venous injection. Circulation 59:379-384, 1979

Goldberg SJ, Allen HD, Sahn DJ: Pediatric and Adolescent Echocardiography. Chicago, Yearbook Medical Publishers, 1975

Giuliani ER, Fuster V, Brandenburg RO, Mair DD: Ebstein's anomaly: The clinical features and natural history of Ebstein's anomaly of the tricuspid valve. Mayo Clin Proc 54:163-173, 1979

Hagler DJ, Tajik AJ, Seward JB, Mair DD, Ritter DG: Wide-angle two-dimensional echocardiographic profiles of conotruncal abnormalities. Mayo Clin Proc 55:73-82, 1980

Henry WL: Evaluation of older children and adults with congenital heart disease by M-mode and cross-sectional echocardiography. Cardiovasc Clin 10:139-171, 1979

Henry JG, Gordon S, Timmis GC: Corrected transportation of great vessels and Ebstein's anomaly of tricuspid valve: Echocardiographic findings. Br Heart J 41:249-252, 1979

Hibi N, Kambe T: Cross-sectional and M-mode echocardiographic study on ventricular septal defect. Jpn Heart J 20:127-139, 1979

Houston AB, Gregory NL, Coleman EN: Two-dimensional sector scanner echocardiography in cyanotic congenital heart disease. Br Heart J 39:1076-1081, 1977
Jaffe CC, Atkinson P, Taylor KJ: Phsical parameters affecting the visibility of small ventricular septal defects using two-dimensional echocardiography. Invest Radiol 14:149-155, 1979
Kinsley RH, Levin SE, O'Donovan TG: Transposition of the great arteries associated with a double left ventricular outflow tract. Br Heart J 42:483-486, 1979
Kronik G, Slany J, Moesslacher H: Contrast M-mode echocardiography in diagnosis of atrial septal defect in acyanotic patients. Circulation 59:372-379, 1979
Leier CV, Call TD, Fulkerson PK, Wooley CF: The spectrum of cardiac defects in the Ehlers-Danlos syndrome, types I and III. Ann Intern Med 92:171-178, 1980
Lieppe W, Scallion R, Behar VS, Kisslo JA: Two-dimensional echocardiographic findings in atrial septal defect. Circulation 56:477-456, 1977
Martin RP, French JW: The role of two-dimensional echocardiography in the evaluation of congenital heart disease. Adv Cardiol 27:266-280, 1980
Matsumoto M, Matsuo H: Echocardiography for the evaluation of the tricuspid valve, right ventricle, and atrium. Prog Cardiovasc Dis 21:1-42, 1978
Mehta S, Hirschfeld S, Riggs T, Liebman J: Echocardiographic estimation of ventricular hypoplasia in complete atrioventricular canal. Circulation 59:888-893, 1979
Meltzer RS, Schwartz J, French J, Popp RL: Ventricular septal defect noted by two-dimensional echocardiography. Chest 76:455-457, 1979
Ostermeyer J, Korfer R, Bircks W: Mitral atresis with normal-sized ventricles, ventricular septal defect, and dextro-transposition of the great arteries. J Thorac Cardiovasc Surg 77:733-737, 1979
Ports TA, Silverman NH, Schiller NB: Two-dimensional echocardiographic assessment of Ebstein's anomaly. Circulation 58:336-343, 1978
Sahn DJ, Henry WL: Clinical applications of real-time two-dimensional scanning in congenital heart disease. Cardiovasc Clin 9:295-316, 1978
Sahn DJ, Allen JD, Lange LW, Goldberg SJ: Cross-sectional echocardiographic diagnosis of the sites of total anomalous pulmonary venous drainage. Circulation 69:1317-1325, 1979
Satomi G, Nakamura K, Imai Y, Takao A: Two-dimensional echocardiographic diagnosis of aorticopulmonary window. Br Heart J 43:351-356, 1980
Schapira JN, Martin RP, Fowles RE, Popp RL: Single and two-dimensional echocardiographic features of the interatrial septum in normal subjects and patients with an atrial septal defect. Am J Cardiol 43:816-819, 1979
Serruys PW, VanDen Brand M, Hugenholtz PG, Roelandt J: Intracardiac right-to-left shunts demonstrated by two-dimensional echocardiography after peripheral vein injection. Br Heart J 42:429-437, 1979
Silverman NH, Schiller NB: Apex echocardiography: A two-dimensional technique for evaluating congenital heart disease. Circulation 57:503-511, 1978
Silverman NH, Snider AR, Rudolph AM: Evaluation of pulmonary hypertension by M-mode echocardiography in children with ventricular septal defect. Circulation 61:1125-1132, 1980
Snider AR, Silverman NH: Suprasternal notch echocardiography: A two-dimensional technique for evaluating congenital heart disease. Circulation 63:165-173, 1981
Snider AR, Ports TA, Silverman NH: Venous anomalies of the coronary sinus: Detection by M-mode, two-dimensional, and contrast echocardiography. Circulation 60:721-727, 1979
Snider AR, Roge CL, Schiller NB, Silverman NH: Congenital left ventricular inflow obstruction evaluated by two-dimensional echocardiography. Circulation 61:848-855, 1980
St. John Sutton MG, Tajik AJ, Mercier LA, Seward JB, Giuliani ER, Ritman EL: Assessment of left ventricular function in secundum atrial septal defect by computer analysis of the M-mode echocardiogram. Circulation 60:1082-1090, 1979
Tonkin IL, Sansa M, Elliott LP, Bargeron LM Jr: Recognition of developing left ventricular

outflow tract obstruction in complete transposition of the great arteries. Radiology 134:53-59, 1980
Way RC, Bloom KR, Izukawa T: Aortic valve prolapse associated with ventricular septal defect: Echocardiographic features. Can Med Assoc J 121:62-64, 1979
Werner JA, Schiller NB, Prasquier R: Occurrence and significance of echocardiographically demonstrated tricuspid valve prolapse. Am Heart J 96:180-186, 1978
Williams RG, Tucker CR: Echocardiographic Diagnosis of Congenital Heart Disease Boston, Little, Brown 1977
Yoshida Y, Fukuda M, Tanaka M, Terasawa Y: Diagnosis of persistent truncus arteriosus by two-dimensional echocardiography: A case study. Tohoku J Exp Med 125:53-57, 1978

CHAPTER 11: Prosthetic Heart Valves

Alam M, Madrazo AC, Macilligan DJ, Goldstein S: M-mode and two-dimensional echocardiographic features of porcine valve dysfunction. Am J Cardiol 43:502-509, 1979
Behi F, Chang S, Welch T: Malfunction of Cutter-Smeloff prosthesis: An echocardiographic diagnosis. J Thorac Cardiovasc Surg 75:313-316, 1978
Hetzer R, Hill JD, Kerth WJ: Thrombosis and degeneration of hancock valves: Clinical and pathological findings. Ann Thorac Surg 26:317-322, 1978
Kisslo J, VonRamm OT, Haney R, Jones R, Juk SS, Behar VS: Echocardiographic evaluation of tricuspid valve endocarditis: An M mode and two dimensional study. Am J Cardiol 38:502-507, 1976
Martin RP, French JW, Popp RL: Clinical utility of two-dimensional echocardiography in patients with bioprosthetic valves. Adv Cardiol 27:294-304, 1980
Rajah SM, Rao S, Ahmad R, Watson DA: Near fatal puerperal thrombosis on Bjork-Shiley mitral valve prosthesis, letter. Br Heart J 41:630, 1979
Salem BI, Pechacek LW, Leachman RD: Major dehiscence of a prosthetic aortic valve: Detection by echocardiography. Chest 1979; 75:513-5
Schapira JN, Martin RP, Fowles RE, Rakowski H, Stinson EB, French JW, et al: Two dimensional echocardiographic assessment of patients with bioprosthetic valves. Am J Cardiol 43:510-519, 1979
Schapira JN, Martin RP, Fowles RE, Rakowski, Stinson EB, French JW, et al.: Two-dimensional echocardiographic assessment of patients with bioprosthetic valves. Am J Cardiol 43:510-519, 1979
Skorton DJ, Child JS, Eber LM: Non-invasive diagnosis of prosthetic mitral valve malfunction. Radiology 131:185-186, 1979

CHAPTER 12: Left Ventricular Function by Two-Dimensional Echocardiography

Crawford MH, Grant D, O'Rourke RA, Starling MR, Groves BM: Accuracy and reproducibility of new M-mode echocardiographic recommendations for measuring left ventricular dimensions. Circulation 61:137-143, 1980
Folland ED, Parisi AF, Moynihan PR, Jones DR, Feldman CL, Tow DE: Assessment of left ventricular ejection fraction and volumes by real-time, two-dimensional echocardiography: A comparison of cineangiographic and radionuclide techniques. Circulation 60:760-766, 1979
Kisslo, JA: Evaluation of the left ventricle by two-dimensional echocardiography. Acta Med Scand, Suppl 627, pp 112-119, 1979
Moynihan PF, Parisi AF, Folland ED, Jones DR, Feldman CL: A system for quantitative

evaluation of left ventricular function with two-dimensional ultrasonography. Med Instrum 14:111-116, 1980

Rakowski H, Martin RP, Popp RL: Left ventricular function: Assessment by wide angle two-dimensional ultrasonic sector scanning. Acta Med Scand, suppl 627, pp 105-111, 1979

Schiller NB, Acquatella H, Ports TA, Drew D, Goerke J, Ringertz H, et al.: Left ventricular volume from paired biplane two-dimensional echocardiography. Circulation 60:547-555, 1979

Appendix F
Abbreviations

AAW	anterior aortic wall
ALW	anterolateral free wall—left ventricle
AML, AMV	anterior leaflet of the mitral valve
AO	aorta, ascending
APM	anterior papillary muscle
ARV, AR	anterior wall right ventricle
AWRV	anterior wall of the right ventricle
AR	aortic root
ATL, ATV	anterior leaflet of the tricuspid valve
AV	aortic valve
AVS	atrioventricular sulcus
CS	coronary sinus
CW	chest wall
DA	descending aorta
ECG, EKG	electrocardiogram
EN, endo	endocardium
EP	epicardium
I	inferior
IAS	interatrial septum
IVC	inferior vena cava
IVS	interventricular septum
L	left
LA	left atrium
LAA	left atrial appendage
LAD	left anterior descending coronary artery
LAW	left atrial wall
LCA	left circumflex coronary artery
LCC	left coronary cusp of the aortic valve
LM	left main coronary artery
LPA	left pulmonary artery
LPV	left pulmonary vein
LSS	left side of septum
LV	left ventricle
LVOT	left ventricular outflow tract
LVPW	left ventricular posterior wall
MA	mitral annulus
MB	moderator band
MO	mitral orifice
MPA	main pulmonary artery

MS	membranous portion of the interventricular septum
MV	mitral valve
NCC	noncoronary cusp of the aortic valve
PA	pulmonary artery
PAW	posterior aortic wall
PE, PER, EFF	pericardial effusion
PER, peri, P	pericardium
phono	phonocardiogram
PML, PMV	posterior leaflet of the mitral valve
PMPM	posteromedial papillary muscle, mitral valve
PPM	posterior papillary muscle
PTL, PTV	posterior leaflet of the tricuspid valve
PV	pulmonic valve
PW, PLVW	posterior wall of the left ventricle
R	right
RA	right atrium
resp	respiratory pneumogram
RAA	right atrial appendage
RCA	right coronary artery
RCC	right coronary cusp of the aortic valve
RPA	right pulmonary artery
RPV	right pulmonary vein
RSS	right side of the septum
RV	right ventricle
RVAW	right ventricular anterior wall
RVOT	right ventricular outflow tract
RVW	right ventricular free wall
S	superior
STL	septal leaflet of the tricuspid valve
SVC	superior vena cava
TV	tricuspid valve
VS	interventricular septum

Appendix G
Glossary*

Accessory subvalvular aortic leaflets. Congenital reduplication of the aortic cusp attached to the interventricular septum and anterior mitral leaflet; a form of subvalvular aortic stenosis. Distortion of the aortic valve causes aortic insufficiency.

A-mode. Mode of operation in which the display records a vertical spot deflection for each pulse delivered from the receiver.

Akinetic. Without motion. In reference to the heart, a segment of myocardium without movement.

Aortic insufficiency. Abnormality of the aortic valve, either congenital or acquired, causing leakage of blood during diastole into the left ventricle.

Aortic root. The proximal ascending aorta, including the aortic valve ring.

Aortic valve stenosis. Abnormality of the aortic valve causing obstruction to left ventricular outflow; may be congenital or acquired.

Apical. Pertaining to or located at the apex. In reference to the heart, the most inferior portion of the cardiac chambers.

Apical four-chamber view. View obtained by positioning the echocardiographic transducer at the apex or at a subcostal location in a plane parallel to the chest wall.

Atrial fibrillation. Disorder of atrial rhythm characterized by chaotic atrial activity and an irregular ventricular response.

Atrial septal defect. Congenital defect in the interatrial partition; it allows oxygenated blood to return to the right heart, causing volume overload of the right ventricle. The defect may be low in the interatrial septum (ostium primum), high in the atrial septum (ostium secundum), or at the border of the interatrial septum with the superior vena cava (sinus venosus).

Atrioventricular sulcus. Groove on the surface of the heart between the atrium and ventricles in which the coronary sinus, the circumflex artery and veins are carried.

Autonomic nervous system. A specific portion of the human nervous system that regulates functions of body organs, including the heart.

Catecholamine excretion. Excretion of the metabolic byproducts of the hormone epinephrine (norepinephrine), which is produced by the autonomic nervous system and the adrenal glands.

---

*Some definitions taken from *Dorland's Illustrated Medical Dictionary,* ed 25. Philadelphia, WB Saunders, 1978

Cathode-ray tube. Display device that produces an image by scanning an electronic beam over a phosphor-coded screen.

Caudad. Directed inferiorly; toward the feet.

Cavities. Used in reference to cardiac chambers: e.g., left ventricle, left atrium.

Chordae tendineae. Thin, fibrous strands that attach leaflets of the atrioventricular valve to the papillary muscles of the ventricle.

Clip. Echoscope recorder control that adjusts the intensity of the individual echoes.

Coarse gain. Echoscope control used to adjust the amplitude of all received ultrasound signals equally.

Complete atrioventricular canal. Defect in the endocardial cushion—the fibrous body to which the mitral and tricuspid valves attach laterally, the interatrial septum superiorly, and the interventricular septum inferiorly. A defect in this structure produces an atrial and ventricular septal defect with structural abnormalities in the mitral and tricuspid valves. Frequently, the anterior mitral and anterior tricuspid valves form one continuous structure.

Congenital aortic stenosis. Aortic valve stenosis in which the aortic valve may have only one cusp (unicuspid) or two cusps (bicuspid).

Congenital bicuspid aortic valve. Aortic valve abnormality in which there are two valve cusps instead of the usual three. The bicuspid valves are unequal in size and frequently are accompanied by aortic regurgitation.

Constrictive pericarditis. Hemodynamic state of the heart in which relaxation of the heart is hindered by a thickened pericardium.

Coronary sinus. Venous structure, located in the atrioventricular groove, that receives venous blood from the cardiac veins and empties into the right atrium.

Coupling gel. Aqueous gel that ensures air-free contact between the patient's skin and the transducer for ultrasound examination.

Damping. Echoscope control used to adjust the power of the transmitted ultrasound impulse. Also the process of reducing pulse duration.

Delay. Echoscope control used to begin the oscilloscope scan from a certain depth after the ultrasound pulse is transmitted and thus eliminate unwanted echoes from chest wall and subcostal structures.

Depth. Echoscope control used to control the amount of tissue between the crystal artifact of the transducer and the lung—with the heart interposed.

Depth compensation. Echoscope control that suppresses the amplification of signals near the transducer and amplifies distant signals.

Depth display. Echoscope control that depicts gradation in the penetration of the ultrasound beam from the transducer. Usually standardized at 0.5-cm or 1.0-cm gradations.

Diastole. Relaxation phase of the cardiac cycle.

Discrete subaortic stenosis. Obstruction to left ventricular outflow in which a membrane or a muscular tunnel hypertrophy exists just below the aortic valve. A gradient of pressure between the left ventricle and aorta is found just below the aortic valve cusps.

Doppler principle (effect). Relationship of the apparent frequency of sound waves to the relative motion of the source of the waves and the observer; the frequency increases as the two approach each other and decreases as they move apart.

Dyskinetic. Abnormal motion that is opposite the normal motion. Refers to a segment of the heart muscle whose motion is paradoxical.

Ebstein's anomaly. Abnormality of the tricuspid valve in which the valve is abnormally displaced and attached within the cavity of the right ventricle. This enlarges the right atrium, which forms an atrialized portion of the ventricle.

Eccentricity index. Abnormally displaced closure point of the aortic valve due to unequal cusp size, such as in a bicuspid or unicuspid valve.

ECG amplitude. Echoscope control that adjusts the electrical height of the ECG QRS complex.

ECG lead. Lead that depicts atrial and ventricular depolarization (usually lead II) during an echocardiographic examination.

ECG position. Position of the ECG on the oscilloscope or on the recording paper; usually at either the top or the bottom of the display.

Echocardiographic size. Echoscope recorder control that adjusts the vertical height of the echocardiographic recording.

Echo display position. Echoscope recorder control that allows the M-mode picture to be positioned on the paper at the desired level.

Echoscope controls. Front-panel control switches, or dials, for regulation of the echocardiographic module.

Embolize. To propel a solid particle or object within a vessel to a peripheral vessel or organ.

End diastole. End of the relaxation phase of the cardiac cycle. A frequent point for measurements, usually taken at the onset of the QRS complex of the ECG.

Endocardial cushion. See Complete atrioventricular canal.

Endocardium. Endothelial membrane lining the heart and the connective tissue bed on which it lies.

Epicardium. Layer of serous pericardium on the surface of the heart.

Excrescences. Abnormal outgrowth of morbid origin.

Externa. Outermost structure or layer, usually a blood vessel.

Exudate. Proliferation of fluid, protein, and white blood cells which can accumulate in any body cavity, such as a pleural or pericardial cavity. Because of the accumulation of protein and cells, the density of this liquid exceeds that of other body fluids.

Fractional shortening. Percentage of minor-axis shortening of the left ventricle during systole.

Fossa ovalis (foramen ovalis). Patent opening in the interatrial membrane caused by incomplete covering or closure of the septum primum over the septum secundum. Anatomically but not functionally patent.

Gain. Ratio of output to input electrical power.

Gain-dependence. The thickness of a line is a function of gain setting.

Hematomas. Localized collection of blood, usually clotted, in an organ, space, or tissue; due to a break in a blood vessel.

Hertz. Unit of frequency, one cycle per second; unit of pulse repetition frequency, one pulse per second. Abbreviation: Hz.

Holosystolic prolapse. Sagging of the valve leaflets into another chamber during all of systole.

Hyperadrenergic. Increased tone or discharge activity of the sympathetic autonomic nervous sytem.

Hyperkinetic. Increased motion. With reference to the heart, generally a segment of the myocardium with exaggerated or increased wall motion.

Hypertrophy. Increased size of individual cells, usually due to a stimulus. Sustained, increased pressure within a chamber will cause thickness of that chamber wall.

Hypokinetic. Decreased motion. In reference to the heart, a segment of the myocardium with decreased or diminished wall motion.

Idiopathic hypertrophic subaortic stenosis. Disorder of the left ventricular outflow tract, in which an asymmetrically thickened interventricular septum and abnormally displaced anterior mitral leaflet obstruct left ventricular outflow during systole.

Infundibular pulmonary stenosis. Congenital hypertrophy or thickening of the right ventricular outflow tract musculature; causes pulmonary outflow obstruction in the sub-pulmonary valve region.

Initial gain or **near gain.** Ratio of output to input of electrical power of the proximal ultrasound beam. Echoscope control that adjusts ultrasound wave amplification from the chest wall to the point where depth compensation takes effect.

Intensity. Power divided by the beam area—the light-giving power of a source.

Intensity control. See Clip.

Interlacing. Method of echoscope two-dimensional display in which reflected ultrasound lines are reduplicated, providing a more dense cross-sectional display.

Intima. Innermost structure.

Intercostal. Situated between the ribs.

Late-systolic prolapse. Prolapse of the atrioventricular valves in late systole.

Leading-edge method. Method used for measuring the dimension of a structure—from the most anterior margin of a line representing the anterior surface of the structure to the most anterior margin of a line representing the posterior surface of that structure.

Left pleural effusion. Transudate or exudate of fluid located in the left plural space between the lung and its lining. In echocardiography, it is usually seen as an echo-free space behind or posterior to the parietal pericardium.

Left ventricular end-diastolic dimension. Diastolic dimension of the ventricle taken at the onset of the QRS complex.

Left ventricular septum. The interventricular septum or partition separating the right from the left ventricle.

Left ventricular systolic dimension. Systolic dimension of the left ventricle, taken at the most anterior position of the posterior wall or most posterior position of the interventricular wall during systole (at end of T wave of ECG).

Linear-array echocardiography. Two-dimensional display with an array mode made up of rectangular elements in a line.

Long-axis view. View obtained by positioning the echocardiographic transducer parallel to the long axis of the heart (base to apex).

Lymphomas. General term applied to any neoplastic disorder of the lymphoid tissue.

Mechanical echocardiography. Two-dimensional display produced by either oscillating or rotating transducers.

Mediastinal cysts. Congenital cyst within the mediastinum—a partition between the right and left lung that contains the heart and great vessels in its middle portion, the thymus glands and portions of the thyroid gland in the anterior portion, and the esophagus and descending aorta in the posterior portion.

Megatertz. One million hertz. Abbreviation: MHz.

Microcavitation. Microbubbles within a medium.

Midsystolic prolapse. Prolapse of the atrioventricular valve into an atrium, beginning in midsystole.

Mitral annular calcification. Calcification of the atrioventricular fibrous ring.

Mitral commissurotomy. Surgical procedure in which fibrosed or stenotic mitral leaflets are separated; fused anterior and posterior mitral leaflets are separated.

Mitral E point–septal separation. Distance or dimension from the point of the anterior mitral leaflet to the left side of the interventricular septum. It is used as an indicator of the left ventricular function.

Mitral valve. A two-leaflet valve separating left atrium from left ventricle.

Mitral regurgitation. Leakage of blood into the left atrium during systole, usually caused by a defect in the mitral valve or subvalvular structures.

Mitral stenosis. Thickening and fusion of anterior and posterior mitral leaflets.

M-mode echocardiogram. Mode of operation in which the display is recorded as a spot brightening for each pulse delivered from receiver. Produces a one-dimensional time display of reflected position or motion.

Mitral valve prolapse. A condition in which a portion of the mitral valve protrudes into the left atrium in systole.

Myxoma. Benign tumor of the heart, usually attached to the interatrial septum, that obstructs left ventricular inflow.

Myxomatous. Describes a disorder of connective tissue, marked by multiple small myxomas, in which there is increased mucopolysaccharide concentration within the tissue.

Nadir. Lowest point or position.

Near zone. Region of a sound beam in which the beam diameter decreases as the distance from the transducer increases.

Near gain. See Initial gain.

Ostium primum atrial septal defect. Congenital opening in the lowest aspect of the septum primum of the embryonic heart.

Ostium secundum atrial septal defect. Congenital opening high in the septum primum of the embryonic heart, in the area of the foramen ovalae.

Overall contrast level. Echoscope control that adjusts the contrast of the entire echoscope display.

Overall gain. See Coarse gain.

Papillary muscle. Pertaining to the papillae. A muscle attachment from the ventricular wall to the atrioventricular valves; that is, the mitral or tricuspid valves.

Paradoxical. Moving opposite. In reference to the heart, abnormal motion of the cardiac wall in which motion is opposite the normal motion. Also, *dyskinetic.*

Paradoxical pulse. Pulse that markedly decreases in amplitude during inspiration; often occurs in constrictive pericarditis and in large pericardial effusions.

Parasternal. Situated next to the sternum.

Parietal pericardium. Parietal layer of the serous pericardium.

Patent ductus ateriosus. Persistence of the ductus arteriosus—the embryonic vessel connecting the left pulmonary artery to the aorta. The vessel generally closes shortly after birth, but may remain patent in premature infants.

Pericardial adhesions. Fibrous strands or attachments within the pericardial sac.

Pericardiocentesis. Placement of an opening in, or surgical puncture of, the pericardial cavity.

Pericardial effusion. Abnormal fluid accumulation in the pericardial sac.

Pericardium. Fibroserous sac surrounding the heart and roots of the great vessels.

Phased-array echocardiography. Linear ray operated by applying voltage pulses to all elements but with small time delays.

Posterior wall thickness. Thickness of the left ventricular posterior wall, usually taken at end diastole.

Pressure overload state. Condition of the ventricles in which abnormal elevated systolic pressure exists, e.g., aortic stenosis.

Pseudo-mitral valve prolapse. False or mimicked mitral valve prolapse. Can be seen in patients with pericardial effusion or when abnormal angulation of the transducer is present.

Pseudo-systolic anterior motion. False or mimicked systolic anterior motion, usually of the anterior mitral leaflets.

Pulmonary hypertension. Elevated pulmonary artery pressure; can be primary or secondary.

Pulmonic valve regurgitation. Leakage of blood from the pulmonary artery into the right ventricle during diastole. May be congenital or acquired.

Pulmonic valve stenosis. Obstruction to pulmonary outflow, usually due to a unicuspic or bicuspid pulmonic valve.

Pulse power. See Damping.

Real-time display. Display that continuously images moving structures.

Reject. Echoscope control that eliminates low-amplitude ultrasound impulses.

Resolution. The ability to perceive two adjacent objects or points as separate.

Right ventricular anterior wall. Anterior free wall of the right ventricle.

Right ventricular cavity dimension. Diastolic dimension of the right ventricle taken at the onset of QRS.

Right ventricular volume overload. Increased blood volume of the right ventricle caused by atrial septal defect, tricuspid regurgitation, or pulmonary regurgitation.

Scan. Sweep of a sound beam to produce an image.

Semilunar. Half-moon shape; usually refers to the aortic or pulmonic valve cusps.

Sensitivity. The quality or state of being sensitive; the percentage of true positives selected correctly by a particular technique.

Short-axis view. Viewed obtained by positioning the transducer perpendicular to the long-axis view of the heart.

Single ventricle. Congenital lesion in which two atrioventricular valves empty into a single common chamber.

Specificity. Quality or state of being specific; the percentage of true negatives selected correctly by a particular technique.

Standard interspace. Intercostal space from which the anterior mitral leaflet is imaged with slight medial, but without superior or inferior, transducer angulation.

Standard plane. Position on the chest wall from which the minor axis of the left ventricle can be viewed.

Sternum. Longitudinal, unpaired plate of bone that forms the middle of the anterior wall of the thorax; articulates above with the clavicles and along the sides with the cartilage of the first seven ribs.

Strip chart. Recording display on paper for time-motion or M-mode echocardiography.

Subcostal. Situated beneath a rib.

Subcostal four-chamber view. A four-chamber view of the heart taken from below the rib cage.

Subpulmonic pulmonary stenosis. See Infundibular pulmonary stenosis.

Subxiphoid. Under the xiphoid process.

Superior vena cava syndrome. Obstruction of the superior vena cava, usually produced by a mass appearing at the superior portion of the vessel. It can obstruct venous inflow into the right heart, causing edema and swelling of the head and neck vessels.

Suprasternal. Situated above the sternum.

Suprasternal notch. An indentation or notch in the superior portion of the sternum.

Swinging heart. Alterations in the cardiac position on alternate cardiac cycles: usually due to a large pericardial effusion.

Switch gain. An echoscope control that highlights reflected echoes from a particular depth, while suppressing reflected echoes from other depths.

Systole. The contraction phase of the cardiac cycle.

Systolic anterior motion. Anterior motion, generally of the mitral valve during systole.

Tetralogy of Fallot. Congenital defect in which there is a large ventricular septal defect, pulmonary valve stenosis, and an overriding aorta; allows unoxygenated blood from the right ventricle to cross the interventricular septum to the aorta.

Thrombus. Blood clot.

Time-compensated gain. Echoscope control that equalizes differences due to reflected depth in received reflection amplitudes.

Time marker. Echoscope recorder control that is used to measure precisely time elapsed.

Time-motion echocardiogram. See M-mode echocardiogram.

Trace contrast. Echoscope recorder control that adjusts the density of the tracing.

Transducer. Device that converts energy from one form to another.

Transducer element. Piece of piezoelectric material in a transducer.

Transposition of the great vessels. Congenital lesion in which the aorta and pulmonary arteries are transposed and arise from the right and left ventricles, respectively.

Tricuspid regurgitation. Leakage of blood back into the right atrium during systole.

Tricuspid stenosis. Obstruction to inflow of the right ventricle; may be congenital or acquired.

T-scan sweep. Sweep with a single-element transducer perpendicular to the long-axis sweep (short-axis sweep).

Ventricular septal defect. Congenital absence of the interventricular septum.

Walls. Myocardial walls.

Window. Echocardiographic position from which cardiac structures can be imaged.

Wolff-Parkinson-White syndrome. Pre-excitation of the ventricle via an atrioventricular bypass tract around the atrioventricular node. Supraventricular tachycardias are commonly associated with this syndrome.

Xiphoid. The most inferior portion of the sternum. It articulates with the lower sternum.

Appendix H
Answers

CHAPTER 1

1-6.1.		Right ventricle, 2.5 cm; left ventricular diastolic dimension, 3.5 cm; left ventricular systolic dimension, 1.9 cm; interventricular septal thickness, 0.9 cm; posterior wall thickness, 0.9 cm.
1-6.2.		Fractional shortening, 46%; ejection fraction, 84%.
1-7.1.		105 cm
1-8.1.		Interventricular septal thickness, 1.5 cm; left ventricular posterior wall thickness, 1.5 cm; left ventricular diastolic dimension, 4.8 cm.
1-9.1.		Left atrium, 5.2 cm; aortic root, 3.5 cm.
1-9.2.		Aortic stenosis. Notice the thickened aortic valve which does not fully open.
1-10.1.	A	The vertical dots seen to the right of the systolic dimension are 1 cm apart and each row of dots is 1 sec apart in this case.
1-10.2.	D	
1-10.3.	A	The fractional shortening (circumferential shortening) of the left ventricle is an indicator of left ventricular performance (normal is considered 30–45%).
1-11.1.	B	
1-11.2.	A	
1-11.3.	B	
1-12.1.	C	Normal aortic root size is 2.0–3.7 cm. The undulating aortic root motion has been shown to be a function of both forward cardiac output and transmitral flow which is diminished.
1-12.2.	C	Normal left atrial size in an adult is less than 4.0 cm. Note the echo "shelf" above the echo marked "LAW." This is often mistaken for the posterior left atrial wall.

1-13.1.	B	
1-13.2.	A	
1-13.3.	B	
1-13.4.	B	This echocardiogram of the left ventricle shows dilatation of that chamber, reduced motion of the interventricular septum and left ventricle posterior wall, and reduced fractional shortening reflecting diminished ejection fraction. The echo might suggest a cardiomyopathy.
1-14.1.	A	Note the relationship of the aortic root to the interventricular septum and mitral valve. The anterior aortic wall is continuous with the interventricular and the posterior aortic wall becomes the anterior mitral valve leaflet.
1-14.2.	A	
1-14.3.	B	

CHAPTER 3

3-1.1.	A	
3-1.2.	B	The posterior mitral valve leaflet remains in a neutral position rather than exhibiting normal antiparallel diastolic motion.
3-1.3.	B	In addition to the loss of the A wave and abnormal posterior mitral valve motion, other findings consistent with the diagnosis include reduced D-E excursion, thickening of the leaflets, and, if seen, enlargement of the left atrium.
3-2.1.	B	There is vibration of the posterior mitral leaflet during systole.
3-2.2.	A	The posterior leaflet of the mitral valve exhibits anterior rather than normal posterior motion, consistent with flail posterior leaflet due to rupture of the chordae tendineae. This patient had bacterial endocarditis.
3-3.1.	B, D	The posterior mitral leaflet moves erratically during diastole, suggesting a flail leaflet. There is loss of the normal antiparallel motion of the posterior mitral leaflet in diastole.
3-3.2.	C	These echoes suggest vegetation of the posterior mitral valve leaflet consistent with endocarditis.
3-3.3.	B	
3-4.1.	B	The echoes seen in the left atrium are portions of the posterior mitral leaflet and / or vegetations swinging into the left atrium during systole.

3-5.1.	A	
3-5.2.	A	
3-6.1.	A	
3-7.1.	B	The patient's cardiac rhythm is atrial fibrillation; the irregular ripples of atrial contraction are transmitted to the aortic root and mitral leaflets, causing these undulations.
3-8.1.	D	In aortic valve insufficiency the blood regurgitating through the aortic valve during diastole strikes the anterior mitral leaflet, causing this fluttering.
3-9.1.	C	Aortic regurgitation causes high-frequency diastolic vibration of the anterior mitral leaflet, greatly hindering initial mitral valve opening (D–E) and lowering the E point.
3-10.1.	D	The dark band of echoes positioned behind the mitral leaflets and ending at the left atrium represents a calcified mitral annulus.
3-11.1.	A, E	
3-16.1.	A, B	
3-17.1.	B, D	
3-20.1.	A, D	
3-21.1.	A, C	

CHAPTER 4

4-1.1.	A	
4-1.2.	D	
4-2.1.	C	The systolic portions of this echo show holosystolic sagging of the mitral valve consistent with mitral valve prolapse. In addition, there is erratic motion of the posterior mitral valve leaflet during diastole, suggesting a flail posterior leaflet produced by ruptured chordae tendineae. This is a rare but important complication of mitral valve prolapse.
4-3.1.	C	There is late systolic prolapse of both the anterior and posterior leaflets; although this occurs less frequently than posterior prolapse, it is not uncommon.
4-4.1.	A, B	Because of the redundancy of the leaflets, systolic anterior motion is first noted, followed by posterior prolapse of the mitral leaflet. This appears due to buckling of the mitral chordal structures into the left ventricular outflow tract.
4-6.1.	B, D	

4-6.2.	A	The presence of other cardiac lesions cannot be overlooked in conjunction with mitral valve prolapse. A congenital bicuspid aortic valve with aortic regurgitation is not uncommon with mitral valve prolapse.
4-7.1.	A	
4-9.1.	C, D	
4-11.1.	B, D	

CHAPTER 5

5-3.1.	D	The diastolic line of closure of the aortic valve leaflets is much closer to the anterior aortic wall. This eccentric closure is suggestive of a bicuspid aortic valve.
5-3.2.	D	
5-4.1.	A	The high-frequency vibrations seen in the aortic root during diastole represent ruptured noncoronary cusp. This patient also had endocarditis.
5-4.2.	B	The left atrium is enlarged and measures 4.6 cm; normal is less than 4.0 cm.
5-5.1.	B	Fluttering of the anterior mitral valve leaflet and the interventricular septum indicates aortic regurgitation.
5-6.1.	D	Rheumatic mitral valve disease is present. The thickened mitral leaflets, reduced E–F slope, reduced D–E excursion, and parallel posterior mitral valve motion suggest mitral stenosis. In addition, the aortic cusps are thickened and probably calcified with decreased separation, suggestive of aortic stenosis. Also noted is enlargement of the left atrium (4.4 cm).
5-8.1.	B	
5-8.2.	D	
5-9.1.	C	
5-10.1.	D	
5-10.2.	C	
5-11.1.	D	

CHAPTER 6

6-10.1.	B	This patient's 2000 cc pericardial effusion caused a greatly enlarged cardiac silhouette on x-ray. Note also the anterior echo-free space consistent with anterior effusion.

6-10.2.	D	
6-11.1.	C	The pericardial effusion in this patient is large, probably greater than 1500 cc. Quantification of pericardial effusion size by M-mode is difficult and carries the expectation of considerable error. A posterior echo-free space is consistent with small-sized pericardial effusion (500 cc). With larger posterior echo-free space and the appearance of anterior echo-free space the effusion should be considered moderate (500–1000 cc).
6-11.2.	C	Due to the motion of the entire cardiac silhouette during systole, an apparent prolapse of the mitral valve is seen.
6-12.1.	C	There is likely pericardial tamponade—in this case due to a malignancy. Also noted is anteroposterior swinging of the heart, with every other beat resulting in the alternating contraction pattern of the ventricular walls and mitral valve and the changing E–F slope of the mitral valve. The anterior right ventricular wall shows an early notch.
6-12.2.	D	There is electrical alternans (alternating changes in the amplitude of the QRS complex). This is also thought to be a result of the swinging heart.
6-13.1.	B	Pseudo-pericardial effusion. At first glance, a pericardial effusion is present behind the left ventricle. However, the left ventricular posterior wall sometimes appears as an echo-free space, as is the case here. The darker echoes above the left ventricular posterior wall are papillary muscle. If these darker echoes were the left ventricular wall, then this wall would be moving normally but thinning in systole—a peculiar situation indeed. This and the other echoes on the page are the tipoff that the echo-free space is actually the posterior left ventricular wall.
6-14.1.	C	Electrical acoustical (heart sounds) alternans is a result of the swinging heart on alternate beats.
6-15.1.	A, D	
6-16.1.	A, B, C, E	
6-16.2.	B	

CHAPTER 7

7-3.1.	C	
7-3.2.	A, B	
7-4.1.	B, C	Paradoxical septal motion and right ventricular enlargement suggest right ventricular volume over-

		load state. However, paradoxical septal motion secondary to open heart surgery has also been noted up to one year following operation.
7-4.2.	E	All of these would cause paradoxical septal motion; however, aneurysm of the interventricular septum can be distinguished from the others by the lack of systolic thickening. Also, atrial septal defect, pulmonic regurgitation, or anomolous pulmonary venous drainage would cause right ventricular enlargement as well.
7-5.1.	A	The septum thickens in systole and thins with diastole, which is normal.
7-5.2.	A	The ECG recorded at the top of the echocardiogram shows a wide QRS with a delta wave (slurred upstroke) suggesting preexcitation (Wolff-Parkinson-White syndrome). The early motion of the left ventricular posterior wall suggests premature excitation of this area due to the bypass tract, located nearby.
7-6.1.	B, C, D	The E-F slope of the mitral valve is diminished. Although this is most commonly thought of in conjunction with mitral stenosis, a state of decreased left ventricle compliance may also yield it. Also noted is systolic anterior motion of the mitral valve.
7-6.2.	C	The findings suggest dynamic left ventricle outflow obstruction. The echocardiogram also suggests asymmetrical thickening of the interventricular septum; however the septum is poorly delineated. Although not noted in this echo, the aortic valve may demonstrate midsystolic closure, suggesting subvalvular aortic obstruction.
7-7.1.	C	The marked thickening of the left ventricular walls without evidence of outflow obstruction suggests the diagnosis.
7-8.1.	A, B, C	Hypertrophy of the interventricular septum is noted. In addition, there is little or no excursion of the left ventricular posterior wall.
7-8.2.	B	Reduced left ventricular posterior wall motion with normal or increased septal motion suggests segmental myocardial disease, the most common cause being ischemic heart disease, inferior wall myocardial infarction.
7-9.1.	A, C	The remarkable change in the two echoes is the reduction in the motion of the interventricular septum, suggesting that a septal myocardial infarction—probably from an embolus of the aortic valve vegetations—has occurred.
7-9.2.	C	

7-10.1.	B	The finding of an enlarged left ventricle with vigorous contractions, as suggested by increased fractional shortening, is consistent with a state of left ventricular volume overload. This may occur in mitral regurgitation, aortic regurgitation, or ventricular septal defect.
7-11.1.	A, C, D	
7-12.1.	B	
7-12.2.	B	
7-12.3.	A	The finding of an akinetic septum without systolic thickening and preservation of normal left ventricular posterior wall motion suggests segmental myocardial dysfunction—most commonly, ischemic heart disease.
7-13.1.	A, B	
7-14.1.	A, C, E	
7-15.1.	C, E	
7-16.1.	C	

CHAPTER 8

8-1.1.	A, B, C, D	
8-1.2.	A	Note the normal E–F slope and excursion of the mitral valve. Rheumatic tricuspid stenosis is usually seen with mitral stenosis, which was not present here.
8-2.1.	C	Notice the posterior motion of the diastolic portion of the tricuspid valve indicated by the arrow.
8-3.1.	C	The interrupted tricuspid valve closure suggests elevated, right ventricular end-diastolic pressure.
8-3.2.	C	The most common cause is elevated right ventricular end-diastolic pressure.
8-5.1.	C	
8-7.1.	C	The pulmonic valve motion may reflect pulmonary artery hypertension or stenosis of the pulmonic valve. The a-wave—motion of the pulmonic valve during atrial systole—is lost in pulmonary hypertension, whereas, in pulmonic stenosis, it may be exaggerated.
8-8.1.	D	
8-8.2.	C	
8-10.1.	A, D	The vegetation is seen on the pulmonic valve during systole and falls into the right ventricular outflow tract during diastole. It is less likely to be seen on the pulmonic valve during diastole.

8-11.1.	A, B, C, D	Marked dilitation of the left ventricle with reduced septal motion is noted. The increased E point-septal separation and reduced fractional shortening are consistent with reduced ejection fraction. The undulating echoes from the right ventricular outflow tract are from a Swan Ganz catheter.

CHAPTER 9

9-1.1.	A	Vegetations characteristically (though there are exceptions) are seen only during one portion of the cardiac cycle (systole or diastole). Note that in the third or fourth complex there is erratic motion of the posterior leaflet, suggesting a flail leaflet.
9-2.1.	D	
9-2.2.	C	
9-2.3.	D	
9-2.4.	A	
9-3.1.	B	
9-3.2.	A	
9-3.3.	C	
9-3.4.	B	
9-4.1.	C	
9-4.2.	A	The characteristic findings of a left atrial myxoma, in addition to the dense echoes appearing between the leaflets in diastole, include a mitral diastole clear space representing the time interval just before the myxoma hits the mitral valve ring. A reduced E-F slope of the mitral valve is noted as well.
9-5.1.	B	
9-5.2.	A, B, C	
9-6.1.	B	Two-dimensional echocardiography is helpful for localization of lesions, but M-mode echocardiography is helpful in the detection of vegetations.
9-9.1.	A, D	
9-10.1.	D	
9-12.1.	B	
9-14.1.	A	

CHAPTER 10

10-2.1.	D	The finding of partial systolic closure of the aortic valve is consistent with the diagnosis of subvalvu-

		lar aortic stenosis. The degree of closure seen here and the systolic aortic valve fluttering are consistent with discrete membraneous subvalvular aortic stenosis.
10-3.1.	D	
10-4.1.	D	The large a-wave in the pulmonic valve is consistent with the diagnosis of pulmonic valve stenosis.
10-5.1.	B	
10-7.1.	A	
10-8.1.	B	The motion of the interventricular septum is paradoxical.
10-8.2.	A	Right ventricular enlargement with paradoxical septal motion indicates right ventricular volume overload.
10-8.3.	A	A history and physical exam would help to ascertain the etiology of the abnormality.
10-10.1.	C	The finding of left ventricular volume overload pattern with normal left ventricular wall thickness in this patient is most consistent with a ventricular septal defect; an atrial septal defect alone would not be connected with left ventricular volume overload.
10-11.1.	C	
10-12.1.	B	This child has an overriding aorta with right ventricular enlargement. A ventricular septal defect cannot be seen.
10-13.1.	A, B, C	
10-17.1.	B	Primum atrial septal defect (atrioventricular canal defect) is present. The finding of right ventricular enlargement and paradoxical septal motion is consistent with an atrial septal defect. The mitral valve seen here appears to traverse the interventricular septum, suggesting a primum rather than secundum atrial septal defect.
10-18.1.	C	There is paradoxical septal motion and right ventricular enlargement, suggesting right ventricular volume overload. The echo seen within the left atrium is actually not in the left atrium at all but is a dilated coronary sinus with an a-wave and a c-venous wave behind the left atrium, suggesting anomalous pulmonary venous drainage. Secundum atrial septal defect would not be expected to have a partition in left atrium. Cor triatriatum should not have right ventricular volume overload.
10-19.1.	A	

CHAPTER 11

11-10.1.	A, B, D
11-11.1.	A, B
11-12.1.	E
11-13.1.	B
11-14.1.	A, B, D
11-15.1.	E

Index

In this index, page numbers are provided only for those pages on which an entry is defined or is discussed in detail.

a b c d e f g h i j
8 2